Advanced Acupuncture
A Clinic Manual

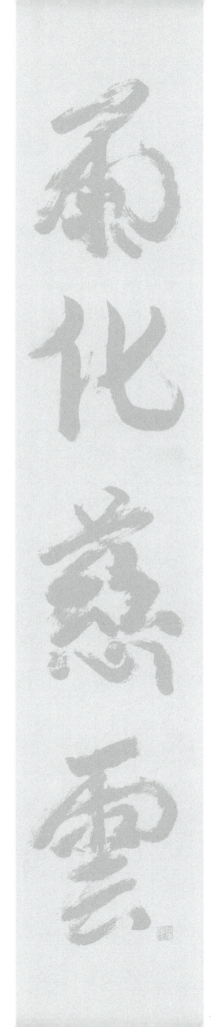

Advanced Acupuncture
A Clinic Manual

Protocols for the Complement Channels
of the Complete Acupuncture System:
the Sinew, Luo, Divergent and
Eight Extraordinary Channels

Includes drawings of the Primary Channels

Ann Cecil-Sterman

Illustrations by Pat Didner

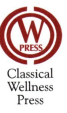

Classical Wellness Press

Copyright © 2012 Ann Cecil-Sterman
New York, NY 10001

www.classicalacupuncture.com

First edition

All rights reserved. Printed in the United States of America. This publication is protected by Copyright under the authority of the Constitution of the United States of America and subject to the jurisdiction of the Federal Courts or other courts of competent jurisdiction as well as other foreign jurisdictions enforceable locally through current or subsequent treaty and the permission should be obtained from the Publisher prior to any prohibited reproduction, translation, storage in a retrieval system, or transmission in any form or by any means, electronic, mechanical, photocopying, recording, or likewise—without the prior written permission of the Publisher and Author, except for brief attributed quotations embodied in critical articles, scholarly publications and reviews.
No patent liability is assumed with respect to the use of the information contained in this book.
Although every precaution has been taken in the preparation of this book, the Publisher and the Author assume no responsibility for errors or omissions. Classical Wellness Press, Ltd. assumes no liability for damages resulting from the use of the information contained herein. For information regarding permission(s), write to Classical Wellness Press, Ltd., Rights and Permissions Department,
214 West 29th Street, Suite 901, New York, NY 10001.

Disclaimer and Note: The information presented in this book is a compilation of existing public and non-proprietary information related to the subject of what is known in the Eastern Medical Community as "Traditional Chinese Medicine" and "Classical Chinese Medicine" and is intended solely for the use by Licensed Acupuncturists and students under the supervised study of acupuncture through an accredited educational institution. Under no circumstances is the information in this work to be used or acted upon by an unlicensed, untrained or unsupervised individual. The Author and Publisher do not advocate or endorse self-diagnosis, self-medication or treatment by unlicensed individuals under any circumstances. Chinese Medicine is a regulated profession and subject to the jurisdiction of the individual states as well as local and national professional and accrediting organizations. Individuals are strongly encouraged to perform their own due diligence and seek guidance and referrals from these organizations or other licensed professionals.

The teachings in this book come from the oral tradition
through the gracious generosity of my principal teacher, Daoist Master, Dr. Jeffrey Yuen.
Any mistakes, however, are mine. A.C.S.

Illustrations: Pat Didner
Cover design, book design, graphic design and diagrams: Cody Dodo
Front cover calligraphy: "The gentle rains of heaven cleanse us of our illnesses."
Gift of Dr. Jeffrey Yuen to the Classical Wellness Center, 2008.

ISBN: 978-0-9837720-0-2

for Ravi and Miriam

A thought from Ravi at four years of age: "Mommy, what can you see if you sit right on the edge of the universe? ...I think I can see the medicine."

A thought from Miriam at three years of age: "Mommy and Daddy, listen! We just have to remember that everything is perfect all the time!"

"There are no incurable diseases, only incurable people."

"The patient must bind to your belief in your system. Your belief must be strong."

*"The more you know, the more confused and the less effective you become.
Know less, but resonate it. Have confidence and invite your patient into the vibrational confidence that they can be healed."*

"Reincarnation is caused by inaction."

*"Medicine should be rich, it should not be absolute.
Chinese Medicine is a constant reminder that we must always have the humility to accept that there are many ways of seeing the world."*

"If someone expects you to direct them, it's not infringement."

Dr. Jeffrey Yuen

*"Practice witnessing your patient. Practice witnessing your mind.
Practice witnessing your mind's reaction to your patient. Yield. Surrender.
Accept their path. Cultivate non-assertive action."*
Chapter 11, Su Wen

*"If the patient doesn't believe in the treatment, the treatment will not work…
If the clinician doesn't believe in the treatment, the treatment will not work."*
Chapter 14, Su Wen

"The person who says it cannot be done should not interrupt the person doing it."
Chinese Proverb

Contents

xix	List of Illustrations
xxi	List of Tables, Abbreviations
xxii	Acknowledgments
xxv	Introduction
xxxv	Nomenclature
xxxvii	A Note on the Illustrations
xxxviii	Author's Note

PART ONE: PREPARATION — 1

Needles and Needling Techniques — 2

2	The Nine Needles of Classical Acupuncture
3	A Word about Insertion
3	Needling Techniques and Cultivation
4	Needling Techniques and Intention According to the *Ling Shu*
4	The Breadth of the *Ling Shu* Needling Techniques Discussion
5	Needling Techniques as an Extension of Tui Na
5	The Four Categories of Needling
6	Needling Techniques Derived from Tui Na
7	General Advanced Acupuncture Needling Techniques
7	Tonification and Reduction
9	Needling in Relation to Depth
10	Needling for Directionality
10	Needling Techniques for the Round-Sharp Needle
10	Contraindications for Needling
11	Metals: Gold, Silver and Stainless Steel
11	Needling Techniques of the Complement Channels
11	Sinew Channel Needling
12	Luo Channel Needling
12	Divergent Channel Needling
13	Alternative Divergent Channel Needling
13	Eight Extraordinary Channel Needling

Diagnosis and Treatment — 14

14	Classical Pulse Taking
15	Engendering the Qi of the Pulse Treatment (Sheng Mai)
15	Point Location by Palpation and Movement
15	Frequency and Duration of Treatment
17	Unilateral versus Bilateral Needling
17	Physiological Responses to Unilateral Needling
18	Scars: Treatment, Protocol and Frequently Asked Questions
20	Ease of Use of the Complement Channels

PART TWO:
THE APPLICATION OF THE COMPLEMENT CHANNELS　　21

- 22　Aspects of Latency of a Pathogenic Factor
- 23　The Achievement of Latency of a Pathogenic Factor
- 24　The Organization and Terrain of the Complement Channels
- 24　The Terrain of the Channels

SINEW CHANNEL TREATMENTS　　26

- 26　Historical References to the Sinew Channels
- 26　Sinew Channel Theory
- 28　Sinew Channel Illustrations
- 40　Sinew Channel Indications
- 40　Etiology
- 40　Objective
- 40　Prerequisites
- 40　Explanation
- 41　Treatment of the Underlying Deficiency
- 41　Treatment Tool Kit
- 42　Sinew Needling Technique
- 43　Sinew Treatment Protocol
- 45　Tonifying the Sinews
- 45　Frequency of Treatment
- 45　Classical Prescription
- 45　Essential Oil Treatment of the Sinew Channels
- 46　Follow-Up Recommendation
- 46　Healing Events
- 46　Troubleshooting
- 47　Frequently Asked Questions
- 48　Case Study

LUO TREATMENTS　　50

- 50　The Arising of the Luo Channels
- 51　Historical References to the Luo Channels
- 51　Longitudinal and Transverse Luo Terminology
- 52　Definitions: Visible Luo Vessels and Luo Channels
- 53　Luos in the Complement Channel Sequence
- 54　Luo Channel Indications
- 55　Full and Emptied Luo Terminology
- 57　Luo Channel Diagnosis
- 58　Luo Treatment Principles
- 58　Luo Needling Technique
- 59　The 15 Luo Points and the 16 Luo Channels
- 59　Locating Luo Points
- 60　Bleeding Luos Unilaterally

60	Longitudinal Luo Channel Trajectories	
62	Points Beyond the Luo Point, Along the Longitudinal Trajectory	
65	Luo Channel Illustrations	
81	Luo Treatment Toolkit	
82	Treatment Protocols	
82	Full Luo Protocol	
82	Emptied Luo Protocol	
83	Treatment Course	
83	Subjective Observations Associated with Luo Treatments	
84	Healing Events	

The Psychosocial Luo Model   84

    84   The Development of Luo Pathology

The Luos of the First Energetic Level   85

    85   The Lung Luo Channel Progression
    87   The Significance of the Sequence of the Luos

Luo Channel Signs, Symptoms and Treatment Protocols   88

    88   Lung Luo Channel Progression
    88   Treatment
    89   Large Intestine Luo Progression
    89   Treatment
    90   Stomach Luo Channel Progression
    90   Treatment
    91   Spleen Luo Channel Progression
    91   Treatment

The Luos of the Second Energetic Level   92

    92   Heart Luo Channel Progression
    92   Treatment
    93   Small Intestine Luo Channel Progression
    94   Treatment
    94   Bladder Luo Channel Progression
    95   Treatment
    95   Kidney Luo Channel Progression
    96   Treatment

The Luos of the Third Energetic Level   96

    96   Pericardium Luo Channel Progression
    97   Treatment
    97   Triple Heater Luo Channel Progression
    98   Treatment
    98   Gallbladder Luo Channel Progression
    99   Treatment

99	Liver Luo Channel Progression	
100	Treatment	
100	Ren Luo Channel	
101	Treatment	
101	Du Luo Channel	
101	Treatment	
102	Great Luo of the Spleen	
102	Treatment	
103	Great Luo of the Stomach	
103	Treatment of the Great Luo of the Stomach	

Longitudinal Luo Essential Oil Treatments   104

105	Essential Oil Application Method
105	Essential Oils for Application on Luo Points

TRANSVERSE LUO TREATMENTS   107

107	Definition
107	Importance of the Transverse Luo
107	The Arising of the Transverse Luos
109	The Transverse Luos can take several possible paths
111	The Effect of Transverse Luo treatments
111	Acute versus Chronic
111	The Luos and Psychology and Psychiatry
111	Transverse Luo Signs and Symptoms
112	Transverse Luo Signs and Symptoms, Theoretical Sequence
113	Treatment of Transverse Luos
113	Transverse Luo Treatment Intention
113	Transverse Luo Diagnosis and Treatment
114	Examples
115	Transverse Luo Treatment Protocols
116	Permutations of the Progression of Luo Latency
117	Constitutional Acquisition of Pathology
118	Other Transverse Luo Applications
119	Narrative Model Examples
119	Other Uses of the Luo Channels
120	The Simple Three Level Emotional Luo Model
120	The Levels of the Pathological Emotions
121	Diagnosis in the Simple Three Level Emotional Luo Model
122	Protocol for the Simple Three Level Emotional Luo Model
122	Musculoskeletal Luo or Injury Luo Treatment
122	Etiologies
123	Musculoskeletal Luo Treatment Protocol
124	Frequently Asked Luo Questions and Troubleshooting

DIVERGENT CHANNEL TREATMENTS — 130
- 130 Historical References to the Divergent Channels
- 130 Description of the Divergent Channels
- 133 The Six Divergent Confluences
- 134 Divergent Channel Needling Technique and Intention
- 135 To Perform the Deep-Superficial-Deep technique
- 135 To Perform the Superficial-Deep-Superficial technique
- 136 Indications of the Divergent Channels

CLINICAL APPLICATION OF DIVERGENTS — 136
- 136 The Divergent Channel Toolkit
- 136 Divergent Confluent Points and their Classical Names

Unblocking Wei Energetics — 139
- 139 Ensuring the Routes of Elimination are Open
- 139 Ensuring Scars are Freed

Clinical Notes — 139
- 139 Divergent Treatment Duration
- 139 Divergent Course Duration
- 140 Clarity of Treatment

BASIC TREATMENT PRINCIPLES — 140
- 140 The First Confluence
- 141 The Second Confluence
- 141 The Third Confluence
- 141 The Fourth Confluence
- 142 The Fifth Confluence
- 142 The Sixth Confluence

Preparation for Diagnosis — 143
- 143 Views of the Divergent Confluent Sequence

Diagnosis — 144
- 144 Divergent Pulse Diagnosis
- 145 Pulse Positions of the Divergents
- 148 Divergent Channel Signs and Symptoms
- 149 Key Phrases for the Divergent Channels
- 150 Single Divergent versus Complete Confluence (two Divergents)

Advanced Treatment Principles — 151
- 153 Deep-Superficial-Deep and Superficial-Deep-Superficial Treatment Protocols

Deep-Superficial-Deep Divergent Treatment Protocol — 153
- 153 Deep-Superficial-Deep Order of Insertion
- 154 Order of Withdrawal of Needles in DSD Treatments

Superficial-Deep-Superficial Divergent Treatment Protocol — 154
- 154   The Divergent Loop
- 155   Jing-Well Point Function and the Loop
- 155   Superficial-Deep-Superficial Order of Insertion
- 157   Order of Withdrawal of Needles in SDS treatments
- 157   Blockages
- 157   Healing Events
- 157   Troubleshooting
- 159   Frequently Asked Questions

DIVERGENT CHANNELS IN DETAIL — 160

BLADDER DIVERGENT CHANNEL — 160
- 160   Key Phrases
- 160   Trajectory Signs
- 160   Wei Signs
- 160   The Bladder Shu Points
- 160   Points

Bladder Divergent DSD Treatment Protocol — 161
- 161   Order of Insertion

Bladder Divergent SDS Treatment Protocol — 161
- 161   Order of Insertion
- 162   Bladder Divergent Channel Illustrations
- 164   Frequently Asked Questions Related to Bladder Divergent Channel

KIDNEY DIVERGENT CHANNEL — 166
- 166   Key Phrases
- 166   Trajectory Signs
- 166   Wei Signs
- 166   Mediumship Depletion Signs
- 166   Points

Kidney Divergent DSD Treatment Protocol — 166
- 166   Order of Insertion

Kidney Divergent SDS Treatment Protocol — 167
- 167   Order of Insertion
- 168   Kidney Divergent Channel Illustrations
- 170   Point Location and Clinical Tips

GALLBLADDER DIVERGENT CHANNEL — 171
- 171   Pulses
- 171   Key Phrases
- 171   Trajectory Signs
- 171   Wei Signs

- 171   Mediumship Mobilization Signs
- 171   Mediumship Depletion Signs
- 172   Points

Gallbladder DSD Treatment Protocol   172
- 172   Order of Insertion

Gallbladder Divergent SDS Treatment Protocol   172
- 172   Order of Insertion
- 173   Gallbladder Divergent Channel Illustrations
- 174   Point Location and Clinical Tips
- 174   Notes
- 174   Questions

LIVER DIVERGENT CHANNEL   175
- 175   Pulses
- 175   Key Phrase
- 175   Trajectory Signs
- 175   Wei Signs
- 176   Mediumship Depletion Signs
- 176   Points

Liver Divergent DSD Treatment Protocol   176
- 176   Order of Insertion
- 177   Liver Divergent Channel Illustrations

Liver Divergent SDS Treatment Protocol   178
- 178   Order of Insertion
- 178   Point Location and Clinical Tips

STOMACH DIVERGENT CHANNEL   179
- 179   Pulses
- 179   Key Phrases
- 179   Trajectory Signs
- 179   Wei Signs
- 179   Mediumship Mobilization Signs
- 180   Mediumship Depletion Signs
- 180   Points

Stomach Divergent DSD Treatment Protocol   180
- 180   Order of Insertion
- 181   Stomach Divergent Channel Illustrations

Stomach Divergent SDS Treatment Protocol   182
- 182   Order of Insertion

SPLEEN DIVERGENT CHANNEL — 183
- 183 Pulses
- 183 Key Phrase
- 183 Trajectory Signs
- 183 Wei Signs
- 183 Mediumship Depletion Signs
- 183 Points

Spleen Divergent DSD Treatment Protocol — 184
- 184 Order of Insertion

Spleen Divergent SDS Treatment Protocol — 184
- 184 Order of Insertion
- 185 Spleen Divergent Channel Illustrations
- 186 Point Location and Clinical Tips

SMALL INTESTINE DIVERGENT CHANNEL — 186
- 186 Pulses
- 186 Key Phrases
- 187 Trajectory Signs
- 187 Wei Signs
- 187 Mediumship Mobilization Signs
- 187 Mediumship Depletion Signs
- 187 Points

Small Intestine Divergent DSD Treatment Protocol — 188
- 188 Order of Insertion
- 189 Small Intestine Divergent Channel Illustrations

Small Intestine Divergent SDS Treatment Protocol — 190
- 190 Order of Insertion
- 190 Frequently Asked Questions

HEART DIVERGENT CHANNEL — 191
- 191 Pulses
- 191 Key Phrase
- 191 Trajectory Signs
- 191 Wei Signs
- 191 Mediumship Depletion Signs
- 192 Points

Heart Divergent DSD Treatment Protocol — 192
- 192 Order of Insertion

Heart Divergent SDS Treatment Protocol — 192
- 192 Order of Insertion
- 193 Heart Divergent Channel Illustrations

TRIPLE HEATER DIVERGENT CHANNEL — 194

- 194 Pulses
- 194 Key Phrases
- 194 What's going on at the level of Triple Heater Divergent Channel?
- 195 Trajectory Signs
- 195 Wei Signs
- 196 Triple Heater Divergent Channel Illustrations
- 197 Mediumship Mobilization Signs
- 197 Mediumship Depletion Signs
- 197 Points

Triple Heater Divergent DSD Treatment Protocol — 198

- 198 Order of Insertion

Triple Heater Divergent SDS Treatment Protocol — 198

- 198 Order of Insertion
- 199 Clinical Tips

PERICARDIUM DIVERGENT CHANNEL — 199

- 199 Key Phrase
- 199 Trajectory Signs
- 199 Wei Signs
- 199 Mediumship Depletion Signs
- 200 Points
- 201 Pericardium Divergent Channel Illustrations
- 200 Opening the Neck and Pelvis
- 202 10 Windows to the Sky Points
- 202 12 Doorways to the Earth Points

Pericardium Divergent DSD Treatment Protocol — 202

- 202 Order of Insertion

Pericardium Divergent SDS Treatment Protocol — 203

- 203 Order of Insertion

LARGE INTESTINE DIVERGENT CHANNEL — 204

- 204 Pulses
- 204 Key Phrases
- 204 Trajectory Signs
- 204 Wei Signs
- 204 Mediumship Mobilization Signs
- 204 Mediumship Depletion Signs
- 205 Large Intestine Divergent Channel Illustrations
- 206 Points

Large Intestine Divergent DSD Treatment Protocol — 206
- 206 Order of Insertion

Large Intestine Divergent SDS Treatment Protocol — 207
- 207 Order of Insertion

LUNG DIVERGENT CHANNEL — 208
- 208 Pulses
- 208 Key Phrase
- 208 Trajectory Signs
- 208 Wei Signs
- 208 Mediumship Depletion Signs
- 209 Lung Divergent Channel Illustrations
- 210 Points

Lung Divergent DSD Treatment Protocol — 210
- 210 Order of Insertion

Lung Divergent SDS Treatment Protocol — 211
- 211 Order of Insertion

Essential Oils and Divergent Channel Treatments — 212
- 212 Essential Oil Complementary Treatments (Simple)
- 212 Essential Oil Complementary Treatments (Complex)

Zonal Divergent Channel Treatments — 213
- 213 A Zonal Divergent Channel Treatment

The Cutaneous Regions — 214
- 215 Zonal Divergent Protocol
- 215 Frequently Asked Questions about Zonal Divergents and the Cutaneous Regions

EIGHT EXTRAORDINARY CHANNEL TREATMENTS — 218
- 218 Historical References to the Eight Extraordinary Channels
- 219 Mechanisms of the Eight Extraordinary Channels
- 221 Indications for the Use of the Eight Extraordinary Channels
- 222 The Names of the Eight Extraordinary Channels
- 222 The Three Ancestries
- 223 Considerations when Beginning any Eight Extraordinary Treatment

Eight Extraordinary Channel Treatment Tool Kit — 223
- 223 Opening Points
- 224 Opening Point Principles
- 224 Trajectory Points
- 225 Coupled Pairs
- 225 Eight Extra Needling Techniques

226	Duration of Treatment	
226	Treatment Course	
226	Unilateral Needling in the Eight Extraordinary Channels	
227	Combining Eight Extraordinary Channels	
227	Points Added to Eight Extraordinary Treatments	
227	Moxa in Eight Extraordinary Treatments	
227	Strong Connections between the Eight Extra Channels and the Curious Organs	
228	Diagnosis of the Eight Extra Channels	
228	Pulse Diagnosis of the Eight Extraordinary Channels	
229	Essential Oil Complementary Treatments (simplified)	
230	Essential Oil Treatment Protocol for the Eight Extra Channels	

Eight Extraordinary Channel Treatment Protocol — 230

- 231 Opening Points, First Points, Landmark Points Reference List
- 232 Frequently Asked Questions about Eight Extra Channel Treatments

CHONG MAI TREATMENTS — 233

- 233 Mechanisms of Chong Mai
- 235 Prenatal and Postnatal Chong
- 235 Chong Signs and Symptoms
- 235 Psychological Presentation
- 236 Needling the Opening Point
- 236 Coupled Pair
- 236 The Five Chong Trajectories

Chong First Trajectory — 237

- 237 Indications of Chong - First Trajectory
- 237 Points of Chong - First Trajectory
- 237 Point Translations and Indications of Chong - First Trajectory
- 238 Chong Channel - First Trajectory Illustration
- 239 Treatment Principles for Chong - First Trajectory
- 239 Point Selection Method for Chong - First Trajectory
- 239 Example of Point Selection for Chong - First Trajectory
- 240 Needling Technique for Chong - First Trajectory
- 240 Treatment Protocol for Chong - First Trajectory

Chong Second Trajectory — 241

- 241 Mechanisms of Chong - Second Trajectory
- 241 Indications of Chong - Second Trajectory
- 242 Chong Channel Second Trajectory Illustration
- 243 Points of Chong - Second Trajectory
- 243 Point Translations and Indications of Chong - Second Trajectory
- 244 Treatment Principles of Chong - Second Trajectory
- 245 Example of Point Selection for Chong - Second Trajectory
- 245 Treatment Protocol for Chong - Second Trajectory

Chong Third Trajectory — 246
- 246 Chong Channel Third Trajectory Illustration
- 247 Mechanisms of Chong - Third Trajectory
- 247 Indications of Chong - Third Trajectory
- 247 Points of Chong - Third Trajectory
- 247 Treatment Principles for Chong - Third Trajectory
- 248 Example of Point Selection for Chong - Third Trajectory
- 248 Coupled Pair Choices
- 248 Treatment Protocol for Chong - Third Trajectory

Chong Fourth Trajectory — 249
- 249 Mechanisms of Chong - Fourth Trajectory
- 249 Indications of Chong - Fourth Trajectory
- 249 Points of Chong - Fourth Trajectory
- 249 Coupled Pair
- 249 Treatment Principle of Chong - Fourth Trajectory
- 249 Treatment Protocol for Chong - Fourth Trajectory
- 250 Chong Channel Fourth Trajectory Illustrations
- 251 Frequently Asked Question

Chong Fifth Trajectory — 251
- 251 Mechanisms of Chong - Fifth Trajectory
- 252 Chong Channel Fifth Trajectory Illustration
- 253 Indications of Chong - Fifth Trajectory
- 253 Points of Chong - Fifth Trajectory
- 253 Coupled Pair
- 253 Treatment Principles of Chong - Fifth Trajectory
- 253 Treatment Protocol for Chong - Fifth Trajectory

REN MAI TREATMENTS — 254
- 254 Mechanisms of the Ren Mai
- 256 Non-Pathological State of Ren Mai
- 256 Pathological State of Ren Mai
- 256 Indications of Ren Mai
- 257 Physical Indications of Ren Mai
- 257 Psychological Indications of Ren Mai
- 259 Ren Channel Illustrations
- 260 Points of Ren Mai
- 260 Ren Mai First Trajectory
- 260 Ren Mai Second Trajectory
- 260 Opening Point of Ren Mai
- 260 Point Translations and Indications - Selected Points of Ren Mai
- 262 Treatment Principles of Ren Mai, First and Second Trajectories
- 263 Differentiating between the First and Second Trajectories of Ren Mai

263 Point Selection Method for Ren Mai
264 Needling Techniques for Ren Mai
264 Needling the Opening Point of Ren Mai
264 Example of Point Selection for Ren Mai
264 Treatment Protocol for Ren Mai

DU MAI TREATMENTS — 265

265 Mechanisms of Du Mai
266 Non-Pathological State of Du Mai
266 Pathological State of Du Mai
266 Indications of Du Mai
266 Physical Indications of Du Mai
267 Psychological Indications of Du Mai
268 Opening Point of Du Mai
268 Main Points of Du Mai
268 Point Translations and Indications of the Main Points of Du Mai
271 Du Channel First Trajectory Illustrations

Du Mai First Trajectory — 272

272 Du Mai First Trajectory Characteristics
272 Du Mai First Trajectory Points
272 Du Mai First Trajectory Pathology
272 Du Mai First Trajectory Treatment Principle
272 Du Mai First Trajectory Sample Point Selection

Du Mai Second Trajectory — 272

272 Du Mai Second Trajectory Characteristics
273 Du Mai Second Trajectory Illustrations
274 Du Mai Second Trajectory Points
274 Du Mai Second Trajectory Pathology
274 Du Mai Second Trajectory Treatment Principle
274 Du Mai Second Trajectory Sample Point Selection

Du Mai Third Trajectory — 274

274 Du Mai Third Trajectory Characteristics
274 Du Mai Third Trajectory Points
274 Du Mai Third Trajectory Pathology
275 Du Mai Third Trajectory Illustrations
276 Du Mai Third Trajectory Treatment Principle
276 Du Mai Third Trajectory Sample Point Selection

Du Mai Fourth Trajectory — 276

276 Du Mai Fourth Trajectory Characteristics
276 Du Mai Fourth Trajectory Points
276 Du Mai Fourth Trajectory Pathology

276	Du Mai Fourth Trajectory Treatment Principle
276	Du Mai Fourth Trajectory Sample Point Selection
276	Selecting Trajectories in Du Mai Treatments
277	Du Mai Fourth Trajectory Illustrations
278	Treatment
278	Landmark Points of Du Mai
278	Point Selection for Du Mai
279	Children with Wind
279	Treatment Protocol for Du Mai

The Wei Channels — 280

YIN WEI MAI TREATMENTS — 281

281	Mechanisms of Yin Wei Mai
282	Non-Pathological State of Yin Wei Mai
282	Pathological State of Yin Wei Mai
282	Indications of Yin Wei Mai
282	Physical Indications of Yin Wei Mai
283	Psychological Indications of Yin Wei Mai
284	Yin Wei Mai Illustration
285	Points of Yin Wei Mai
285	Opening Point of Yin Wei Mai
285	Xi-Cleft Points as Eight Extra Emergency Points
285	Xi-Cleft Point of Yin Wei Mai
285	Point Translations and Indications - Selected Points of Yin Wei Mai
287	Treatment
288	Treatment Principles of Yin Wei Mai
288	Needling the Opening Point of Yin Wei Mai, PC-6
288	Treatment Protocol for Yin Wei Mai
289	Frequently Asked Questions

YANG WEI MAI TREATMENTS — 289

289	Mechanisms of Yang Wei Mai
290	Non-Pathological State of Yang Wei Mai
290	Pathological State of Yang Wei Mai
291	Indications of Yang Wei Mai
291	Physical Indications of Yang Wei Mai
292	Psychological Indications of Yang Wei Mai
293	Yang Wei Mai Illustrations
294	Points of Yang Wei Mai
294	Alternative Trajectories of Yang Wei Mai
294	Opening Point of Yang Wei Mai
294	Xi-Cleft Point of Yang Wei Mai
294	Point Translations and Indications - Selected Points of Yang Wei Mai
297	Treatment

297	Treatment Principles for Yang Wei Mai
298	Example of Point Selection for Yang Wei Mai
298	Needling the Opening Point, TH-5
298	Treatment Protocol for Yang Wei Mai

YIN QIAO MAI TREATMENTS   299

299	Mechanisms of Yin Qiao Mai
300	Differentiating between Ren Mai and Yin Qiao Mai
300	Differentiating between the Wei Channels and the Qiao Channels
300	Non-Pathological State of Yin Qiao Mai
300	Indications of Yin Qiao Mai
301	Yin Qiao Channel Illustrations
302	Physical Indications of Yin Qiao Mai
302	Psychological Indications of Yin Qiao Mai
303	Yin Qiao Mai and Yin Luo Channel Connection
303	Points of Yin Qiao Mai
303	Opening Point of Yin Qiao Mai
303	Xi-Cleft Point of Yin Qiao Mai
303	Point Translations and Indications - Selected Points of Yin Qiao Mai
307	Treatment
307	Treatment Principles of Yin Qiao Mai
307	Needling the Opening Point of Yin Qiao Mai, KI-6
308	Needling Yin Qiao Mai
308	Example of Point Selection for Yin Qiao Mai
308	Treatment Protocol for Yin Qiao Mai

YANG QIAO MAI TREATMENTS   309

309	Mechanisms of Yang Qiao Mai
310	Non-Pathological State of Yang Qiao Mai
310	Indications of Yang Qiao Mai
310	Physical Indications of Yang Qiao Mai
311	Psychological Indications of Yang Qiao Mai
312	Yang Qiao and Yang Luos Connection
312	Points of Yang Qiao Mai
312	Opening Point of Yang Qiao Mai
312	Xi-Cleft Point of Yang Qiao Mai
313	Yang Qiao Channel Illustrations
314	Point Translations and Indications - Selected Points of Yang Qiao Mai
316	Treatment Principles of Yang Qiao Mai
316	Needling the Opening Point of Yang Qiao Mai, BL-62
317	Pain in the Context of Yang Qiao Mai
317	Choosing between Yin and Yang Qiao Mai for unilateral Bi-Obstruction
317	Example of Point Selection for Yang Qiao Mai
317	Treatment Protocol for Yang Qiao Mai

DAI MAI TREATMENTS 319

- 319 Mechanisms of Dai Mai
- 320 Comparison of the Two Dai Mai's
- 321 Consolidating Dai Mai
- 322 Dai Channel Illustrations
- 323 Indications of Consolidating Dai Mai
- 323 Choosing between Consolidating and Draining Dai Mai
- 323 Points of Consolidating Dai Mai
- 323 Needling Technique for Consolidating Dai Mai
- 323 Treatment Principles of Consolidating Dai Mai
- 323 Treatment Protocol for Consolidating Dai Mai
- 324 Draining Dai Mai
- 325 Indications of Draining Dai Mai
- 325 Physical Indications of the Dai Mai's
- 325 Psychological Indications of the Dai Mai's
- 326 Points of Draining Dai Mai
- 326 Opening Point of the Dai Mai's
- 326 Translations and Indications of the Points of Dai Mai
- 327 Pairing Dai Mai with Yang Wei Mai
- 327 Treatment Principles of Draining Dai Mai
- 327 Consolidating Prior to Draining Dai Mai
- 327 The Importance of Releasing the Five Pillars before Treating Dai Mai
- 328 Point Selection Method of Dai Mai
- 328 Differentiating between GB-27 and GB-28
- 329 Needling the Opening Point of Dai Mai
- 329 Treatment Protocol for Draining Dai Mai
- 330 Frequently Asked Questions About Dai Mai

DA BAO and BAO MAI 331

- 331 Comparison of Draining Da Bao and Consolidating Da Bao
- 332 Signs and Symptoms of Da Bao
- 332 Signs and Symptoms of Bao Mai
- 332 Points of Da Bao
- 333 Da Bao Channel Illustrations
- 334 Bao Channel Illustrations
- 335 Points of Bao Mai
- 335 Point Selection, Da Bao and Bao Mai
- 336 Treatment Principle for the Use of Da Bao, Draining Bao Mai and Dai Mai Together
- 336 Treatment Protocol for Connecting Da Bao to Bao Mai and then Dai Mai

APPENDIX I 337

- 337 The Primary Channels Including their Internal Pathways

APPENDIX II 366
366 Divergent Confluent Point Functions

APPENDIX III 375
375 Healing Events

APPENDIX IV 377
377 Safety

APPENDIX V 379
379 Equipment Essential for Advanced Acupuncture Treatments

APPENDIX VI 382
382 Cultivation

Bibliography 387

Index 388

List of Illustrations

8	Tonification and Reduction
9	Needling in Relation to Depth
23	The Achievement of Latency of a Pathogenic Factor
24	The Terrain of the Channels
28	Bladder Sinew Channel
29	Gallbladder Sinew Channel
30	Stomach Sinew Channel
31	Small Intestine Sinew Channel
32	Triple Heater Sinew Channel
33	Large Intestine Sinew Channel
34	Spleen Sinew Channel
35	Lung Sinew Channel
36	Kidney Sinew Channel
37	Heart Sinew Channel
38	Liver Sinew Channel
39	Pericardium Sinew Channel
51	Longitudinal and Transverse Luo Terminology
56	Luo Channel Pathology Progression
65	Lung Longitudinal and Transverse Luo Channels
66	Large Intestine Longitudinal and Transverse Luo Channels
67	Stomach Longitudinal and Transverse Luo Channels
68	Spleen Longitudinal and Transverse Luo Channels
69	Heart Longitudinal and Transverse Luo Channels
70	Small Intestine Longitudinal and Transverse Luo Channels
71	Bladder Longitudinal and Transverse Luo Channels
72	Kidney Longitudinal and Transverse Luo Channels

73	Pericardium Longitudinal and Transverse Luo Channels
74	Triple Heater Longitudinal and Transverse Luo Channels
75	Gallbladder Longitudinal and Transverse Luo Channels
76	Liver Longitudinal and Transverse Luo Channels
77	Ren Luo
78	Du Luo
79	Great Luo of the Spleen
80	Great Luo of the Stomach
85	Energetic Levels of the Luos
110	Pathways of the Transverse Luos
117	Routes of Luo Pathology to the Source Point
131	Divergent Channel Diverts Pathogen
134	Divergent Channel Needling Intention
140	Divergent Channels move Pathology away from Organs
162	Bladder Divergent Channel
168	Kidney Divergent Channel
173	Gallbladder Divergent Channel
177	Liver Divergent Channel
181	Stomach Divergent Channel
185	Spleen Divergent Channel
189	Small Intestine Divergent Channel
193	Heart Divergent Channel
196	Triple Heater Divergent Channel
201	Pericardium Divergent Channel
205	Large Intestine Divergent Channel
209	Lung Divergent Channel

Chong Mai

238	First Trajectory
242	Second Trajectory
246	Third Trajectory
250	Fourth Trajectory
252	Fifth Trajectory

259	Ren Mai, First and Second Trajectories

Du Mai

271	First Trajectory
273	Second Trajectory
275	Third Trajectory
277	Fourth Trajectory

284	Yin Wei Mai
293	Yang Wei Mai
301	Yin Qiao Mai
313	Yang Qiao Mai
322	Consolidating and Draining Dai Mai

333	Consolidating and Draining Da Bao
334	Bao Mai, Bao Mai with Da Bao and Dai Mai
338	Lung Primary Channel
341	Large Intestine Primary Channel
342	Stomach Primary Channel
344	Spleen Primary Channel
347	Heart Primary Channel
349	Small Intestine Primary Channel
351	Bladder Primary Channel
355	Kidney Primary Channel
356	Pericardium Primary Channel
359	Triple Heater Primary Channel
363	Gallbladder Primary Channel
365	Liver Primary Channel

List of Tables

15	Frequency and Duration of Treatment
17	Unilateral versus Bilateral Needling
24	The Organization and Terrain of the Complement Channels
60	Longitudinal Luo Channel Trajectories
123	Principles of Diagnosis and Treatment Techniques
136	Divergent Confluent Points and their Classical Names
137	Opening Points of the Divergent Channels
143	Mobilization of Mediumship by the Divergent Channels
202	Windows to the Sky, Doorways to the Earth
212	Essential Oils for the Divergent Channels (simple)
213	Essential Oils for the Divergent Channels (complex)
228	Pulse Diagnosis for the Eight Extraordinary Channels
229	Essential Oils for the Eight Extraordinary Channels
231	Openings, First Points, Landmark Points Reference List
263	Point Selection Method for Ren Mai

Abbreviations

DC - Divergent Channel.

SDS - Superficial-Deep-Superficial.

DSD - Deep-Superficial-Deep.

In this book, the terms channel, pathway and meridian are interchangeable. The term vessel is used to denote visible Luo Channels.

Acknowledgments

A book like this by its very nature is a collection of the insights and work of countless contributors, many of them unknown geniuses of medicine. If I've done my job well there is very little original work here except the gathering of pieces of the puzzle that have not been presented together before. All credit goes to the innovators in this complex medicine and the great minds who have transmitted the oral as well as written traditions.

Closer to home, there are too many individuals who have contributed than I could name, including teachers, colleagues, students, and of course, patients. It is through my patients that I have truly come to know the depth of this medicine and the utter importance of its living transmission to the future. To all of them I owe a continuing debt of gratitude.

This book would not have been possible without **Pat Didner, Kristin Carnahan, Cody Dodo,** *and* **Dr. Linda Puckette,** *each of whom played a major part in its creation.*

Pat Didner worked tirelessly for over three years to produce these beautiful and very important drawings, towards the end sometimes even with babe in arms.
Kristin Carnahan spent years expertly editing, checking and re-organizing. She ensured the clarity of the work, also with babe in arms.
Cody Dodo, an accomplished acupuncturist and designer, brought both sets of skills together to make this text as beautiful as it is. Apart from designing the entire book, Cody designed the diagrams from my written summaries, clarifying and making visually clear what could have been a relative torrent of words. His work shows great design skill as well as deep understanding and love for Classical Acupuncture's theories and practices.
Dr. Linda Puckette contributed meticulous reading, stimulating and challenging dialogue, expert mark ups of the entire text, and dozens of pages of invaluable feedback, all with deeply warm support.

A big thank you also to:
Rosie O'Shea, who kept me focused on this work and constantly made sure I had all the support needed. Thanks for the firm pushes and the strong assurances, Rosie.
Helder Coelho, co-director of our *Classical Wellness Center* in New York City, for his steady and solid shouldering of the Center as I retreated to write.
Diane Gioioso, for critical reading of the entire text, expert transformative suggestions, dedication to the medicine, and important friendship.
Dr. Sheila George, one of my principal teachers; I'm forever grateful for her expertise and depth. I've been honored to receive her guidance, to teach alongside her, and very much value her generosity and friendship.
Evan Rabinowitz, for his invaluable astuteness and enthusiastic readiness to bounce complex ideas back and forth.
The students of the very last year of Swedish Institute acupuncture classes who shared some important gems of information from the historic final lectures just before that great school was suddenly closed in 2011. Jeffrey taught more densely than ever, which is hard to imagine.
Libbie Rice, whose inspirational lectures first lit the fire of enthusiasm for this medicine in me. When I first heard her teach, I nearly fell off my chair.

Christine Sotmary, who loves the Divergents and taught them in such an engaging way that I never think of certain signs or symptoms without smiling.

Dale Stearn, who so clearly taught the surprisingly elusive art of classical point location.

Paula Chin, who clearly taught classical point location and such skillful tui na.

John Daily, who taught foundational theory and invited me to observe his clinical work once a week early in my training.

Pieter Sommen, who taught deeply effective classical tui na protocols for the Complement Channels.

All my teachers of all disciplines at the Swedish Institute, who taught freely and generously.

Brian Cullman, for reading the text with his author's eye, for enlightening feedback and for his very warm support.

Ross Rosen, for his warm-hearted collegial generosity.

Hope Hathaway, for reading the entire final draft with her expert and eagle eye.

Richie Vitale, for proofing the plethora of minutiae.

David Cecil, for reading, guidance and feedback, and editing the introduction.

Betsy Sterman, for reading the entire text and for her expert suggestions relating to the use of language and punctuation.

Erin Telford, for doing the important job of reading the text as a TCM-trained practitioner and her invaluable feedback.

Gabrielle Zlotnik, for caring so well for the Classical Wellness Center, for constant encouragement, proofreading and friendship.

Josephine Spilka for lively Complement Channel chats, and for her friendship.

Michele Stupka for her unique, indispensable help.

Nancy SantoPietro for her immensely helpful guidance.

Margaret, Sue, Holly, Tammy, Amanda, Priya, Jordana, Patti, Linda, Belinda, Michael, Bao, Melpi, Pat, Rosie, Gabrielle, Erin, Cody, Carrie, Leah, Jin Young, Eleonore, Danelle, Jessica, Rachel, Adrienne and those yet to come, for being with us at the Classical Wellness Center and for their dedication to Acupuncture.

Grace Devlin, who gave wise counsel and whose quiet and deep grasp of this medicine is inspiring.

Lynn Redman and Patrick Lynch, for writing time in the country and great friendship.

Francesca Biryukov, Dean of the Swedish Institute Acupuncture School, who nurtured the Classical Acupuncture program and extended its legacy with her staunch support of the teachings. And for her friendship.

Paula Eckardt, for creating and maintaining a truly unique treasure of a school which will be shown in retrospect to have been the catalyst for a deep shift, not only in the way medicine is practiced, but in the health of our entire society.

Cissy Majebe, for her tireless dedication to the medicine and her generosity and love for my family. Every country, *every county* needs a Cissy.

Philip Glass, for his deeply wise counsel, encouragement, and friendship.

Marjorie and Noel Cecil, for their vast teachings, especially that anything is possible.

Andrew Sterman, my partner in life and collaborator in thought. A font of engaged encouragement, he cheerfully read five years of drafts.

Dr. Jeffrey Yuen, our teacher: a living *Zhen-Ren* whose quiet and powerful presence is a fathomless gift. I am more grateful to Jeffrey than I could ever express.

About the Author

For many years, Ann Cecil-Sterman, MS, L.Ac, taught Advanced Clinical Observation and was a senior clinic supervisor at the School of Acupuncture which was founded by Dr. Jeffrey Yuen in 1997 at the Swedish Institute College of Health Sciences in New York City. Ann is currently an associate faculty member of the Chinese Herb program at the Maryland University of Integrative Health. She graduated from the Swedish Institute and is a long-time student of Dr. Yuen, having extensively studied acupuncture, diet, Chinese medical history, herbs, qigong, essential oils and philosophy with him across North America. Ann is the Director of The Classical Wellness Center in Manhattan where she practices acupuncture and teaches classes on advanced diagnosis, as well as the theory and application of Classical Chinese Medicine. Her patients—children and adults of all ages—come from all over the United States and regularly from Europe, Russia, Asia and Australia, presenting with chronic degenerative diseases, psychological issues, digestive disorders, organ failure or end-stage disease. Her practice features the Complement Channels of acupuncture, and is augmented with Classical Chinese dietary therapeutic guidance. She travels frequently to teach the application and methodology of the Complement Channels, and the art of pulse diagnosis. Ann's books are available at www.classicalacupuncture.com. She lives in Manhattan with her husband and two children.

About the Illustrator

Pat Didner, MAcOM, L.Ac, is an acupuncturist board certified in Chinese herbal medicine and a graduate of the Academy of Oriental Medicine at Austin Graduate School of Integrative Medicine. She has done extensive Asian bodywork training in tui na with Yongxin Fan as well as training in Qigong Anma with Devon Hornby. A long-time practitioner of tai chi and qigong, Pat continues training with Sifu Fong Ha and studies Classical Chinese Medicine with Ann-Cecil Sterman. Pat specializes in the treatment of chronic conditions, pain, emotional and stress-related concerns, family and women's health, including infertility, using acupuncture, bodywork, Chinese herbal medicine and nutritional counseling. Pat has an art and art history background and enjoys drawing. She lives with her family and practices in New York City.

INTRODUCTION

In 2010, my family and a group of long-time students accompanied our teacher, Dr. Jeffrey Yuen, on his first trip back to central China, his first trip back to one of the homes of Daoist medicine, the home of his teacher (his grandfather, the great master Yu Wen), and the majestic Hua Shan, one of the five sacred mountains of Daoism. Master-physicians, (including Yu Wen, 86th generation holder of the Jade Purity School of Daoism and its incredible medical lineage) had lived on Hua Shan for generations, since before the medicine began to be notated in the 2nd century BCE. In 1905, Jeffrey's grandfather had visions of what was to happen mid-century, and decided to leave the mountain. As the Cultural Revolution unfolded in the 1960s and 70s causing so much upheaval and destruction, the last of the Daoist doctors also left Hua Shan, never to return.

During our travels in China we visited many temples and monasteries famous in the history of Chinese Medicine. We visited Sun Si Miao's mountain retreat and put our hands in the pools he used for washing herbs. We stood by Hua To's tomb. I personally was looking forward very much to the experience of Hua Shan. What would it feel like to be on this mountain, in my mind the center-point of the medicine's collected lineages and mastery?

Hua Shan is stunningly beautiful and awesome in its quasi-inaccessibility. It rises 7000 feet in impossibly sheer rock faces, many of which still have the old chiseled footholds visible, points from which many a climber has fallen over the centuries. To climb it is to walk on ancient paths, holding only somewhat improved safety chains as you rise through the clouds to the five peaks, each crowned with ancient monasteries devoted to different traditions of Daoism. Much of the mountain is covered in extraordinary groupings of herbs. It is said that if you become ill on Hua Shan, the appropriate herb can be found within a circle made by one large footstep from where you are standing. The herbs grow not in large concentrations of one type, but seem evenly and magically distributed over the mountain. A square meter might have a few dozen different herbs in it. Monkeys, mugwort, giant Reishi mushrooms, and all things in between reside there. But the medical lineage does not. Of course we knew that this was the case before we arrived; the medical practice had been gone since the 1960s, but the extraordinary absence of almost anything Daoist was arresting on a very profound level. The ancient Daoist temples are either destroyed or have become resting hostels for vacationers. A few monks tend the grounds and a handful of hermits continue to practice in solitude, but the thriving culture of masters passing on fully intact teachings to younger practitioners is irrevocably gone. All things change; what was thriving for two thousand years in this place has moved on. The medicine, once part of the full curriculum of Daoist studies in these very monasteries, is now nomadic, at best.

At dawn in the monastery on Hua Shan's West peak, my long period of hesitation over completing a Manual for the acupuncture practice of this medicine vanished and I found myself feeling a need to deliver. I am keenly aware that Sun Si Miao was 70 years of age before he wrote his first book, and that many of the greatest masters worked under a vow not to write, in order to honor the fluidity of the Dao. While I recognize that it takes lifetimes to thoroughly explore this rich and vast medicine, after that experience I felt compelled to at least record and share the way in which I practice, to record an encapsulation of my understanding of what I have been given.

The Complement Channels

Choosing what material to write about first posed no problem. My practice favors Complement (also known as Secondary) Channel treatments, and most of the questions I am asked while teaching relate to these channels and their practice. The Complement Channels can be complex and challenging, but with careful and methodical study they can be practiced with utmost certainty. With acupuncture now well established in the West, focus on the Complement Channels seems both timely and needed.

Acupuncture is a broad field with many historical styles and branches. Without doubt, the most important qualifications for all acupuncturists are two: strong intention for the healing of their patients and the coherent application of the branch of acupuncture in which the practitioner has been trained. Great treatments do not need to be greatly complicated. Because the Complement Channels are far less commonly used in modern acupuncture, their use can seem more complicated than it is. There is a variety of historical reasons why the Complement Channels are not a large part of many people's acupuncture training. For many good practitioners who had only brief introduction to these channels, or for those whose exposure to them never fully "clicked", they remain too obscure for practical use, seeming the epitome of complicated or esoteric practice. In truth, the Complement Channels of acupuncture belong to the trunk of the acupuncture tree itself; they are part of the Classical practice from which all branches of acupuncture emerged. They are part of everyone's lineage. Once clearly understood, their theory and application are no more complex than that of any other familiar treatment protocol. What had seemed obscure, complicated, esoteric, or only hypothetical, can then be like discovering another source of very welcome well water beneath your feet: deep, clear, ancient and freely available to all who wish to drink from it.

The Complement Channels have no limit to their application, and are the channels that acupuncture utilizes to understand and then to reverse the course of chronic degenerative diseases. They are the key to a detailed understanding of how the body deals with a pathological encounter that it was unable to fully handle at the time of invasion. They explain the mechanisms of visceral protection that follow in the body during the progression of disease. The Complement Channels are also a model for understanding (and even altering) personal evolution, including our personal emotional journey and its impact on our physiology.

Disease Nemesis Theory

The human body recognizes that the disease of an internal organ is the most serious of all illnesses. Using very sophisticated strategies (described by the Complement Channels), the body shifts a pathogen out of the Primary Channels to ensure the safety of the organs or, in the case of the Sinew Channels, prevents penetration of the Primary Channels altogether. In the presence of a potentially life-threatening disease the Complement Channels move the illness away from the Zang Fu, and can create a different disease so that the viscera are preserved; they shift an acute condition into latency or they create a "slower" disease. The Complement Channels are present literally to preserve humanity.

A practitioner of these channels, through the examination of pulses, tongue and palpation, determines which channel is being employed to keep the pathogen at bay and then decides whether the body needs more help to do so (accentuating the body's command of the channel in its suppressive capacity), or whether it's time to give the body a directive to expel the pathogen (encouraging the body to engage the channel in its releasing capacity), or to move the pathogen to a different channel altogether. Whether known as Advanced Acupuncture (because the Channels are beyond the curriculum of many Acupuncture schools) or Classical Chinese Medicine (because the channels are described in the Classical texts) the theoretical knowledge and confident practice of the Complement Channels is potentially available to practitioners of any style of acupuncture today.

Pathogens are many but in Chinese Medicine we use a simple taxonomy of Cold, Heat and Dampness. In Western terms this could be understood as including viruses, bacteria and molds/yeasts/funghi, respectively. In Classical Medicine an enormous focus is placed on Cold and Wind-Cold. The Classics say that Wind is the origin of a thousand diseases. (Wind is a transporter or precipitator of pathogenic Cold or Dampness.) Ninety percent of the *Shang Han Lun* (*The Treatise on Damage Due to Cold*) is devoted to Wind-Cold invasion. In Manhattan's Chinatown even today, regardless of the season, you'll see the older generation walking about with scarves around their necks. The idea that the invasion of a simple virus (including the common cold) must be avoided has pervaded Chinese culture for thousands of years. The reason is that if the body lacks sufficient resources to create a fever and a brief sweat to push that Cold out straight away, the pathogen will lodge in the body and illness will occur. The body must then engage a Complement Channel to contain that Cold so that it cannot reach the organs.

A very common example of that process is an individual with arthritis which arose after a common cold penetrated through the Sinews, then perhaps the Luo's, and eventually lodged in the joints, where it proceeded to irritate, inflame and disintegrate the bone. Western medicine acknowledges that strep throat (throat Bi-Obstruction), which occurs when the Wei Qi is unable to defend the interior, can eventually penetrate the Pericardium and lead to Heart disease. This is an example of the failure of the Divergent Channel mechanism to prevent the pathogen from reaching the viscera. Although a number of such disease progressions are acknowledged in Western medicine, Chinese Medicine has exquisitely and methodically explored the underlying complexities of these disease processes, both theoretically and practically, to understand the disease progression and give instructions in multiple modalities for its reversal and healing, often rolling back decades of disease and degeneration.

Often, the progression goes something like this: the patient gets a bad cold that they just can't defeat. They were out in poor weather without the right coat or scarf and the Wind carried Cold into the Sinew Channels. The pathogen was very strong, or they were too dehydrated to sweat and/or too tired to muster the Yang to make heat for a fever, so the Sinew Channels, the first line of defense for pushing the pathogen up and out, failed. The Primary Channels (also known as the waterways) could not foster the transformation of Ying Qi to Wei Qi to produce a sweat to push it out. Perhaps there was also taxation on the Blood due to lack of good sleep, failure to hydrate well, prolonged stress, or emotional upset, so there was inadequate Blood to move

Wind via the Blood, (an action of the Longitudinal Luo's).

The Lungs are then at risk of insult since the first defenses have failed, and now coughing begins. Coughing is a form of rebellious Qi enacted to push the pathogen away from the Lungs, or literally out of the Lungs if the pathogen has penetrated them. If there is inadequate Qi to create a cough, or if the Lungs have become sticky due to deficient Fluids, the scene is set for the body to reach more deeply, creating a Divergent Channel to shift the pathogen away from the Lung organ. The body then moves the pathogen into the places in the body which have the densest, most Yin material capable of making a pathogen relatively quiet—the major articulations/joints.

Now the individual has developed achy joints and is feeling miserable. The nose is still running, still trying to push the cold out, the head and neck are tense trying to prevent further invasion, making the patient tired. Their head feels as though in a vice because the cold is compressing toward the center, but the person keeps working hard, keeps staying up late or traveling, refusing to miss commitments. All the while, the Divergent Channels are ensuring containment of the pathogen in the joints. Once that containment is assured, latency is achieved and the symptoms fade away—the patient appears to get better and life goes back to normal.

Meanwhile, that pathogen remains trapped in the joints, having been diverted away from the Lungs. A hidden, latent condition is thereby substituted for what might have become an acutely dangerous case of pneumonia. After a couple of decades, as the Jing declines because the patient never really rests properly, or doesn't eat well, or never really addresses their high-stress lifestyle, they start to notice that their joints are aching and stiff in the mornings and they feel as though they're getting old. Although this is commonly seen as simply part of the aging process, it is occurring because the complement of Jing at the level of the bones is declining, making the individual unable to maintain that latency; the old pathogen is slowly being revealed.

In the case of arthritis, this is usually the point at which the patient seeks acupuncture. The strategy of the clinician could be one of two broad options: to help enable the patient to contain the pathogen for a longer period of time because they lack the resources to push it out, or to help the patient build those resources. After the resources are gathered and the individual is considerably stronger, the practitioner can then embark on a series of Divergent treatments to pull that pathogen out of the joints, at which time the original severe cold will re-emerge from its long sleep in a relatively brief healing event that feels similar to the original illness but resolves itself surprisingly quickly. The resulting freedom of illness in the joints seems miraculous to the patient, but it's merely using the theory explained in Chapter 63 of the classical text, the *Su Wen* of the *Huang Di Nei Jing*. Case histories such as this, described in acupuncture as Disease Nemesis Theory, can be told about all the Complement Channels: the Sinews, the Luo's, the Eight Extras, as well as the Divergents. Disease Nemesis Theory explains Latency (Fu Qi) also known as Dormant, Latent or Hidden Qi.

Although a part of acupuncture theory and practice since the earliest days of Chinese Medicine (as demonstrated by their featured inclusion in the foundational Classics of Chinese Medicine), the Complement Channels are often not included in the curriculum of modern acupuncture schools. Many acupuncturists I meet have been introduced to some level of knowledge of the Complement Channels but say they lack the confidence to use them. This book is intended to fill this gap, to be a comprehensive introduction to the Complement Channels and to be a guide to their use in the clinic. It is a book of suggested treatment protocols, not official ones—or, more accurately, not the only official ones because official protocols in truth are all those that adhere to the spirit and instruction of the Classical texts. There are myriad ways to apply a given channel, and each practitioner will develop their own style, their own way of owning the medicine and working with patients. That being said, I have tried to keep my own developments away from this Manual, or at least to a minimum. I've used the treatments described in this Manual thousands of times in my own practice and I urge everyone to continue ongoing study (as I certainly do), making their own clinic manual as they go.

Transmission

In the mountain monasteries, medicine was one part of the complete Daoist monastic curriculum along with the other monastic arts: ritual, meditation, philosophy, divination, geomancy, martial arts, cooking, calligraphy and poetry, and qigong. Every practitioner was expected to become proficient in all of them. To receive medical care in a monastery (or by one of its traveling master physicians) meant being treated on a physical, emotional and spiritual level. The Complement Channels were a key part of the monastic medical training in acupuncture. The theory and practice of the Complement Channels was widespread at various stages in history, but beginning in the Song Dynasty acupuncture increasingly focused on the Primary Channels. After the Song, the practical knowledge of the Complement Channels was effectively held only in family or monastic family lineages. To receive transmission of this information required a formal initiation. It was reserved for select family members or students who had proved themselves especially capable. Many lineages were held this way. The lineage of Dr. Yuen's transmissions involved the entire monastic curriculum of the Jade Purity Sect. Along with the many disciplines (listed above) it featured a vast medical training and with it the oral tradition of acupuncture. Dr. Yuen's mastery is a combination of his incomparable reading of the Classical medical texts and the rich oral tradition that he transmits as the 88th generation of the Jade Purity Daoist tradition.

The intact oral tradition of this medicine is key to the detailed understanding of the *Ling Shu* and its more general partner, the *Su Wen*, including their discussions of the Complement Channels. One needs guidance by an initiate to make practically applicable the instructions coded in the Classical texts. Often, in commentaries or commentaries on the commentaries, a writer will remark that the language used in these texts is arcane, that the texts are disorganized, inconsistent or in many parts simply impenetrable. This is because the medicine was intentionally written in a kind of code, protecting it by keeping it available only to trained individuals in the master/disciple tradition. In the mid-twentieth century with the traumatic dissolution of old China and the development of modern China, the monastic system of learning seemed destined to be lost along with the destruction of monastic life. This has turned out not to be the case because Dr. Yuen has decided not to train a sole disciple (as is customary), but to offer the decoded classical medical teachings to any serious student. This tradition is still fully based in the spiritual cultivation of Daoism but no longer requires formal religious initiation. It is an experiment in the history of Chinese Medicine to bring these teachings forward in an open setting. The result is that although the medical Classics and their implications are deeply complicated, they can be clearly understood. For example, in Chapter 63 of the *Su Wen*, we are instructed to "needle the Divergent Channel three times". A reader of a literal translation (which is also essential study) will wonder: three times a day? Three times a week? Three times in total? None of those is the answer. A point on a Divergent Channel is needled with three different intentions at different depths without letting go of the needle. In relaying this knowledge to us, a master teacher holding the intact oral teachings from the master/disciple transmission can make the seemingly impenetrable language of the texts crystalline in its clarity.

The protocols contained here are a part of what I have gathered from years of dense study with Dr. Yuen. Although his teaching is always immensely generous and thorough, this Manual is compiled from countless teaching sessions spread out in time and place. The Manual is a gathering I made for myself (and later, my students), a working picture of the practical implementation of the Complement Channels—a piece of the puzzle answered here, another piece years later. Perhaps the pieces are not meant to be presented all in one place in so linear a fashion, but this approach has proven very helpful for my students and colleagues (and our patients). Naturally, no book alone is sufficient to learn and practice complex medical theories and protocols. Personal instruction is essential. It is an axiom of any tradition that there is an enormous difference between learning something from a book and being taught that same thing from a living teacher. This book is intended to greatly support that process, filling in gaps, adding protocols, clarifying theory and the essence of the teachings for practitioners and students. I believe that the organization of the teaching transmission in this manner does no harm to the essence of this medicine. To me it's a heavy honor to be a recipient of these transmissions. It's also a hefty responsibility: if we are entrusted with the medicine—such rare and important teachings with such unfettered access—the least we can do is hold it as precious and help disseminate it responsibly.

Although we may not be studying this medicine within the context of a complete spiritual practice, to study, contemplate, and digest these teachings is itself a practice of self-transformation. It is my hope that reading each sliver of information will awaken that knowledge within us as if it has always been there. These teachings are intended to be studied with great involvement, and then brought to the treatment table, not to be studied with detachment or as mere historical information. They are to be taken to Heart, then applied for the powerful benefit of real patients on their healing journeys.

Books and the Oral Tradition

It should be noted that this book is extremely condensed and concise. A book of this size could be written about a single aspect of any class of Complement Channels. A whole tome could be devoted to the use of the Divergent Channels to treat the somatization of emotional trauma: the Luo Channels for the treatment of cardiovascular disease or blood-borne diseases or digestive disorders, the Sinew Channels for the treatment of skeletal misalignment due to misuse, the Eight Extra Channels for treatment of geriatric diseases, just to name a tiny few. Although it may seem relatively large, I have truly left out more than has been included. All four categories of the Complement Channels appear together in one volume here because it's essential to study all of them; a treatment in one category of channel can cause healing shifts in another category of channel, shifts that must be addressed. The Complement Channels are really like an enormous self-contained network, deeply interconnected. To study one class of channels without the others would be like studying reproductive hormones without studying thyroid hormones or adrenaline—they're in the same interactive loop; what happens to one affects the others.

And, of course, the most important thing of all is regular and diligent study of the principal Classics of Chinese Medicine, the *Su Wen, Ling Shu, Nan Jing, Jia Yi Jing, Shang Han Lun* and *Mai Jing*. If we cannot say with commitment that our treatments are conceived and performed according to the teachings in the Classical texts, we cannot say we yet have a living relationship with the roots of our art.

This text is not particularly intended to function in the classroom. The role of the classroom is to impart medical theory and principles, as well as the derivation of acupuncture practice from the Classical texts. This text is intended to be a helpful companion in the clinic.

Due to the incredible vastness of the medicine (and its development over long periods of time and across wide variations in political geography), when different master teachers transmit the oral tradition, or even when the same master teaches on multiple occasions, the teachings can seem quite different. There will be variations between what appears in this Manual and other material that has been and will be transmitted in the future. This is part of the nature of Chinese Medicine; it is not a fixed science. I have no intention to convey that anything contained in this Manual is fixed in stone. Information taken out of context can seem to be in direct contradiction with other information. It cannot be otherwise; channels are applied in many different ways depending on the patient, the practitioner, the presentation of the illness at the time of treatment and the historical period being referred to in a specific teaching. Rather than being the final word on any topic included here, each entry in this manual could easily be further developed at great length. Therefore, it's my hope that this manual serves as a springboard for more discussion, for discourse, blogs, papers, and books. Together, let's create a larger library of precious books on this limitless subject. Let's discuss and debate, engage in meaningful, constructive dialogue, all the while stimulating ourselves, our colleagues and our students to practice the broadest and most comprehensive acupuncture possible, for the sake of all those who might choose us to guide their healing journeys.

Every single day I am awed, deeply grateful, and truly astonished by the unlimited possibilities of this medicine. It is my sincere hope that this Manual helps other practitioners in some way to enjoy the same exhilarating and deeply rewarding experience of the medicine, and spur the realization that Advanced Acupuncture will someday become mainstream medicine. I am humbled to think that this Manual may help other clinicians bring the benefits of Classical Acupuncture, and the sophisticated use of the Complement Channels in particular, to countless patients for what can be their indescribable benefit.

May every day be one of meaningful and profound healing and wellness.

Ann Cecil-Sterman
NYC, 2012

Nomenclature

The *Nei Jing* explains the Complete Acupuncture System of Channels and Collaterals, a vast system comprising five classes of channel: Sinew, Primary, Luo, Divergent and Eight Extraordinary. Of these, the Sinew, Luo, Divergent and Eight Extraordinary Channels are named as such in the Nei Jing (although translations vary somewhat: Divergent is sometimes translated as Distinct or Separate, and some scholar-practitioners understandably prefer Curious to Extraordinary).

However, in these source texts of acupuncture what we call the Primary Channels are never referred to as "primary." Rather, each of them is referred to by its formal name individually: Leg Tai Yang, Arm Shao Yin, Leg Jue Yin, and so forth. In English translations, these 12 channels have become collectively referred to as Primary. The term Primary in this context accurately indicates the primary necessity of these channels, which are responsible for the movement of Qi and Blood, thereby enabling the organs to operate, sustaining basic physiological function on a moment-to-moment basis.

After the attribution of the term Primary to these 12 channels, the remainder of the Complete Acupuncture System (the Sinew, Luo, Divergent and Eight Extraordinary Channels) became known collectively as the Secondary Channels, a term coined in the 1970s by the British practitioner and author, Royston Low. The grouping of the non-Primary channels is pedagogically very useful, but they are by no means of secondary importance. These channel classes are described in the *Nei Jing*, but are not grouped together or seen in any way as counterpoised to the Primary Channels.

The non-Primary Channels as a group provide the remainder of the complete energetic picture of the body. The Collaterals (the Sinews, Luos and Divergents) move pathology into and out of latency ensuring the preservation of life through their often complex mechanisms. The Eight Extraordinary Channels allow life to unfold to its full potential while also absorbing pathology that has entered the Yuan level. Together, these four classes of channel complete the Acupuncture System. Hence, here they are collectively called the Complement Channels.

In the presence of pathology the Complement Channels allow the uninterrupted functioning of the Primary Channels. A Complement Channel can quickly become one of prime importance; if one or other of them were to fail to intercept a pathogen, an individual's condition could quickly become life-threatening. Therefore the Complement Channels can assume a level of importance equal to that of the Primary Channels. For example, one could say that if going outside with wet hair in a strong wind, the Sinew Channels are primary. After a vaccination, the Luos are primary. In the case of failure of the Sinew Channels, the Divergent Channels are primary. Whatever channel system must be called upon in that moment to ensure preservation of the organs and free organ function is equal in importance to the Primary Channels.

The Complement Channels are utterly necessary for a complete understanding of the energetics of the full acupuncture system and its clinical application.

This book explores the importance of the Complement Channels—the Sinew, Luo, Divergent and Eight Extraordinary channels—considering all five classes of channel of equal importance in the Complete System of Acupuncture. Once confident with all classes, there are no conditions that cannot be successfully treated. Modern acupuncture has made tremendous inroads around the world, mostly based on Primary Channel protocols. Once we understand the other channels and see them not as Secondary but as essential to the Completion of the acupuncture system as presented in the Nei Jing and in the various oral traditions, their use will no longer seem arcane or mystifying, but in the best and most profound sense, simple.

A Note on the Illustrations

Four years ago I sent out a group email asking whether there was an acupuncturist out there who also happened to be an artist. The same day, I received a reply from my colleague (and now friend) Pat Didner. She shared excitement about the project, understood its importance and was soon at work. The illustrations took three years to complete. Pat has an amazing and quick eye and a ready and deep intuitive sense. I'm certain this book would not have been possible without her. The Primary and Complement Channels are extremely complex and there were many aspects to consider during the countless hours of discussions between us. Pat developed a unique way of conveying vital information and the result is deeply meaningful and beautiful. The most wonderful thing to me is that the drawings truly are art.

We decided to put nearly every channel on a separate page as a way of showing that the tiniest and simplest channel is just as important as the longest one with the most branches.

These drawings present some information about the channels that has not been shown before. The Sinew Channels, for example, are shown with their actual width, that is, covering the entire surface of the body and overlapping with one another. Pat has achieved this beautifully, devising a way to show the real width and complexity of the Sinews and the clarity of the bindings without losing the definition of the trajectories.

The organs are generally not shown in the drawings for the simple reason that when the Classical texts refer to the treatment of an organ, they are referring to a point that has access to that organ since the organs themselves cannot be directly needled. The Mu and Shu points have this function and they are shown in order to facilitate visualization of the completed treatment and its connection with the viscera.

Although the scope of this manual does not encompass treatment protocols for the Primary Channels, we felt the book would not be complete without a set of illustrations of those channels drawn according to the descriptions in the Classical texts. The inclusion of the Primary Channels drawn this way will also help in determining Transverse Luo and Emptied Luo diagnoses.

Author's Note

The purpose of this book is to assist practitioners in focusing their intention during an acupuncture treatment utilizing the Complement Channels. As we all know to be the case in any healing in any modality, the most important component of treatment is intention. Of course all practitioners in the healing arts have the intention to provide the path for healing. In Complement Channel treatments the roadmap of the channel being treated, along with an understanding of the process in which the body is engaged, enables the clinician to focus their intention in a more powerful and very precise way. The clinician then has a clear view of what the body needs help doing or undoing and a clear view of the way in which he or she is using needles to achieve that. This clarity is held foremost in the clinician's mind as the treatments are performed.

Chinese Medicine is underpinned by the idea that we cannot make blanket statements and rules. Chinese Medicine eschews absolutism and dogma in order to protect and honor the uniqueness of each individual. The passage an illness takes through the body will be different for every individual and is determined by their weaknesses and strengths, their history, their psyche, their physiognomy and perhaps even their astrology. It's impossible to determine what path a pathology will take without encountering the patient and then taking their pulses. Therefore it should be noted that this book contains protocols selected from the countless conceivable possibilities which adhere to the principles explained in the Han Dynasty texts.

Part One: Preparation

Needles and Needling Techniques

The Nine Needles of Classical Acupuncture

The First Needling System: Chapters 1, 7 and 78 of the Ling Shu

Acupuncture has its roots in massage which is as ancient as human touch. In pre-history, moxibustion preceded bleeding which in turn preceded the development of various types of stone needles. The earliest needle yet discovered is a lance needle from the Neolithic period. By the time of the Han Dynasty there were nine needles, each of which performed a distinct function. Today we have one type of needle and various techniques to replace the needles that are no longer in use. Below is a list of the nine original needles of Classical Acupuncture and their techniques.

1. **Chisel** needle. Maximum depth: 1.6 cun. Commonly used at a shallower depth. Moves Yang Qi and stimulates Wei Qi to treat Wind-Cold and Wind-Damp. Chiseling is the technique of the Sinew Channels and of the superficial level of the Divergent Channels. The entire arm is held straight from the shoulder, (straight elbow, straight wrist). The needle is lifted and thrust with a very small amplitude.

2. **Round** needle. (Round-tipped needle.) 1.6 cun long. The elbow and the wrist are rounded. Used to bring something deep to the surface, for example, when needling GB-41 to dredge Dai Mai. Also used for Bi-Obstruction. This needle did not pierce the skin.

3. **Spoon** needle. Spoon *(gua)* is the same character as in gua sha, to scrape. 3.5 cun long. Wrist movements are used to stimulate Qi at the surface or to entice something to the surface. Stimulates Yang Qi to support Wei Qi. This needle did not penetrate the skin and was used like a small gua sha tool.

4. **Lance** needle. (The three-edged needle.) 1.6 cun long. Used to scatter or let blood. Treats chronic Bi-Obstruction resulting from unresolved pathogenic factors. Brings Yang to the area. The modern lancet and the plum blossom replace the lance needle.

5. **Sword or knife** needle, or **Skin** needle. 4 cun long. Circling technique is used to open the point. The circles can be large or small. This needle was used to pierce to allow pus to exit from boils or abscesses. Insert and circle, then drag needle out. This needle was only inserted 2.5 fen (0.25 cun).

6. **Round-sharp** needle. *(Today's needle.)* 1.6 cun long. Seizes the Qi. Once you get *De Qi*, the needle grips. Treats Bi-Obstruction. The capacity of the practitioner to get that Qi to let go, or to invite it to behave in a way appropriate to the treatment depends on self-cultivation (for example, through tai chi or qigong). It comes from

the clinician's capacity to relax their own body. Self-cultivation is the single most important factor in the ability to effectively use the round-sharp needle.

7. **Hair** needle. 3.6 cun long. Used for threading: connecting one point to another with very shallow insertion. The skin is pinched up and the needle slipped in and kept just beneath the surface. Used for nourishing. Direct the needle toward what you want to nourish. For example, SP-6 to LR-5 to nourish Blood, SP-6 to KI-3 to nourish Yin. Expels pain, treats numbness. Long retention (hours or days) for chronic numbness.

8. **Long** needle. 7 cun long. For numbness, or paralysis in the low back. For the treatment of atrophy and numbness when humors are stagnant. For fleshy areas and for conditions deep in the abdomen. Used to treat Wind in the joints.

9. **Big** needle. 4 cun long. A big wide needle like a wood chisel. Drains Dampness near the major joints. For Bi-syndrome and deep pathological factors.

A Word about Insertion

The manner in which a needle is inserted is extremely important. The techniques and channels used in acupuncture are potent and can create strong sensations as Qi is directed within the channel. If the technique of insertion is startling, the patient can be overwhelmed and resistant before the real work is done. Although not necessary (and certainly not available in classical times), I highly recommend using guide tubes. If the guide tube is firmly pressed into the skin, the needle can be gently pressed or squeezed into the point. With this technique, most often the patient will not mind the introduction of the needle. Techniques of insertion that involve tapping or flicking are so aggressive that Wei Qi automatically comes to the defense. If your intention is to shock stagnant Wei Qi, that is a technique that can be used, but the vast majority of techniques in acupuncture work best when the patient and their Qi are quietly and unobtrusively invited to accept the needle and its work in the channel. To elicit a defensive stance from the patient's Qi can utterly ruin a treatment.

Needling Techniques and Cultivation

The *Ling Shu* emphasizes that the mastery of needling techniques requires cultivation.

> **"The ordinary guards the gate; the cultivated controls intentional power."**
> —Chapter 1.

> "Ordinary skills will maintain the physical, cultivated skills will maintain the spirit." —Chapter 3.

> With any needling technique, the most important thing is to engage the Qi. The Qi must be felt in the needle, like a biting fish. This is called *De Qi*[1] and its engagement is confirmed by the practitioner, not the patient. The patient might not feel the work in the point or the channel at the time the Qi is first engaged, but if the practitioner feels the needle connect with Qi, it has occurred. Once the Qi is engaged, the manipulation can happen. Acupuncture involves connecting with Qi through a needle and then directing that Qi with one's intention. This is what makes acupuncture a healing *art*. Inserting needles quickly and walking away is not a part of Classical Acupuncture.

Needling Techniques and Intention According to the *Ling Shu*

> "Hold the needle like a tiger firmly in one's grasp." —Chapter 54.

> "If an acupuncture point is accurately needled, the sensation will be transmitted to the passages." —Chapter 4.

This statement means that after manipulation of the point, the sensation of Qi should travel up the channel, e.g., needling LI-4 should result in a sensation beyond the wrist, elbow and hopefully even the shoulder.

> "Check the pulse after insertion." —Chapter 1.

Only by checking the pulse after needling can we be sure that our intention has taken effect at the point and in the channel.

The Breadth of the *Ling Shu* Needling Techniques Discussion

A full discussion of the needling techniques explained in the *Ling Shu* would make a very large treatise. The nine needles and their specific techniques appear in chapters 1, 7 and 78, and needling technique discussion appears in chapters 3, 4, 23, 45, 51, 52, 54, 62 and others. Much of this needling theory is beyond the scope of this manual, specifically techniques for the antique points, the back Shu points, distal locations, the Primary Channels, blood vessels, the Xi-Cleft points, abscesses, threading, needling

---

[1] Chapter 67 of the *Ling Shu* states that the capacity of the patient to experience De Qi depends on the individual's constitution and spirit.

the side of the body opposite the complaint, Cold Bi (hot needle technique). Chapter 7 discusses needling styles: front and back needling, chasing the Wind, ah shi points, spreading and *uniform* needling, needling by lifting the skin, needling for fevers, bone Bi, and spasms, simultaneous left and right needling, treating Bi using a laterally inserted neighboring needle, needling painful swellings and much more. Chapter 7 also gives specific details on the needling of the Lung, Heart, Liver, Spleen and Kidney Primary Channels. Chapter 5 discusses basing the choice of needling technique on the pulses, which could also be a book on its own.

Needling Techniques as an Extension of Tui Na

Acupuncture is an extension of the sophisticated massage technique known as *An Qiao*, which later developed into tui na. Like acupuncture, massage is a complete medical system and was a rigorous ten year study in ancient China. The hand techniques of massage were developed to move Qi in a particular way. These have been integrated into acupuncture and are accomplished with specific needle techniques. There are 28 methods of needling that fall into four categories.

The Four Categories of Needling

- **Jian**: to rid factors that are weakening the organs, for example, ridding Damp to tonify the Spleen.
- **Yi**: to benefit the Qi, for example, helping Spleen transform and transport; to reinforce the direction. This technique generally refers to Lung and Spleen. Includes scraping up or down the handle of the needle. To delineate any organ direction, scrape up. To strengthen any organ, scrape down. For example, to descend Stomach Qi, scrape the handle with an upward motion. To strengthen the Spleen to drain Damp, scrape down.
- **Hui**: relates to the Kidneys. To tonify in order to return something to where it belongs. Thrust and twirl until the skin puckers around the needle. This technique is used to astringe Yin in order to anchor Kidney Yang.
- **Zhuang**: to invigorate Yang. For example, in impotence and fertility cases. Use a hot/fire needle to bring Yang Qi inwards. Needle superficially, lift and thrust, obtain De Qi, push to the moderate level, lift and thrust, push to the deep level.

Needling Techniques Derived from Tui Na

1. *Na* (to grasp.) Lifting and thrusting. A foundational technique which enters any of the three layers of Qi (Wei, Ying or Yuan.)
   a. To tonify, hold the wrist off the body. Be gentle; to tonify is to nurture. Use slow actions.
   b. To reduce, rest the wrist on the body. The Qi reacts to the heaviness on the surface and releases. Use rapid actions.
   c. Used to nudge something to the surface. Can be used in any of the three layers.
2. *Cha* (to scrub.) Twirling and rotating. The entire arm participates. Used for scattering. Used on Jing-Well and Ying-Spring points to scatter external conditions.
3. *Gua, Tui* (to scrape.) Needle and then place thumb on top of the needle and the index finger behind the handle. Scrape the exposed part of the handle with the thumbnail of the other hand. Support the back of the needle with a finger of your other hand as you scrape, so the needle does not move. Scrape upwards to tonify. Scrape downwards to reduce (disperse). Used most often on abdominal points. *Note:* This is scraping, in which the needle is held firmly in place, not scratching which has no resistance meeting the force of the scraping, allowing the needle to bend. Scraping imparts intention of directionality to the needle which is very important for Lung and Stomach points. If scraping doesn't cause the patient to feel the sensation of direction, vibrate the needle instead.
4. *Pai* (to tap.) Hold the needle and tap the top of it until the needle reaches the desired depth. Or, hold the needle tightly and tap without allowing the needle to move and use your intention to reach the desired depth. This technique breaks up Bi-Obstruction.
5. *Tan* (to flick.) Flick the handle of the needle while the needle is inserted. To quicken the Qi, especially to quicken the Blood. Used especially at SP-10. Used with deeper, more Yin points, such as He Sea's. Flick to enhance the effect of the point. Brings mediumship to the surface. Quickens Yin humors. For example, in a faint person, flick the handle of a needle inserted at LI-4 and blood rushes to the face, or flick the handle of a needle inserted at CV-3, CV-4, or CV-6 to invigorate Qi for impotence.
6. *Fei* (to fly.) Twirl the needle and let go: the fingers fly. Use if difficult to get Qi. Use for deep level where the Qi is harder to engage. Also spreads sensation. Use for paralysis. Used to disperse Lung Qi at LU-7.
7. *Pun* (to circle.) Hold and stir with needle, making a circle with the elbow. Small circles are tonifying. Large circles are dispersing. In relation to the midline of the body go clockwise to tonify and counterclockwise to disperse. Can be done with lift-

ing and thrusting. Focus on lifting to disperse. Focus on thrusting to tonify. To push Qi, make a tornado with the described action as you pull the needle up. To drain downwards, stir as you push. Circling technique can be used to disperse "gummies" or nodules.

8. *Chan* (to vibrate.) Hold the base of the actual needle at the skin, lean the needle to the left or right and vibrate (finely shake) the needle. Shake to the (patient's) left to tonify Yang Qi and shake to the (patient's) right to tonify Yin Qi. Or, shake towards the midline to tonify, away from the midline to reduce. Or, shake in the direction of the channel to tonify, against the direction of the channel to reduce. Used for stagnation.

9. *An* (to press.) Insert the needle. Hold the end of the handle and bend the needle so that the handle is perpendicular to the skin. Press down on the handle so that the point experiences pressure. This technique stabilizes Qi in a point.

10. *Tui* (to push, to sweep.) As the needle is twirled, sweep the other hand firmly along the skin, up toward the point to draw energy into the point for tonification. For reduction, sweep the hand away from the point as the needle is twirled. The technique enhances the flow of Qi in the point and also helps direct Wind away and out of the body.

General Advanced Acupuncture Needling Techniques

Tonification and Reduction

1. **By turning the needle.**

    There are many ways to tonify or reduce a point. When these techniques are talked about in terms of turning a needle, the following often-mistranslated rule applies.

    To tonify a point, the needle is turned toward the midline of the body.
    To reduce a point, the needle is turned away from the midline of the body.
    The following examples are given as though the practitioner is face-to-face with the patient.
    To *tonify* ST-25 on the right side of the body, the needle is turned *clockwise*.
    To *tonify* ST-25 on the left side of the body, the needle is turned *counterclockwise*.
    To *reduce* ST-25 on the right side of the body, the needle is turned *counterclockwise*.
    To *reduce* ST-25 on the left side of the body, the needle is turned *clockwise*.
    This rule also applies to the back where the spine, of course, is on the midline.

To tonify a point,
the needle is turned toward the midline
of the body.

To reduce a point,
the needle is turned away from the
midline of the body.

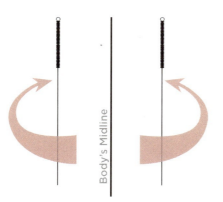
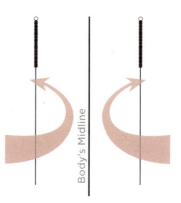

When tonifying, focus on the thumb and turn less than 180 degrees toward the midline. When dispersing, focus on the index finger and turn more than 360 degrees away from the midline.

Note: If you're needling the Gallbladder Channel on the lateral midline of the body, only then does the idea of clockwise for tonification and counterclockwise for reduction apply.

If ever it seems unclear on leg or arm points, imagine that the handle is pointed straight to the floor or the ceiling, whichever is closer, and treat according to its relation to the midline.

2. **Using speed of insertion.**

    Chapter one of the *Ling Shu* gives the following instruction:

    To tonify: insert the needle slowly and withdraw quickly.

    To disperse: insert the needle quickly and withdraw slowly.[2]

    This technique is applied to the action of lifting and thrusting. When tonifying, every thrusting action is slow and every lifting action is fast. When dispersing, every thrusting action is fast and every lifting action is slow.

    Chapter 3 of the *Ling Shu* cautions us that if not treating a condition of excess, quick insertion and slow withdrawal will produce a deficiency.

3. **By opening or closing the hole.**

    Chapter 54 of the *Ling Shu* says that when treating excesses, leave the hole open upon withdrawal. When treating deficiency, close the hole upon withdrawal. Classically, this technique was performed by holding the finger against the shaft of the needle as it was being withdrawn and seamlessly sliding the finger onto the insertion site.

---

[2] The *Nan Jing* gives the opposite instruction.

4. **By directionality of breath.**[3]

   Chapter 62 of the *Ling Shu* gives the following instruction:

   To disperse: the practitioner concentrates on the point and inhales during insertion and exhales upon withdrawal, leaving the point open.

   To tonify: the practitioner concentrates on the point, exhales during insertion and inhales during withdrawal.

Needling in Relation to Depth

- *Cooling technique*: Reach into the cool level of Qi, engage the Qi and bring it up to the superficial level to cool a fever.
- *Fire Mountain technique:* Needle the superficial level, engage the Qi and move it down to a deeper level to warm the interior.
- *Clearing Internal Heat:* Needle into the Yin (cool) level, engage the Qi and draw it up to the moderate level, re-engage the Qi and draw it up to the superficial level as patient breathes out. This technique is used to clear Internal Heat.
- *Tonifying Yang:* For example, Kidney Yang at KI-3. Needle superficially, engage the Qi, push to the moderate level, re-engage the Qi, push to the deep level.
- *Tonifying Yin:* For example, Kidney Yin at KI-3, 6, or 9, needle deeply, engage the Qi, pull up to the moderate level, re-engage the Qi, pull up to the superficial level.
- *Tonifying Qi:* Lift and thrust at the moderate level.
- *Raising Qi:* Squeeze skin up as the needle is inserted.
- *Descending Qi:* Insert needle as patient breathes in and then press the flesh down around the needle.
- *Ascending Qi:* Insert needle as patient breathes out and then grasp the skin around the point.

Chapter 3 of the *Ling Shu* warns us that needling too deeply can cause perverse Qi to move more deeply.

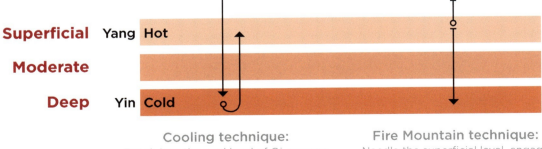

Cooling technique:
Reach into the cool level of Qi, engage the Qi and bring it up to the superficial level to cool a fever.

Fire Mountain technique:
Needle the superficial level, engage the Qi and move it down to a deeper level to warm the interior.

---

[3] These instructions are consistent in all texts.

Needling for Directionality

To direct the Qi:
- Scrape the handle of the needle in the direction you intend the Qi to go. (Important for Lung and Stomach points.)
- Needle, vibrate the point with the hand surrounding the point. The patient should feel a sense of direction.

Needling Techniques for the Round-Sharp Needle to Simulate the Nine Needles of Classical Acupuncture

Today we use the round-sharp needle, (needle 6 on page 2). In order to create the distinct effect of each of the nine needles, different techniques are now applied to the round-sharp needle. These techniques are best learned one-to-one, teacher and student side by side. According to chapter 45 of the *Ling Shu*, they require the shoulders, elbows and wrist to be cultivated and opened to allow adequate Qi to flow to the hands. An excellent way to develop this openness is serious practice of the art of calligraphy.

1. To simulate the chisel needle, chiseling technique is used. The arm is held as one straight unit from the shoulder to the needle (the elbow is kept straight) and small up and down movements are made from the shoulder only.
2. To simulate the round needle, a rolling technique is used. The focus of movement is at the elbow and wrist in a hook-like motion.
3. To simulate the spoon needle, turn the round-sharp needle upside down and scrape with the handle using movements at the wrist.
4. The lancet and plum blossom replace the lance needle.
5. To simulate the techniques of the sword needle and big needle, use shaking technique (moving rapidly from side to side).
7. and 9. To simulate the hair and the big needle, the round needle is threaded in series. Additional needles are added to create a continuous line of threading.
8. Long round sharp needles replace the long needle.

Note: The list numbers above correlate to the list numbers on p. 2.

Contraindications for Needling

Chapter 23 of the *Ling Shu* warns against needling if the following signs appear during a febrile disease:

1. Absence of sweat with red cheeks and dry heaving.
2. Abdominal distention with diarrhea.

3. Cloudiness of the eyes with unrelenting fever.
4. Fever with a distended abdomen.
5. Absence of sweat with vomiting of blood.
6. Ulcers at the root of the tongue with unrelenting fever.
7. Absence of sweat, coughing blood and nosebleeds.
8. Fever in the Marrow.
9. Fever with convulsions, crooked spine, lockjaw and absence of speech.

Chapters 51 and 52 caution not to damage any anatomy and not to puncture the organs or major arteries (including those in the inner thigh, the feet, and near the eyes).

Metals: Gold, Silver and Stainless Steel

Gold needles tonify. Silver needles reduce/disperse. Stainless steel needles require cultivation on the part of the practitioner in order for the needle to effectively engage and direct the Qi.

Entitic Invasion During Needling
If concerned about taking on an entity during needling, use scalenes as stabilizers and clamp jaw firmly shut. If an entity is felt entering, simply clamp jaw, firm the wrist and the hand and push it back. Certainly the most effective method of avoiding an entity is cultivated detachment from the energy of the patient.

Needling Techniques of the Complement Channels

Here follows a selection of techniques essential for the performance of the treatments of the Complement Channels outlined in this book.

Sinew Channel Needling

The technique for the Sinew Channels is called "chiseling". The elbow and the wrist are kept absolutely straight and lifting and thrusting movements are made from the top of the shoulder. The lifting and thrusting movement is kept within the Wei level so the movement of the tip of the needle is very small. Needles are not retained.

Alternative technique: Insert the needle only the distance the tube allows. Turn the needle a little until it grabs the skin and pull it straight out. Don't touch the hole; allow the Wind to escape. This technique is not comfortable and should be used quite judiciously.

Luo Channel Needling

These treatments involve "lancing" or pricking the skin and allowing a drop or two of blood to be let. Sometimes the point requires a gentle squeeze after lancing to encourage the blood to emerge. Lancing is best performed with a fine lancet.

An alternative method to lancing is plum-blossoming. The practitioner lightly taps the skin with a disposable, long-handled tool that has five or seven embedded needles. I find this technique far more invasive than lancing.

Divergent Channel Needling

These treatments require engaging Wei Qi either at the Wei level or at the Yuan level, dragging it to the respective opposite level and back again. The technique is called "deep-superficial-deep" (DSD) or "superficial-deep-superficial" (SDS).

1. To perform the SDS technique:
    a. Insert the needle into the Wei level with a tube. That means it's pressed into the point the depth the tube allows and not inserted further. (BL-1 and GB-1 are always inserted freehand with a half inch needle. For these points, the Wei level is relative to the depth of the point: very shallow.)
    b. Lift and thrust within the Wei level to engage Qi. This means the tip of the needle is moving up and down with very small movements. Keep holding the needle.
    c. Push the needle in deeply relative to the point and lift and thrust at the Yuan level to engage the Qi. Keep holding the needle.
    d. While the Qi is engaged, drag the needle back up to the Wei level and lift and thrust at the Wei level. Leave the needle inserted. It should be so shallow that it's almost falling over.

2. To perform the DSD technique:
    a. Insert the needle deeply into the point, relative to the point and lift and thrust at that level. Keep holding the needle.
    b. Drag the needle up to the Wei level and lift and thrust at that level. Keep holding the needle.
    c. Push the needle back down and lift and thrust again at the Yuan level. Leave the needle at the Yuan level.

If you lose the Qi on the way up or down, go back to the point where you lost the Qi, lift and thrust to re-engage the Qi and continue with the larger movement of the needle.

You'll know if you've lost the Qi because the "dragging" sensation (which is normal when Qi is engaged and moved) disappears. When the Qi is not engaged, the needle feels as though moving through butter.

Note: It is not possible to engage Wei Qi with a silicone-coated needle.

Alternative Divergent Channel Needling Techniques

Instead of lifting and thrusting at the Wei and Yuan levels (which takes a great deal of control), use circular technique in the Wei level and vibrating technique in the Yuan level.

1. To perform the Superficial-Deep-Superficial technique:
    a. Insert needle into Wei level and engage Qi with circular technique.
    b. Keep holding on to the needle.
    c. Push the needle to the Yuan level and vibrate until Qi is engaged.
    d. Pull needle back up to the Wei level and use circular technique.

2. To perform the Deep-Superficial-Deep technique:
    a. Insert needle into Yuan level and engage Qi with vibrating technique.
    b. Keep holding onto the needle.
    c. Pull the needle up to the Wei level and use circular technique.
    d. Push needle back down to the Yuan level and use vibrating technique or no technique at all at this final stage, just simply return to the deep level.

Eight Extraordinary Channel Needling

These channels are needled with "vibrating" technique. When I learned this from my teacher, the movement he used was imperceptible, so fine was the frequency of vibration.

a. Needle relatively deeply to access the Yuan level.

b. While still holding the needle, vibrate it as finely and quickly as possible and imagine a deep hum, like a subway train traveling underground below your office building, or like a distant bee. The movement should be virtually imperceptible. The capacity to perform this vibration is attainable through cultivation using qigong and tai chi practice. Use standing technique:
    i. While standing, vibrate from the legs, ankles and heels.
    ii. Stop vibrating physically, standing still, sensing the vibrations continuing internally.

After much practice of both steps, use the second step when using vibrating technique with a needle. See Cultivation appendix on page 382.

Diagnosis and Treatment

Classical Pulse Taking

Pulse-taking is arguably the most important aspect of acupuncture training. Accurate diagnosis through analysis of the pulses is essential in determining the correct treatment.

To learn pulses well one needs practical instruction. The traditional method is learning by apprenticeship. There are some great teachers of Classical pulse-taking who offer classes and practical tutorials. Practitioners all over the country have formed study groups. To refine your pulse-taking technique ask very advanced practitioners for permission to observe in their clinics, calibrating your readings with theirs.

Chinese Medicine is often thought of as various modalities such as acupuncture, herbal medicine, tui na, etc., but the essence of this medicine is beyond its varying modalities and lies in its theoretical framework and its diagnostic methods. The theoretical framework is the knowledge of health and illness, including the detailed understanding of the progression of illness and mechanisms of healing. Diagnosis is the art of identifying which progression is underway and where a particular patient is in such a progression in the context of their individual complexities.

Diagnosis within Chinese Medicine is done through feeling the pulses, looking at the tongue, listening to the patient (including both the tone and content of what they tell us), watching their quality of movement, and so forth. The art of pulse-taking has been consistently emphasized through all periods of the medicine. Tongue diagnosis became popular and developed only in the Ming Dynasty. Prior to the Ming, the tongue was not a diagnostic tool; the state of the tongue as a whole was merely regarded as a sign.

Pulse-taking has a long history and includes many styles and specialities. There are specific pulse diagnosis techniques for all the categories of channels. Methods will naturally vary according to the practitioner's lineage and intention. Whatever the method, be it Classical or modern TCM, the initiation of the healing process occurs in earnest not with the insertion of the needles but during the taking of the pulses, which is a genuine opportunity to engage and direct the patient's energy.

Engendering the Qi of the Pulse Treatment (Sheng Mai)

If there is difficulty locating pulses, the following treatment will summon them.
CV-12, ST-25, CV-17, LU-1, BL-12, all tonified.

Point Location by Palpation and Movement

In Classical practice, acupuncture points are seen as *living events*. They change and move. They can even move by several cun. Very often, the correct location of a point in terms of the *living anatomy* of the individual patient differs considerably from the standardized text book location, (although textbook locations are also extremely important to know). The fact that acupuncture points move doesn't mean that there's more margin for error. Quite the contrary. For example, Xi-Cleft points are literally in clefts in the anatomy. With that in mind, locating ST-34 is a very different experience to simply remembering the textbook location. The results of needling in the location of the living anatomy are comparably different. If you stretch out your hands and make a circle with your index fingers touching at the top and your thumbs touching at the bottom, that's the range of possible location for many points on the body. Obviously, BL-1 occurs within a tiny area, but points like ST-30 and GB-37 and many others could be far from the textbook location.

Locating points using the *living anatomy* involves moving the body in various ways to reveal a point. For example, BL-10 is found by extending the head, BL-40 by flexing the leg, GB-30 by flexing the hip, TH-10 by flexing the elbow, LI-15 by raising the arm, LI-5 by extending the thumb, etc.

Frequency and Duration of Treatment

The frequency and duration of acupuncture treatments varies according to the category of channel treated.

Channel Category	Basic Frequency of Treatment	Duration of treatment
Sinew	Every day for three to five days. No more than 10 days.	No retention of needles.
Luo	Every other day for 21 days (eleven treatments).	No retention of lances or blood regulating needles.

Channel Category	Basic Frequency of Treatment	Duration of treatment
Primary	Varies between every other day and every five days depending on the organ emphasis of the treatment, (Lung Primary Channel treatments are at the every other day end of the spectrum and Liver Primary Channel treatments are at the every five day end of the spectrum), for 30 days. Points from no more than three channels can be used in a single treatment.	Twenty minutes and few needles for tonification treatments. Forty minutes and more needles for reduction treatments.
Divergent	Three days on and three days off for 18 days.	Twenty minutes for SDS. Forty minutes for DSD. The time starts from the insertion of the last of the meeting points.
Eight Extras	Once a week for twelve weeks. If progress is rapid, the treatments can be reduced to weeks 1, 2, 3, 4, 6, 8, and 12.	Forty minutes from the completion of the needling of the landmark points.

In today's style of practice patients generally come to see us once a week when they have a complaint. It's fine to do any type of treatment (even Sinew treatments) once a week, but technically speaking that does not constitute a true Classical treatment of that channel, except in the example of the Eight Extras.

On the occasions where I have done a course of treatments according to the stipulations above the results have been extraordinary. However, with practice, a weekly treatment of any class of channel can be extraordinary. There's no need to worry about these prescribed frequencies if they seem impractical. They are important to know for context and for respectful formality.

Unilateral versus Bilateral Needling

Category of Channel	Side
Sinew	Needle the side of the body which has the complaint.
Luo	Lance the Luo point on the side opposite the pulse, e.g., ST-40 is lanced on the left, LR-5 is lanced on the right. Then treat the remainder of the Luo Channel bilaterally, beginning on the side of the treated Luo point.
Primary	Unilateral or bilateral.
Divergent	Bilateral for meeting/Confluent points, unilateral for Jing-Wells, unilateral or bilateral for opening and trajectory points.
Eight Extra	Unilateral. (Li Shi Zhen says it is disrespectful to needle the Eight Extras bilaterally.) Needle Opening point on the right for females, left for males, except for the Ren and Du, which are reversed.

Physiological Responses to Unilateral Needling

The discussion about unilateral and bilateral needling is a complex one. Nowadays in my practice I needle unilaterally whenever permissible. I find unilateral needling to be far more powerful than bilateral needling. This is because the action of the needle at a point elicits a very potent response, and the body's desire to be symmetrical or balanced is also very strong. Therefore when you create an effect in an acupuncture point on one side of the body, the body immediately tries to generate the same effect in the same point on the opposite side of the body. Once that happens, the body's capacity to heal itself is enormously accelerated because it's not having the treatment served up on a platter. Instead, it's working hard to produce the healing on its own. This is one of the most incredible things to witness—a patient shifting from within, turning the corner right there on the table.

Scars

Scars create breaks in the channels of energy and therefore prevent the free flow of Qi. Because of this, scars can impede the effectiveness of acupuncture treatments. To maximize the effectiveness of acupuncture treatments, scars must be freed.

Scar Treatments

Scar treatments play an essential role in the freeing of the flow of Qi in any channel that the scar crosses. Minor scars can often be dealt with in a Sinew treatment, but if the scar is deeper due to surgery or other trauma, or if the scar is old, a more specific treatment is performed. A scar treatment is necessary when the scar:
1. does not feel flexible when you press it.
2. does not mirror the flexibility of the surrounding skin.
3. appears convex or concave.
4. appears discolored.
5. is inflamed, infected, painful, or in any way bothersome.

Scar Treatment Protocol

1. Examine the scar to establish whether it is concave, meaning sunken below the level of the skin, or convex, meaning raised above the level of the skin.
2. Needling Technique:
    a. All needles are inserted quite superficially and very close to the scar but not directly into it.
    b. The needles around the scar are all inserted with pressure applied to the handle of the needle to cause it to bend into a half-moon shape.
    c. If the scar is concave, the point of the needle pushes up under the perimeter of the scar to pull it up.
    d. If the scar is convex, the point of the needle is inserted curving down onto the perimeter of the scar to direct the scar tissue downward.
3. Take 13 half inch needles. Using the technique described above, insert one needle at either end of the scar orientated toward the other end of the scar. Add another eleven needles to the scar, six on one side, five on the other. These can be evenly spaced, or concentrated in areas of the scar that appear to need more attention.
4. Add the Jing-Well point pertaining to the channel on which most of the scar is situated. If the scar traverses more than one channel, choose the Jing-Well related to the most remarkable part of the scar.

5. Retain needles for 20 minutes. Remove the scar needles first, then the Jing-Well.

6. Give the patient two drops of lavender oil to apply directly on the scar, one drop for each of the following two days. If the scar is very large, you might focus the oil on the most remarkable part of the scar.

7. Repeat the treatment if necessary, in a week. One scar treatment is extremely powerful and can free a scar completely. You'll know because the scar will change noticeably and become pliable or flexible.

Frequently Asked Questions About Scar Treatments

1. *My patient had a tummy tuck and the scar goes all the way across the abdomen. Should I use more than 13 needles? And which Jing-Well should I use?* 13 needles is adequate. The best Jing-Well to use would be ST-45 because the Stomach Channel is most replete with Qi and Blood.

2. *Which Jing-Well is chosen if the scar is on the midline?* If the scar is on the Ren Channel, ST-45 is the Jing-Well point. If on the Du, BL-67.

3. *Is there a limit to the size of scar that can be treated?* No.

4. *How can I get the needle to penetrate the skin around the scar if it is a keloid lesion?* Move away from the scar until you can get the needle in. Don't go so far away that it's easy to insert the needle.

5. *Why did the scar change color and become red during treatment?* This indicates Qi and Blood are flowing to heal the scar.

6. *My 62 year-old patient has a thick ropey scar from an appendectomy at the age of five. Can a scar treatment soften a scar that age?* Definitely.

7. *Can a very small scar really affect the free flow of Qi?* Yes.

8. *How does the treatment protocol change if the scar is tiny?* Use fewer needles. Three would be the minimum.

9. *The scar I'm treating has no ends because it's circular. How does the treatment protocol change for a scar with no discernible ends?* Simply surround the scar with up to 13 needles.

10. *Do I have to use 13 needles for it to be a bona-fide scar treatment?* No. Fewer than 13 is fine.

Ease of Use of the Complement Channels

When learning the Complement Channels, we can get the feeling that it might be very difficult to arrive at a diagnosis in an appropriate length of time in the clinic. While it's quite true that any class of Complement Channel can treat anything, when first practicing the Complement Channels in the clinic it's useful to limit your choices in order to maintain a clearer mind.

I recommend that in the first year or so of practice we limit our choices in one of two ways:

EITHER:

Use the Sinew Channels for acute conditions, the Luo Channels for emotional complaints, the Divergent Channels for chronic, one-side, intermittent complaints and autoimmune issues, and the Eight Extra Channels for issues that began in childhood, or issues in the Yuan level.

OR:

Practice one class of Channel for everything for a set period, then switch to another class of Channel for a time, e.g., one month of purely Divergent Channel treatments followed by one month of Luo Channel treatments, etc.

These two methods of organising thought not only save time but also help generate efficiency and certainty. I prefer the former method but the latter will help develop diagnostic skills quite rapidly. The most important thing is to dive in and use these amazing tools.

Part Two: The Application of the Complement Channels

The Complement Channels perform the common function of keeping pathology away from the Zang Fu. A pathogen will first encounter the Sinew Channels which create sneezes, sweat, coughing, vomiting, diarrhea or frequent urination to release the pathogen. They can also create tightness to hold the pathogen in the exterior until enough resources have been gathered to release it.

Aspects of Latency of a Pathogenic Factor

1. If the Sinews fail, the pathogen moves either to the Divergent or to the Luo Channels. When those avenues are exhausted, the Eight Extra Channels can absorb the pathology. When a pathogen is being held latent in the Luos, Divergents or Eight Extras, there are no signs or symptoms.

2. If the Tai Yang Sinew—the very first line of defense for an external pathogenic factor—fails and the Luo Channels do not absorb the pathogen, the pathogen can enter the He-Sea point of the Bladder Primary Channel. The body diverts the pathogen from the Bladder organ (to which the He-Sea has access) to the joints. The pathogen has entered the Divergent Channel sequence at that point.

3. If the Luo Channels are taxed due to Ying (Blood or Fluid) deficiency, the pathogen can go to the Divergent Channels.

4. If the Sinews fail due to insufficient Yang, the pathogen can go to the joints. As Jing declines, latency is lost (symptoms emerge as the pathogen becomes unhidden in the joints) and arthritis ensues.

5. If Ying is taxed by heat, the Jing will step in and use its cold to hold the pathogen. When latency is lost from the Jing, heat along with the pathology is released, causing the Triple Heater pulse to float as it tries to clear the Jing of pathology. The pathogen then has access to the organs. Therefore the body will try at all costs to find an alternative reservoir of latency.

6. The Luo Channels can empty into the Yuan-Source level if they overflow with pathology and fail to find a neighboring Luo to occupy.

7. The Luos can empty into their related Primary Channel or a neighboring Luo.

8. Pathology in the Luos can find its way to the Eight Extra Channels. The last Yang Luo (the Gallbladder Luo) can empty its pathology to ST-42 which connects to Chong Mai, and the last Yin Luo (the Liver Luo) can empty into the Ren Mai at the end of its trajectory, CV-2, giving entry to the Constitution.

9. The Constitution can pass the pathology to its main reservoir, Dai Mai. When Dai Mai fills, it should drain, but if it cannot, it uses Kidney Divergent Channel to extend its field of latency.

10. Once in a Divergent Channel, the pathogen can then move through the Divergent Channel sequence until it reaches the last confluence, the Large Intestine and Lung Divergent Channels.

11. At the end of the Divergent Channel sequence, the pathogen can enter the Primary Channels at ST-12, but the body will try to push the pathology to the Da Bao at GB-22 which is another point on the Lung Divergent Channel trajectory. GB-22 is also the Great Luo of the Spleen and the pathogen can find latency in the Luo arena there, also.

12. When The Great Luo of the Spleen fills, the pathology can spill down via either the GB Primary Channel or Bao Mai to Dai Mai, a major holding site.

13. At the end of the Divergent Channel sequence, the pathogen can go to Du Mai at GB-8.

14. When the capacity to hold the pathogen in latency is exhausted, the pathogen moves to the organs and the disease becomes terminal.

The Achievement of Latency of a Pathogenic Factor

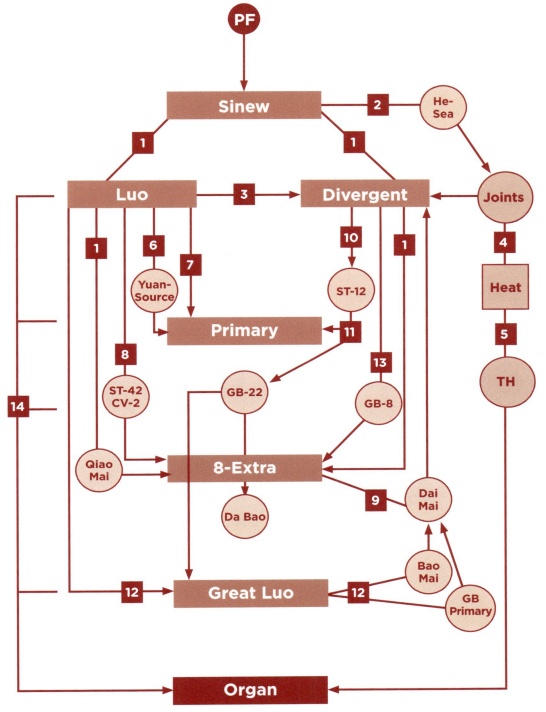

The human body recognizes that the disease of an internal organ is the most serious of all illnesses. Using very sophisticated strategies (described by the Complement Channels), the body shifts a pathogen out of the Primary Channels to ensure the safety of the organs or, in the case of the Sinew Channels, prevents penetration of the Primary Channels altogether. In the presence of a potentially life-threatening disease the Complement Channels move the illness away from the Zang Fu, and can create a different disease so that the viscera are preserved; they shift an acute condition into latency or they create a "slower" disease. The Complement Channels are present literally to preserve humanity.

The Organization and Terrain of the Complement Channels

Channel	Qi Levels		
	Wei	Ying	Yuan
12 Sinew Channels	✓		
6 Cutaneous regions	✓		
12 Primary Channels	✓	✓	
16 Luo Channels		✓	
12 Divergent Channels	✓		✓
8 Extraordinary Channels			✓
2 bisecting or cross-sectioning connections		✓	✓

The Terrain of the Channels

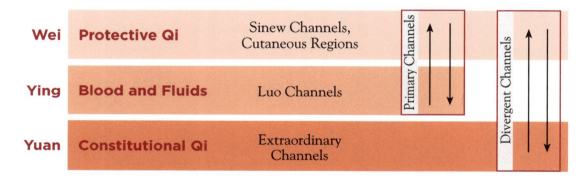

Wei	**Protective Qi**	Sinew Channels, Cutaneous Regions
Ying	**Blood and Fluids**	Luo Channels
Yuan	**Constitutional Qi**	Extraordinary Channels

(Primary Channels; Divergent Channels)

The Sinew Channels

SINEW CHANNEL TREATMENTS

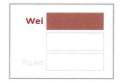

Historical References to the Sinew Channels

Chapter 43 of the *Su Wen* says that Wei-Defensive Qi is formed from food and drinks. It says it cannot travel in the blood vessels but circulates between the skin and sinews. The pathways of the Sinew Channels are given in detail in chapter 13 of the *Ling Shu*. The chapter also says that pathology of the Sinews causes pain, tightness and flaccidity. It then discusses the resulting impairment of movement. Chapter 59 discusses the pathology that results when Wei Qi stagnates and accumulates in the sinews.

Sinew Channel Theory

The Sinew Channels are conduits of Wei-defensive Qi. They cover the entire surface of the body, overlap with their adjacent neighbors, and have one acupuncture point, the Jing-Well. The Sinew Channels exist in the absence of pathology because they are responsible for bringing to the senses information about the external environment. They offer protection from that environment because when they are stimulated by a pathogenic factor (Cold, Wind or Dampness) they instigate a defense by creating a sneeze and a sweat or a fever. Wei Qi is a subset of Kidney Yang; it's warming and moving. It's derived from Gu Qi, specifically the turbid aspect of Stomach Fluids. The distribution of Wei Qi to the surface of the body is governed by the Lungs, and the quality of Wei Qi, its ability to move smoothly, is determined by the Liver. The Sinew Channels are activated at BL-1 upon the opening of the eyes after sleep. Wei Qi flows through the Sinew Channel sequence, taking 24 hours to complete a full cycle.

Sinew Channel Sequence: BL, GB, ST, SI, TE, LI, SP, LU, KI, HT, LR, PC.

When the sinews are initially challenged by an external pathogenic factor, the following sequence of events should occur: the back of the neck tightens and a sneeze ensues with its accompanying micro-sweat, pushing the pathogenic factor back out. If the body fails to produce that response and the pathogen becomes stuck where it entered at the surface of the posterior body, the pathogenic factor is said to have entered the Tai Yang zone (the Bladder or even Small Intestine Sinew). If the body continues to fail to resolve the pathogenic factor, it can move from Tai Yang and be transmitted to any station along the Sinew Channel sequence, from Tai Yang to Shao Yang to Yang Ming to Tai Yin, to Shao Yin and finally to Jue Yin. Each time the pathogen progresses, the location of limitation of movement changes or spreads.

The objective of a Sinew treatment is to free a trapped pathogenic factor and obstructed Wei Qi in a Sinew Channel, either from Tai Yang if it is still in its early stages and hasn't spread or directly from the Sinew Channel to which it has spread. Sinew treatments can also be used to work the pathogenic factor back to Tai Yang from the zone to which it has spread.

When the body experiences an injury, Wei Qi, carried by the sinews, accumulates at the injury site naturally creating swelling to immobilize the area and prevent its use so that it can heal. As Wei Qi accumulates it concentrates resulting in excess heat, but as with swelling, this is a normal response to injury. By concentrating Wei Qi in an area, not only is there more Qi for healing, but the chance of transmission of the injury to its adjacent sinews is reduced. If there is gentle movement, treatment, and much rest, the healing of the injury should be complete. However, in our culture ice is used in the treatment of most injuries. This is extremely harmful as it sends both the Wei Qi and the swelling inward, freezing the healing action of Wei Qi, preventing the smooth flow of Wei Qi once its task of bringing protection has been completed, and compounding the chance of an injury being transmitted to an adjacent Sinew Channel. If an injury has been treated with ice, it's likely that more Sinew treatments will be needed than if no ice had been applied. All use of cold packs and ice must stop altogether for full healing to occur. It's essential to teach patients receiving Sinew treatments about the function of Wei Qi and the way in which ice greatly prolongs injury.

It's important in Sinew Channel treatments to assess the nature of the pain. If the pain is radiating, Wind is the predominant factor. If the pain is stabbing or there are spasms, Cold is the predominant factor. If the pain is fixed, Damp is the predominant factor. Cold and Dampness require the inclusion of moxa in the treatment.

If Wei Qi is insufficient, the injury might not receive a thorough response and so Kidney Yang must be tonified to generate Wei Qi. Deficiency of Wei Qi can result in numbness, weakness and loss of sensitivity. Excess Wei Qi can result in over-sensitivity, redness and pain when touched. This happens when Wei Qi is not moving properly. Sinew treatments correct the flow of Wei Qi.

The great minutiae of the Sinews in general and the internal complexities of the Yin sinews could fill a volume this size. This chapter is a basic overview of Sinew treatments. The illustrations of the Sinew Channels show the central area of the sinews in a dark shade and the parts of the Sinew that overlap with adjacent sinews in a lighter shade. The entire colored area shown on a page comprises a single Sinew Channel.

Bladder Sinew Channel

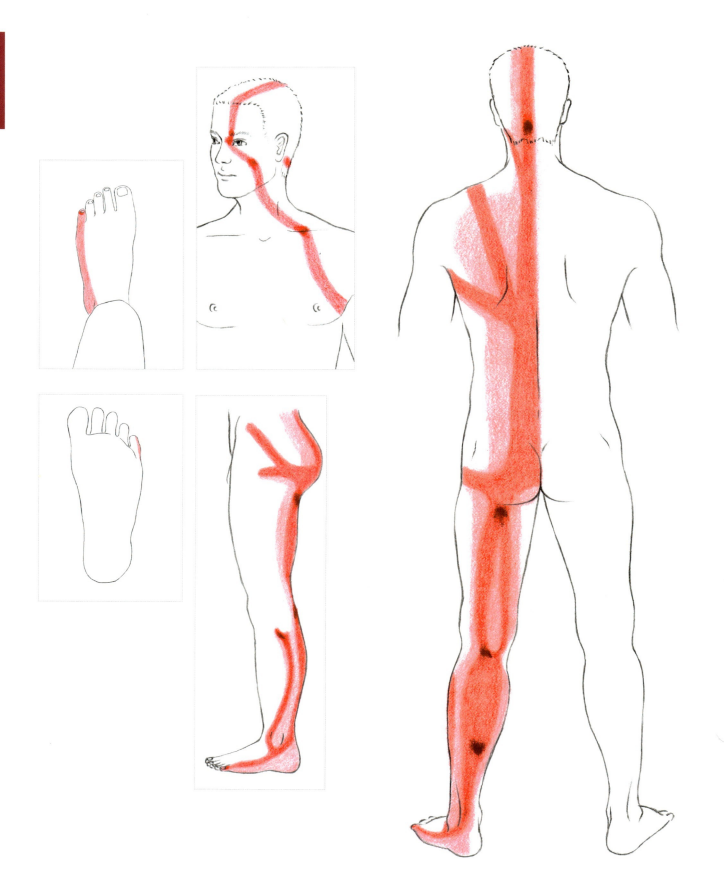

Gallbladder Sinew Channel

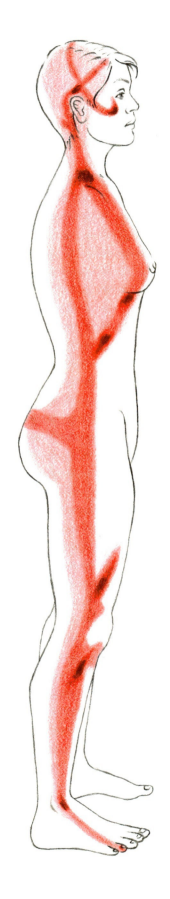
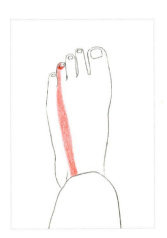
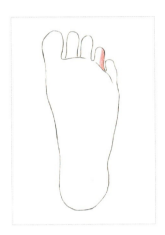
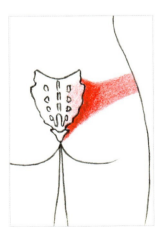

Stomach Sinew Channel

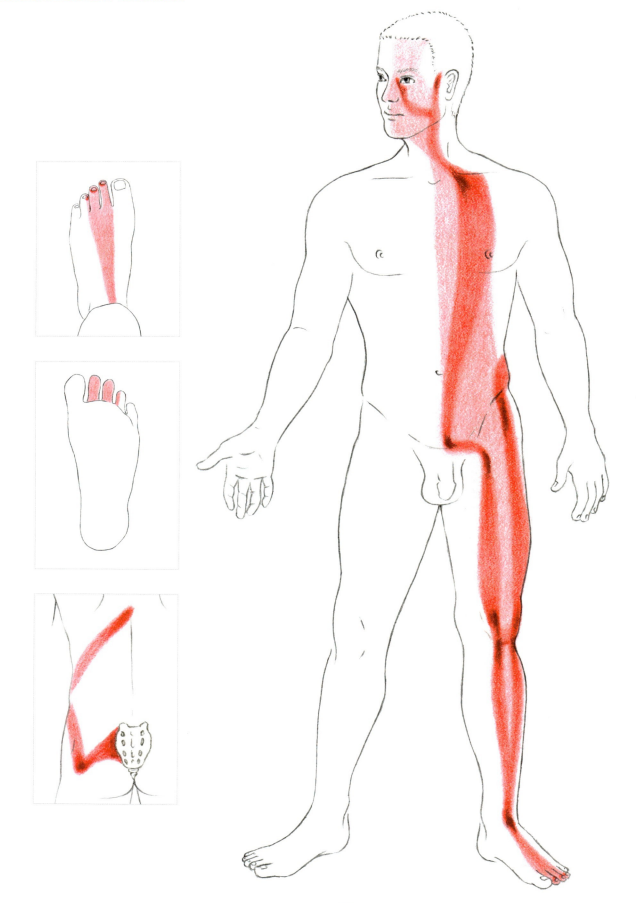

Small Intestine Sinew Channel

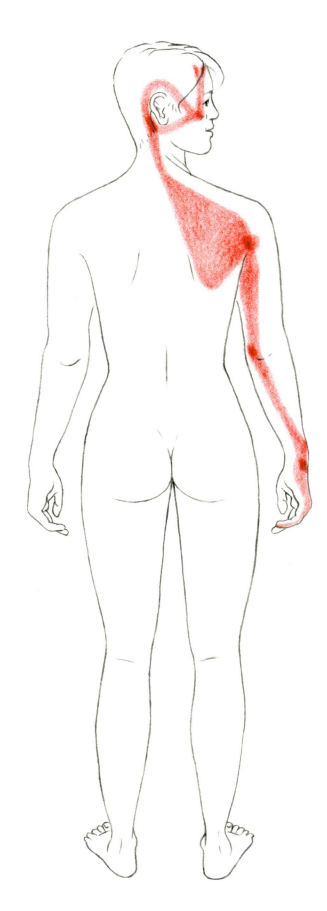
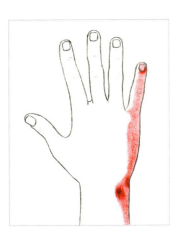

Triple Heater Sinew Channel

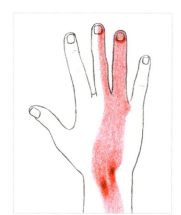
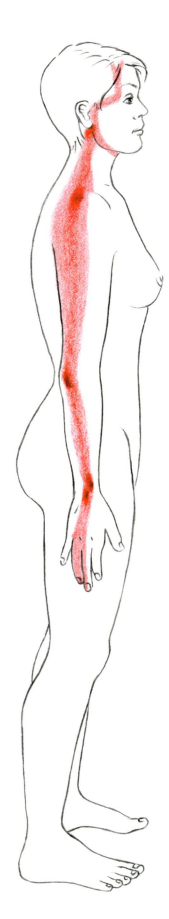

Large Intestine Sinew Channel

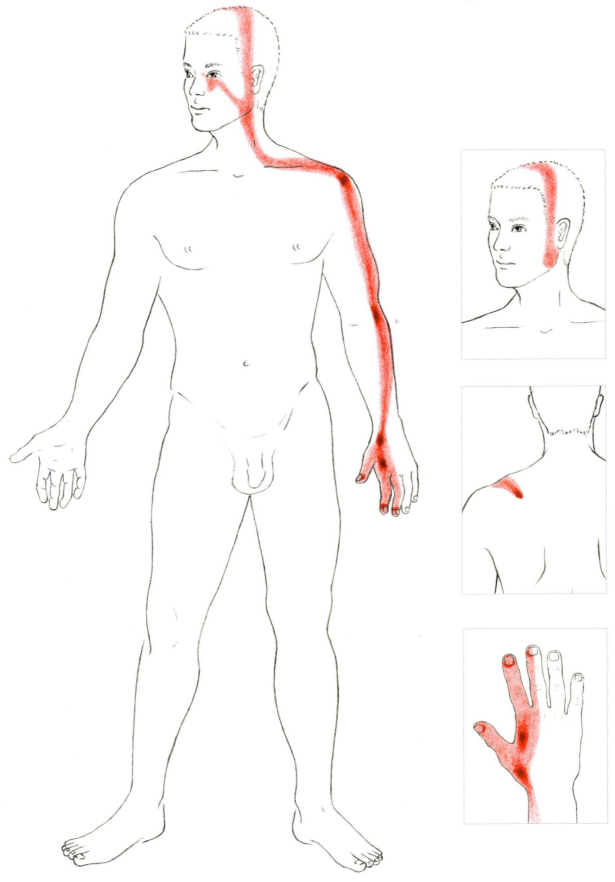

Spleen Sinew Channel

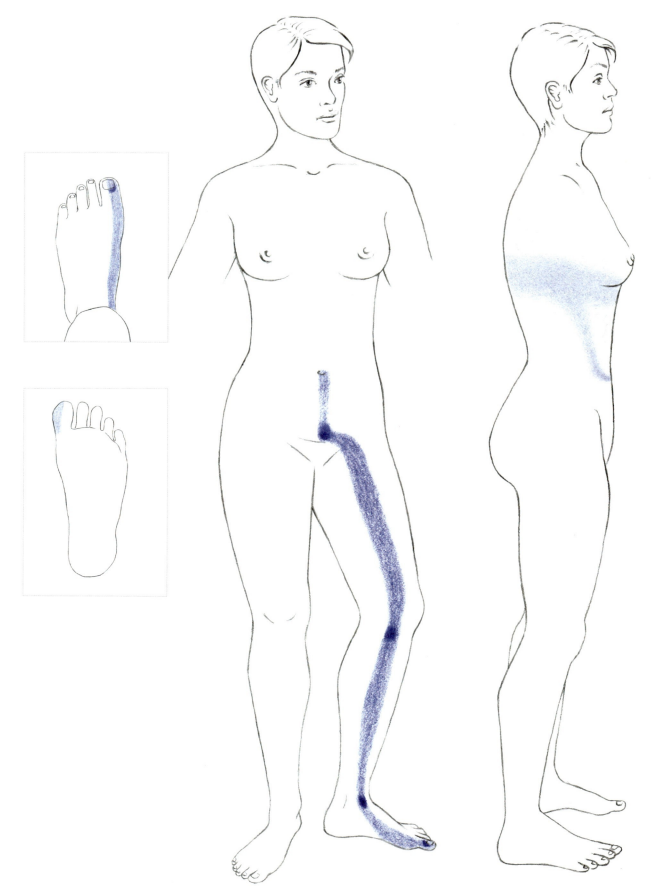

Lung Sinew Channel

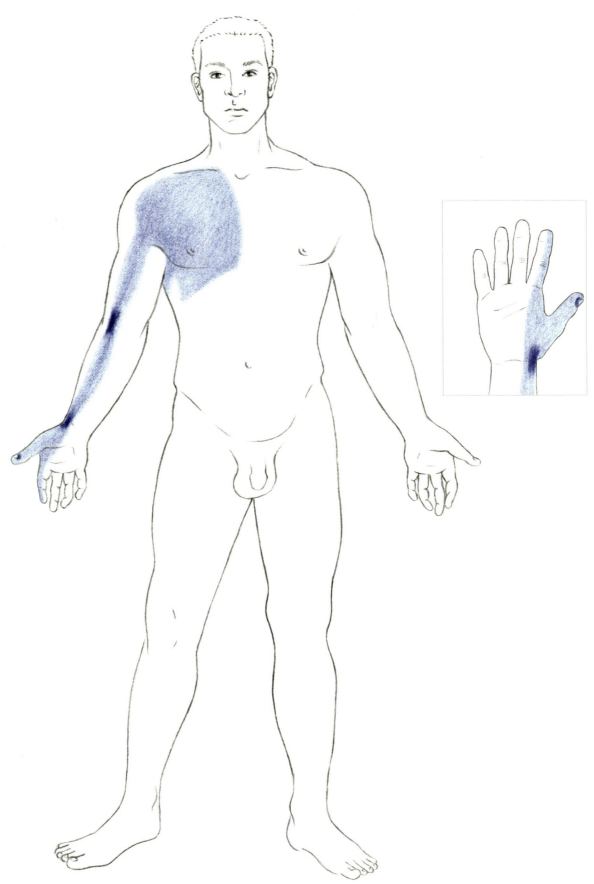

Kidney Sinew Channel

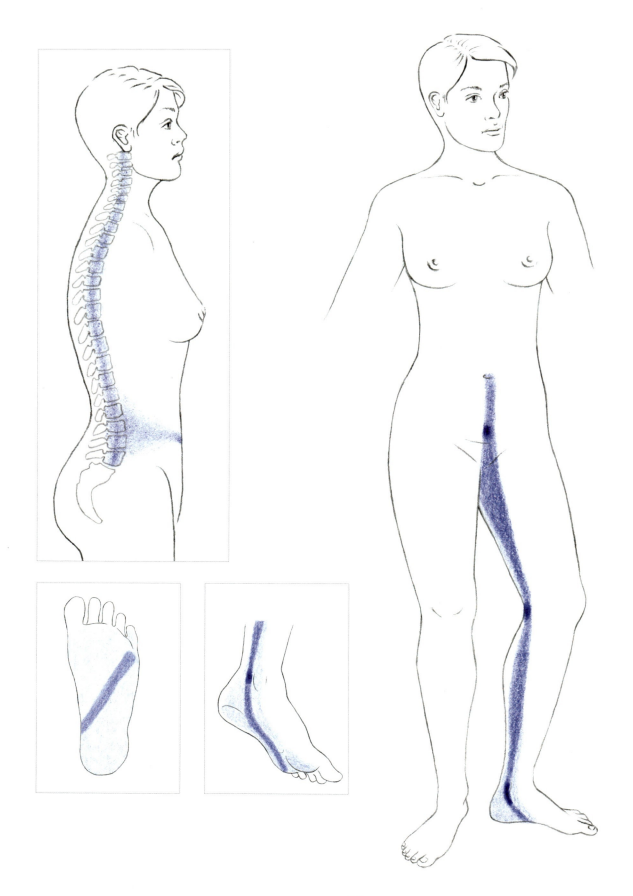

Heart Sinew Channel

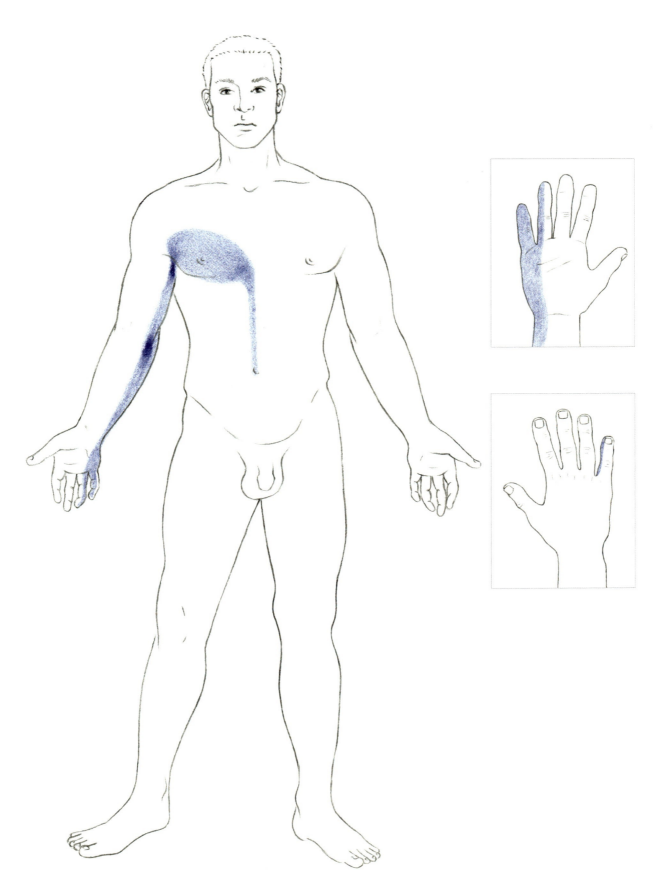

Liver Sinew Channel

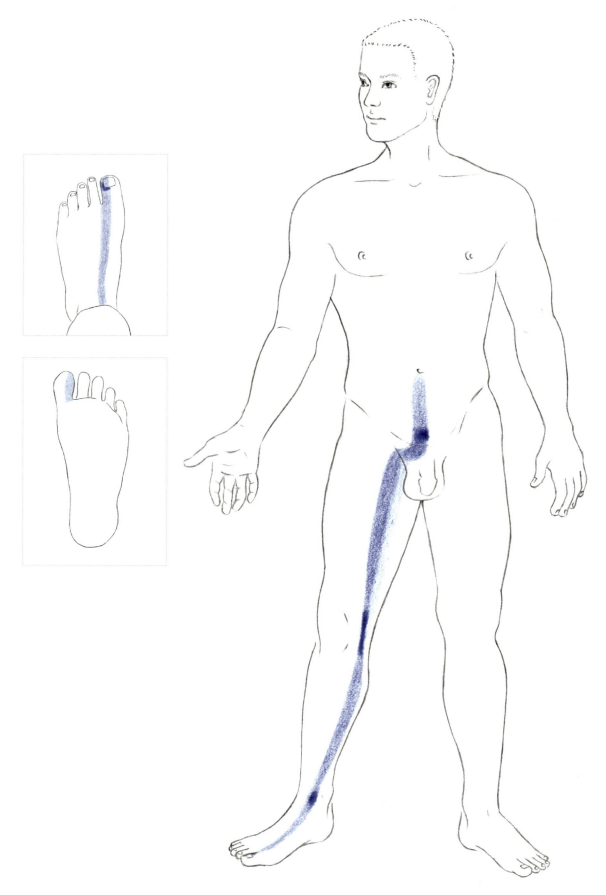

Pericardium Sinew Channel

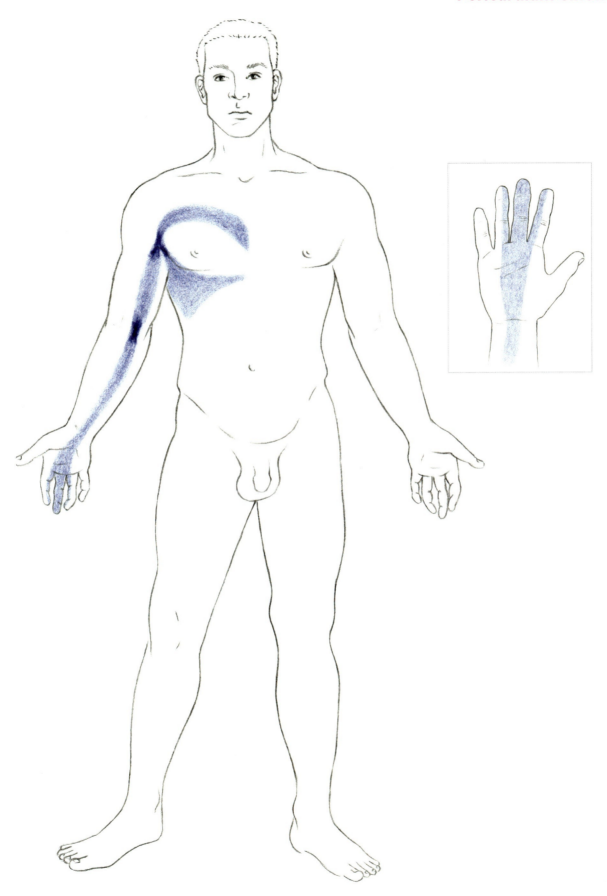

Sinew Channel Indications

- Sinew treatments release any combination of Cold, Damp, Heat and Wind trapped in the Wei level, resulting in pain, stiffness, tightness, weakness, numbness, neuropathy, allergies, digestive issues, mood disorders, hypersensitivity to weather and temperature.
- The Sinew treatment is the most appropriate treatment for acute injuries.
- The Sinew treatment can also be used for chronic injuries; new, old, and very old scars from surgery or burns; and for the misalignment of joints, as in the case of bunions, for example. Sinew treatments dramatically speed recovery after injuries and surgeries, burns, breaks and fractures.

Etiology

Injury, Wind-Cold invasion, or stress-induced injury. Maximum Wei Qi is available for the expulsion of Wind-Cold in the Tai Yang Sinew. If the body was unable to expel the pathogen via Tai Yang, it can spread to other Sinews, causing pain.

Objective

The objective of a Sinew treatment is to expel a trapped pathogenic factor and to free obstructed Wei Qi in a Sinew channel. Sinew treatments relieve pain and restore movement of Qi and Blood and range of motion.

Prerequisites

There are two crucially important requirements for a successful Sinew treatment:

    a. Assessment by movement
    b. Treatment of the underlying deficiency/ies

Explanation

Assessment by movement

Assessment by movement is essential because that alone determines which Sinew is injured. Very often, the Sinew that appears affected is not the location of the injury. The symptoms have transferred to the apparently injured Sinew, but the injury remains in the originally injured Sinew. Treating the apparently injured Sinew— the one showing symptoms—may not yield a successful Sinew treatment. Conversely, the injury may, in fact, *have* traveled to another Sinew and no longer be fully in the originally affected Sinew (although there might be residual pain and swelling in the original Sinew). In either case, assessment by movement gives an accurate reading of the current location of the injury and, therefore, determines the focus of treatment.

Treatment of the Underlying Deficiency

Sinews are most often injured because a deficiency of Qi prevented the body from being able to deflect or quickly eradicate the pathogenic factor.

Treatment Tool Kit

1. Pulse assessment:

Check the status of the four underlying deficiencies most often responsible for a deficiency of Wei Qi:

    a. Kidney Yang: What is the strength of the Kidney Yang pulse?

    b. Stomach Fluids: What is the width of the Spleen pulse at the moderate level?

    c. Freedom of Liver Qi: Is the Liver pulse tight? Is the smooth flow of Wei Qi compromised?

    d. Lung Qi dispersal: Is the Lung pulse dispersing? Does it follow your finger up to the surface as you slowly release it? Can the Lungs disperse Wei Qi to the surface?

    e. Locate the Sinew pulse: Where is the pulse tight and superficial?

2. Assessment by movement:

Determine which Sinew is injured by asking the patient which movement is most difficult to make.

- **Tai Yang** is affected if the most difficult movement to make is **extension**. This includes lateral extension of the arm (abduction) and "forward extension" of the arm which is usually known as flexion. Difficult actions are walking and driving. Pain occurs upon the *movement* of extension.
- **Shao Yang** is affected if the most difficult movement to make is **rotation**. This means turning the head, torso or rotating anything including the hip joint or arms. Lateral flexion of the head indicates Shao Yang.
- **Yang Ming** is affected if the most difficult movement is **stopping or bearing weight.** Gripping and holding, especially with a straight arm, bending over at the hips and standing still are all Yang Ming. The difference between extension pain in Tai Yang and Yang Ming is that the pain that occurs on extension in Yang Ming is while the body is stationary while the pain that occurs on extension in Tai Yang is during movement.
- **Tai Yin** is affected if the most difficult movement to make is **retracting.** Bringing hands, knees or feet towards the body.
- **Shao Yin** is affected if the most difficult movement to make is **rotation with a bent limb**, for example, sitting with the ankle resting on a thigh, or pouring tea.
- **Jue Yin** is affected if there is **pain all the time** or if there is **paralysis** (loss of all movement).

3. The meeting /confluent areas of the Sinew Channels:

The Leg Yang, Leg Yin, Arm Yang and Arm Yin sinews meet in four areas.

The Leg Yang Sinews meet at the cheekbone area.

The Leg Yin Sinews meet at an area above the pubic bone.

The Arm Yang Sinews meet at an area at the temples.

The Arm Yin Sinews meets at an area below the axilla.

4. Ah shi points:
- a. Points that are flaccid
- b. Points that are tight
- c. Points that are cold
- d. Points that are hot
- e. Painful points

5. Binding nexuses along the Sinew Channel:

Refer to the illustrations of the Sinew Channels in this manual. See where the sinews bind to the major articulations: the shoulders, hips, knees, and also the occiput, face, and ankles. All of these regions are marked in a darker shade along the Sinew Channel. The bindings are places where the sinews connect to the bones or ligaments. Cold (tightness) can concentrate in these areas. It's important to release these "fruits of the sinews" during the treatment.

6. Jing-Well points:

These are the only acupuncture points on the Sinew Channels and are extremely important as the gateway for the release of the pathogen. You'll notice in the drawings that the Jing-Wells are not points; they are considered moon-shaped areas for potential release. The optimum point for needling within that area is located by the action of pumping, as you would a well. To locate a Jing-Well point, rest the patient's distal interphalangeal joint on your index finger, and with your thumb resting on the distal end of the patient's nail, pump the nail up and down several times. An area somewhere around the nail bed will turn red. That's the location of the Jing-Well's actual point. LU-11, for example, could be on the medial or lateral side of the finger, or even in the middle of the base of the nail bed.

Sinew Needling Technique

The technique for the sinews is called "chiseling". The needle is inserted the distance the tube allows (very shallow, whether using guide tubes or not). The elbow and the wrist are kept absolutely straight and a lifting and thrusting movement is made from the shoulder only. The lifting and thrusting movement is kept within the Wei level so the movement of the tip of the needle is very small. Keep lifting and thrusting until the Qi is engaged, then withdraw the needle. (Needles are not retained.)

Alternative "twisting" technique (this is what I use most often): Insert the needle only the distance the tube allows. Turn the needle away from the midline until it just begins to grab the skin a tiny bit and pull it straight out. Tenting will occur around the needle. This technique must be learned through demonstration. While astonishingly effective, it can be painful and should not be used if a patient finds it too unpleasant. Chiseling is much less invasive.

Sinew Treatment Protocol

1. *Take the pulses and write down the findings from item one in the toolkit above.*

2. *Ask where the pain is and write it down. Or, if you can see the injury, write down its location.*

3. *Ask about the nature of the pain:*
    a. "Sharp" indicates cold
    b. "Dull" indicates Damp
    c. "Radiating" indicates heat
    d. "Moving" indicates Wind
    e. Wind is the conveyer of all environmental EPFs

4. *Ask the patient which movement is most difficult. This is the most important question in Sinew diagnosis.*

5. *Now you have one or several sinews notated on your chart:*
    The Sinew pulse you found in pulse-taking.
    The Sinew determined by movement assessment.
    The Sinew related to the location of the pain.
    These could all be the same, or two of them could be the same, or they could all be different.

6. *Treat the underlying deficiency or deficiencies determined in your pulse findings. It may be necessary to do one or more of the following depending on your pulse assessment:*
    1. Tonify Kidney Yang
    2. Nourish Stomach Fluids
    3. Release the Liver
    4. Disperse Lung Qi

> **Failure to address any of these four deficiencies if they are indicated will jeopardize the treatment. Verify that you have adequately addressed any deficiencies by checking the pulse before continuing on with the treatment.**

7. *Treat the Sinew that's most interior first. Determine that from the Sinew Channel sequence:*

    Most interior—PC, LR, HT, KI, LU, SP, LI, TH, SI, ST, GB, BL—most exterior

8. *Needle the tightest point in the confluent area with even technique.*

    a. If treating a Leg Yang Sinew, palpate the cheekbone and surrounding area to find the tightest spot.

    b. If treating a Leg Yin Sinew, palpate the area approximately a cun superior to the pubic bone to find the tightest spot.

    c. If treating an Arm Yang Sinew, palpate the temples and the area around ST-8 and GB-13 to find the tightest spot.

    d. If treating an Arm Yin Sinew, palpate the area inferior to the axilla and down to around GB-22 to find the tightest spot.

9. *Palpate the Sinew Channel (whole or in part) from the most proximal location of pain or tightness on the Sinew and progressing to the Jing-Well point, to find the ah shi subjectively (the patient says "Yes, that hurts") or objectively (you find what's flaccid, tight, cold or hot) or both subjectively and objectively.*

10. *Needle the ah shi as you go, using the chiseling or twisting technique.*

11. *Release the bindings as you come to them with the same technique.*

12. *Cup or use sliding cups if necessary to move stagnation.*

13. *Don't retain the needles at all. You're treating Wind.*

14. *Moxa tight, cold and flaccid areas either as as you discover them en route, or after you finish needling the channel. Needle the ah shi point in question, then moxa at the insertion site.*

15. *When you reach the end of the Sinew Channel, needle the Jing-Well point on the Sinew you are treating and remove the needle in order to release the pathogenic factor. Simply insert the needle pointed distally, and remove the needle. Do not use chiseling or twisting technique on the Jing-Well.*

16. *Repeat for all sinews in your diagnosis, working backwards in the order of progression. For example, if the injury is in Tai Yang but has moved to Yang Ming, treat Yang Ming first and Tai Yang last.*

17. *Use the remaining treatment time to go back to the areas that received moxa, to ensure that they remain warmed. If they have not stayed warm, continue to moxa those areas.*

Tonifying the Sinews

If there is flaccidity in the Sinew that is allowing a joint to repeatedly dislocate, or a weakness that is causing a lack of integrity in structure, tonifying the Sinew Channel in question rather than releasing it, may be called for.

1. Needle the Confluent area.
2. Needle the Jing-Well pointed UP (proximally) the channel.
3. Palpate from the Jing-Well proximally up the channel. Find flaccid areas, insert the needle, chisel, then immediately withdraw it and cover the hole with a sliding action so that the opening made by the needle is not exposed at all. Work your way up the entire channel.

Some areas might be excess (Cold, Damp or Heat) in which case, treat those areas as you would in the releasing treatment protocol in the "Sinew Treatment Protocol" section above.

Frequency of Treatment

The injury will improve dramatically during the first treatment. Often it will disappear entirely. If you can only see a patient once a week, the treatment will still be successful but it may take longer. You may want to consider sending them home with a liniment (see below) but it is not necessary if the treatments are performed correctly. (Prescribe liniments if you and your patient resonate with that method.)

Classical Prescription

Sinew treatments should be done three days in a row, up to three times a day.

Practical Note: The patient should be instructed to stay warm and covered, to strictly avoid cold or raw foods, to strictly avoid ice or cold packs, and to take an Epsom salt or sea salt bath. Most often, a single treatment will produce astonishingly successful results. It's possible for decades-old chronic Sinew injury conditions to vanish in a single treatment.

General Expectation: These days, since patients typically see us only once a week, most injuries take a few weekly treatments.

Essential Oil Treatment of the Sinew Channels

Since the Sinew Channels are wide and have only one point per channel, treatment with essential oils is done with liniments. Ideally the liniment is mixed to match the diagnosis, so there would be different liniments for Wind-Cold, Wind-Heat and Wind-

Damp, but it's quite normal for mass-produced liniments to contain the oils for all scenarios. If you're mixing your own, it's best to have all three individual types on hand. Mixing essential oil liniments for Sinew treatments is very complex and not the focus of this book. One must choose the correct oil for all the underlying deficiencies and then the directionalities involved, and whether there's numbness, pain, or Blood involvement. However, for completeness, here's a list of the oils that stimulate the six zones. They are mixed at between 1% and 5% solution with carrier oils carefully chosen for the individual's underlying deficiencies and to suit the diagnosis:

Tai Yang:	Spruce, Basil
Shao Yang:	Rosemary, Celery, Lemon
Yang Ming:	Bitter Orange, Petitgrain
Tai Yin:	Eucalyptus Smithii/Dives, Galbanum
Shao Yin:	Benzoin, Sage
Jue Yin:	Clary Sage, German Chamomile

Follow-Up Recommendation

Sinew treatments are greatly enhanced by Epsom salt or sea salt baths. An entire quart or even a half gallon of Epsom salts in a safely hot bath and a soak of at least twenty minutes is a good follow-up. (Use caution if high blood pressure is present.)

Healing Events

Sinew injuries might travel to an adjacent Sinew. This is more likely if the Confluent point is omitted.

Troubleshooting

The treatment didn't work.

Make sure you've treated the underlying deficiency/ies. Failure to do this is the most common reason a Sinew treatment is not effective. See FAQ section for treatment tips.

There is no improvement (in pain or flexibility) during movement assessment after treatment.

Blood stasis is indicated and must be addressed.

The pain moved, but didn't come out.

Most likely the Confluent point or the Jing-Well point was omitted, or the sinews were not treated in order of most interior to most exterior.

There is significant improvement, but there is still sharp pain.

Most likely, no moxa was used on the areas of pain or tightness. Use moxa and sliding cups and be sure to release the Jing-Well point.

I was unable to get the needle to engage Qi by either turning it or lifting and thrusting in the Wei level.

Most likely the wrong kind of needle is being used. See Equipment appendix, page 379.

Frequently Asked Questions

1. Is it reasonable to expect to be able to treat the underlying deficiency/ies and do the Sinew treatment in the same session?

Yes, with practice, you can successfully treat the underlying cause in the same hour you do the Sinew treatment. Often, not all four deficiencies are present. When first practicing Sinew treatments, schedule more time. Only ask questions relevant to the sinews and take the pulses very early in the consultation.

2. I can't get enough Kidney Yang to emerge in the pulses before I do a Sinew treatment. What can I do?

Moxa GV-4 and GV-14.

3. I can't get enough Stomach Fluids to emerge in the pulses before I do a Sinew treatment. What should I do?

Tonify ST-42 and TH-2. Have a mug of warm water and a bendy straw on hand so patient can sip fluids.

4. I tried but I can't get the Liver pulse to release. What should I do?

Needle BL-17 at the Hua To position bilaterally and moxa. Remove needles, turn the patient, and reduce LR-14. Or, reduce LR-6 and LU-6.

5. I can't get Lung Qi to disperse in the pulses before I do a Sinew treatment. What should I do?

Needle LU-7 with the flying technique.

6. If the Wei Qi is trapped in the joints, how can the needle reach the Wei Qi if it's only inserted a very short distance?

The techniques of chiseling or twisting specifically engage Wei Qi. So even though the needle is not inserted beyond the depth the tube allows it to be inserted initially, the technique "speaks" to the Wei Qi and will pull it to the surface from any depth.

7. What is a "Sinew release" and do I have to do it?

A Sinew release is a classical manual (hands-on) technique involving no needles that releases a set of muscles in the body and is part of the Wai Ke tradition. It's a very difficult technique to put into words because it's supremely subtle. It's very time consuming for the practitioner, but is quite miraculous. For those who are familiar with this technique, releasing the neck (GV-14) and GV-4 with Sinew release technique is very helpful before doing a Sinew treatment. This would be done prior to any needling. However, if the above protocol is followed, Sinew treatments without manual releases are extremely successful.

Case Study

A man presents with an ankle injury. He was stepping onto the sidewalk from the gutter and slipped on the ice, twisting his ankle. He had just showered and was running for the bus, which had caused him to sweat. There is swelling along the lateral leg and foot from BL-59 to BL-62. The pain is sharp. The most difficult movement to make is rotation.

Diagnosis:

Wind-Cold in the Gallbladder and Bladder Sinews.

Rationale:

1. There is visible injury of the Bladder Sinew.
2. Pain elicited by rotation indicates the injury has moved to and is in Shao Yang which means the Gallbladder Sinew Channel is affected.

Treatment:

1. Needle the tightest point (ah shi) in the vicinity of SI-18.
2. Palpate for ah shi along the Gallbladder Channel and treat with chiseling or twisting technique.
3. Moxa the cold, tight or swollen areas as you go.
4. Needle GB-44 and remove.
5. Needle into the swelling along the Bladder Channel and treat with chiseling or twisting technique.
6. Moxa the swelling as you go.
7. Needle BL-67 and remove.
8. Check that the moxa'd areas remain warm. Use the remaining time to moxa those areas.

Note: I like to needle the Jing-Well right after the Confluent point and again at the end. That helps my intention because when the Confluent point and the Jing-Well are both in at the same time, the body understands unequivocally that it is the Sinews Channels that are being activated.

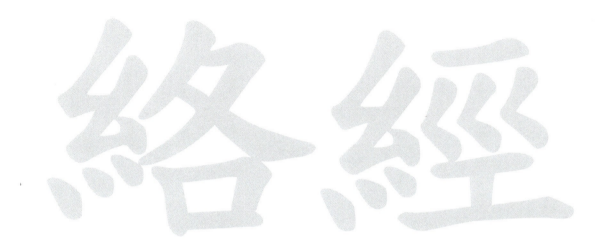

The Luo Channels

LUO CHANNEL TREATMENTS

A discussion of chapters 10, 21, 22, 27, 39, 48 and 62 of the *Ling Shu*, and chapter 18 of the *Su Wen*.

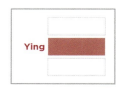

The Arising of the Luo Channels

"The Primary Channels cannot be seen; one must use the pulse at the wrist to diagnose them. The channels that can be seen are the Luo Channels."
—Chapter 22, *Ling Shu*

Luo Channels are collaterals of the Primary Channels. They are visible reservoirs for pathology, and are created by the body in response to a pathogenic factor. They run the gamut from spider veins to varicosities, and can generate swellings and nodules. The function of the Luo Channels is to keep pathology in the Ying level, away from the organs, using the mediumship of Blood.

The Luo Channels (also known as Connecting Channels) do not exist in the absence of pathology. Pathogenic factors are defined as challenges to the body's defense. They include external climatic factors (Wind, Cold, Damp), and internal factors: the effects of poor dietary choices and poor lifestyle choices, ecological factors (pollution, viruses, bacteria, funghi, parasites), toxins (e.g., asbestos, heavy metals) and emotions. Diet and lifestyle-choice related pathology are neither exclusively internal nor external. Emotional factors are internal, meaning they will initially affect the interior, particularly the Luo terrain since Blood carries the emotions. The emotions are: anger, fear (including shock or fright), worry or pensiveness (known in modern times as obsessive thinking), anxiety and sadness.

As a Luo Channel holds pathology and makes attempts to clear it, rebellious Qi results. The body creates heat to move the pathological Qi up and out. We will see in the functions of the Luo Channels a means of treating rebellious Qi (by clearing pathology), internal Heat (by clearing Heat from the Blood and organs), musculoskeletal conditions (via channel pathways), all Blood pathologies (by moving and regulating Blood) and the emotions (as Blood carries the Shen).

Historical References to the Luo Channels

Chapter 10 of the *Ling Shu* describes all trajectories and lists the signs and symptoms of the Luo Channels. It states that the Luos are visible and do not enter the joints. It instructs us to bleed the Luos every second day to release their pathology and cautions us that failure to do so will allow the pathology to empty out of the Luo Channels into the Yuan level to cause rheumatism. Chapter 19 suggests Luo treatments should be performed when Blood is visible, and continued until the disease is concluded.

Chapter 21 discusses the use of Luo points to treat rebellious Qi. Chapter 22 of the *Ling Shu*, a chapter noted for its remarkable language, describes Luo signs and symptoms and treatment protocols. One could base their entire practice on this chapter. Chapter 27 describes the emptying of the Luo Channels, the resulting diseases and the emptied Luo treatment protocol. Chapter 39 explains the various appearances of Blood during treatment and discusses the relationship between Blood and Fluids. It describes Blood that is black and muddy, Blood that shoots or that looks like tree sap, all of which we commonly see in treatment. Chapter 48 refers to prophylactic treatment of the Luo Channels. Chapter 62 says that when the Luos are obstructed, the pathology is kept in the four limbs, blocking the antique points and rendering Primary Channel treatments ineffective. Chapter 18 of the *Su Wen* describes the Great Luo of the Stomach in detail. Chapters 23 and 26 of the *Nan Jing* identify 15 Luo Channels. Chapter 26 says they are found on the side opposite their corresponding Primary Channels.

Longitudinal and Transverse Luo Terminology

The nomenclature of the Luos is in some ways unfortunate because the Luo Channels are each one unit comprising a longitudinal and transverse aspect. Longitudinal Luos and Transverse Luos have different signs and symptoms but they are not separate units. The Transverse section of a Luo Channel is where the disease deepens.

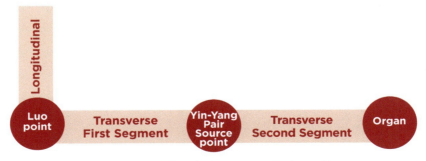

One can imagine the Luos as an "L-shaped" unit with the Luo point at the bend.

The Longitudinal Luos are so named because they originate at the Luo point and have a trajectory of their own, either proximally or distally, along the limbs of the body.

Transverse Luos are so called because the pathology is crossing from the Ying level into the Yuan-Source level because the body is no longer able to find latency for it in the Longitudinal Luo Channel. This movement, when mapped on the body, is often relatively Transverse (see drawings).

Luo Channels run proximally from the Luo point, with the exception of the Lung and Gallbladder. The Lung Luo moves distally in an attempt to move the pathology back out to the exterior. The Gallbladder Luo moves distally to ST-42 at which point it enters the Yuan-Source level via the fifth trajectory of Chong Mai, dumping the emotional and physiological pathology into the Constitution. Conversely, this same opening enables the Gallbladder Luo to pull constitutional pathogens out to the Ying level.

The Transverse Luos are often represented by simple lines we can trace with a finger, for example, from ST-40 to SP-3, but these small trajectories are simply representations of the potential deep internal pathways being made into the Yuan-Source level. Some of these deep pathways are shown in light green in the illustrations.

If Luo pathology is treated anywhere on its path, the process of complete healing can begin as the pathology is reversed along its pathway of progression.

Definitions: Visible Luo Vessels and Luo Channels

Generally, the words *channel* and *vessel* are used interchangeably. In this manual a *Luo Channel* is the entire Luo pathway which begins at the Luo point, and the term *Luo vessel* denotes a visible Blood vessel or discoloration.

A *Luo vessel* can be many things:
- Spider veins
- Varicose veins
- Bruises
- Dark blue, purple, black or dark red Blood vessels
- Protruding Blood vessels
- Areas discolored by occluded Blood (usually red, blue or purple)

> "When the vessels are blue it indicates Cold. When the vessels are red it indicates Heat or fever. When there is Cold in the Stomach, the thenar eminence will be blue. When the thenar eminence is black, the Cold has stagnated and there is much pain." —Chapter 10, *Ling Shu*

> "A Luo vessel may be fine like a needle, or large, like a tendon." —Chapter 39, *Ling Shu*

Luos in the Complement Channel Sequence

In the absence of pathology, natural physiology is maintained under the influence of the Primary Channels. No pathology arises if difficulties are resolved and/or let go as they are encountered.

Most of the acute difficulties the body encounters are dealt with at the level of the sinews. The countless external pathogenic factors we are constantly exposed to through breathing, eating and skin contact such as unwelcome viruses (Cold) and unwelcome bacteria (Heat) are deflected by Wei-Defensive Qi. Wei-Defensive Qi resides on the exterior of the body and in the gut, and is governed by the Sinew Channels. If Wei-Defensive Qi is deficient due to various systemic weaknesses (explained in the Sinew chapter) it can fail to resolve a pathogen, meaning it can fail to produce a healing response to push the pathogen out of the body.

The Sinew Channels begin at the Jing-Well points. If the sinews fail, the pathogen is said to have *penetrated beyond the Jing-Well point*, that is, beyond the level of the Sinews.

Once past the Sinews, the pathogen can then move further into the interior; it travels further along the Primary Channel and encounters the Shu-Stream point: the nexus of the exterior and the interior. The Shu-Stream point is like a dam gate; it can usher a pathogen out. If the pathogen passes beyond the Shu-Stream point, it has moved to the interior.

Note: An external pathogenic factor that has moved to the interior is not the same as an internal pathogenic factor. An internal pathogenic factor is one that originated in the interior, usually described as dietary, emotional or from lifestyle.

At any point early in the process of invasion of the pathology, the Primary Channel can push the pathogen back, but the Primary Channels are not chiefly focussed on pathogenic factors so they very often bring the pathogen to rest in a point with a reservoir quality. The Yuan-Source point is the first such reservoir encountered. If Yuan-Source Qi is unable to resist the pathogen, the pathogen can settle into the Yuan-Source point. However, the body would much prefer not to use the Yuan-Source point as a pool of latency because if the Yuan-Source points were challenged and unable to hold onto the pathogen, the pathogen would have access to the entire Yuan level, and therefore the organs. The organs must be protected at all cost. Therefore the body most often moves the pathogen further along the Primary Channel, past the Yuan-Source point, to the Luo point. The pathogen encounters and enters that Luo point. The body then creates a reservoir of Blood—a (Longitudinal) Luo Channel—to contain the pathogenic factor. The function of the Longitudinal Luos is to keep pathology in the limbs, well away from the organs.

The body's aim here is to use Ying Qi (Blood) as a buffer for the pathogen and to arrest its passage past the Luo point. If it were to move past the Luo point to the He-Sea point, it could reach the organs.

Internal pathogenic factors can be translocated to the Luos, also. Emotions affect the organs. In order to prevent stress or damage to the organs, the body may create Luo vessels and move the emotional pathology into those vessels to keep the organ clear of the stress of the emotion. This may happen whether the emotion is overwhelming in the short term, or unresolved in the long term. Indeed, the Luos are empirical points for any unresolved issue related to Blood. Other internal factors, including dietary, can be moved to Luo vessels. For example, pestilent Qi such as food poisoning from a bad clam which the Stomach might not have sufficient Wei-Defensive Qi to purge may be shifted to a Luo vessel.

> **The Luo vessels are formed**
> - **When the Sinew Channels have failed to defend the body against an external pathogen.**
> - **When an internal pathogenic factor arises, the body doesn't have the resources to expel it, and the body chooses Blood as the buffer between the organs and the pathogenic factor.**

Luo Channel Indications

A Luo treatment might be chosen in cases:
1. where there are visible Blood vessels.
2. where Blood is visibly accumulating causing discoloration (redness or blue/purple hue), or where lymph or Damp is accumulating causing swelling or nodules.

3. where emotional, psychological or psychiatric signs and symptoms are involved, whether acute or chronic, since Blood houses the Shen.
4. of Blood pathology, including diseases of the Blood, fire toxins in the Blood, circulation issues, Blood stagnation, occluded Blood.
5. of Heart pathology.

Full and Emptied Luo Terminology

As the Luo point becomes taxed by holding onto pathology for the long-term, it creates more space for latency by generating spider veins along the channel in the moderate level of the flesh, through the process of angiogenesis. Over time, the spider veins become visible as they "float" up to the surface in an attempt to release (bleed out) their pathology through the Wei level. When the Luo vessels become visible, the diagnosis of *fullness of the Luo* is given.

> **The term *full Luo* does not mean the Luo cannot take any more pathology; it simply means that the Luo vessel has become visible.**

To release the pathology at this time in the progression, a Fullness of the Luo treatment is given. (See detail on page 82.) The Luo point, which is where the Channel wants to release the pathology, must be bled in order to "clear the Luos". A full Luo treatment series will release the pathology to the surface, completely freeing the pathogenic factor at best, or at least, freeing up space in the Luo vessel to make room for more pathology, thereby delaying the progression of the disease state.

If the pathology is not released, the Luo vessel can continue to expand, but at some point it will become overly full and unable to hold more pathology. The pathogen will then return to the Primary Channel. At this point the Luo Channel is said to have emptied. The previously visible Luo vessels (spider veins) can disappear as the Blood in the Luo vessel and the pathology it is holding are dumped into the Primary Channel. The pathology is now loose in the Primary Channel. The body then seeks to protect the Source point of the channel by bringing Yin up through the Yuan-Source point and depositing that Yin in the channel to create nodules to block the flow of more pathology to the Yuan-Source point. Cysts can appear locally at the Luo point, the Source point, distal to the Luo point, or along the entire length of the Primary Channel, as Fluids, (the other component of Ying Qi) congeal to attempt to block the deeper penetration of more pathology. At this point an emptied Luo treatment is given (described in detail on page 82.) During the time the emptying process is occurring there may be signs and symptoms of both full and emptied Luo, as the Luo is "half full and half emptied." Treat emptied Luo in these cases.

The aim of an *emptied Luo* treatment here is to clear space in the Luo Channel and provide enough Yang for the pathology to be syphoned back to the Luo point. The Luo vessels may become visible again (spider veins may reappear) as the pathology is returned to the Luo Channel.

The cysts and nodules keep the pathogen at bay in the Primary Channel; they block the pathology from entering the organs. When the pathology increases and cannot be contained in the Primary Channel by the Damp any longer, Transverse Luo signs and symptoms occur. These are Heat signs which arise as the body recognizes that the capacity for latency has been exhausted and generates heat to try to move that pathology outward. If unsuccessful in that effort, and with Blood and Qi depleted, the heat, along with the pathology, begins to move toward the organ.

Transverse Luo signs and symptoms are signals that the organ is beginning to be affected and that the body is likely to start sending the pathology to another channel altogether. The next choice of latency sites is the Yuan-Source point of the Yin-Yang pair. The aim of a Transverse Luo treatment is to pull the pathology back from the Yuan-Source level and at the same time clear space in the Longitudinal Luo Channel. (Transverse Luos are discussed on page 107.)

The following progression can occur in a matter of hours (in cases of pestilent Qi) or several decades. A great many variations are possible in the scenario below. The pathology can be arrested anywhere along the progression. It could become stabilized at any Luo or Source point in the sequence. Diagnosis is made by analyzing signs, symptoms and pulses.

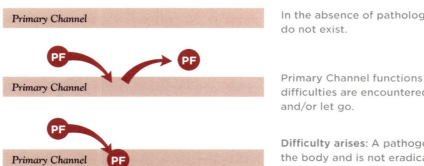

In the absence of pathology, Luo Channels do not exist.

Primary Channel functions normally and difficulties are encountered, resolved and/or let go.

Difficulty arises: A pathogenic factor enters the body and is not eradicated through the Sinew Channels.

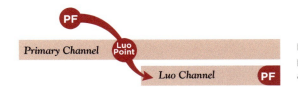

Longitudinal Luo formation: The pathogen progresses to the Luo point where the body creates a reservoir of Blood called a Longitudinal Luo.

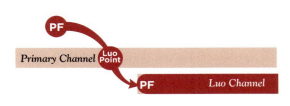

Longitudinal Luo Channel fills up: If untreated and if the pathogenic factor continues to be introduced, the body creates spider veins, or capillaries to contain the Blood which is holding the pathogenic factor latent, either at the Luo point, or anywhere along the Longitudinal Luo Channel trajectory. When the Luo vessels become visible they are said to be "full". Signs and symptoms of "fullness of the Luo" arise. A Full Luo treatment is performed at this point to "clear the Luos" and rid the pathology or allow room for more pathology should the body require it.

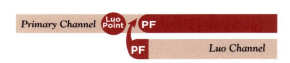

Emptying of the Longitudinal Luo into its own Primary Channel: When the Luo vessel becomes very full and is not capable of holding more pathology, it overflows back into the Primary Channel. The Luo Channel is then said to be "emptied". Cysts, tumors, nodules or swellings form in order to contain the pathology in the Primary Channel and prevent it gaining access to the organs. The spider veins either fully or partially disappear. An Emptied Luo treatment is performed at this point to "clear the Luos and tonify the Primary Channel". This treatment pulls the pathology from the Primary Channel back to the Luo Channel.

Luo Channel Diagnosis

Diagnoses are made by assessing:

1. the location of visible Luo vessels (spider veins, sometimes called visible capillaries) which indicates "fullness" of the Luo Channel. Make this assessment using the drawings of the Luo Channels as your guide. You're looking for spider veins and any other visible Blood vessel or discoloration. Of course not all spider veins are exactly along the trajectory of the channel. The Luo Channels are more like fields. Sometimes you'll find spider veins that lie exactly on the Luo point, or the Yuan-Source point, or on the channel, but sometimes they'll be diffusely arranged or lying in a seemingly random formation. Your task is to decide which Luo Channel pathway is closest. Use the other diagnosic criteria (physiological and psychological, described later) to corroborate your visual findings.

2. the locations of nodules which indicate "emptied" Luos. Nodules occur anywhere on the Primary Channel related to the affected Luo.

3. the mood, emotion or disposition. These assessments are made by correlating the pre-

sentation of the patient with the signs and symptoms of the Luos in the Psychosocial Luo model.
4. pathology according to the presentation of the Longitudinal Luos' classical signs and symptoms. This assessment is made by correlating the presentation of the patient with the signs and symptoms for the Longitudinal Luo.
5. pathology according to the presentation of the Transverse Luos' classical signs and symptoms. The presentation of the patient is correlated to the signs and symptoms of the Transverse Luos.

Luo Treatment Principles

Full Luo: "Clear the Luo"

Emptied Luo: "Clear the Luo and tonify the Primary Channel"

Transverse Luo: "Tonify the Source point of the Yin-Yang paired Primary Channel and clear the Luo," or "Reduce the Yuan-Source point of the Yin-Yang paired Primary Channel and tonify (bleed and moxa) the Luo."

Luo Needling Technique

Luo treatments involve "lancing", best performed with a fine lancet. Some lancets on the market are too thick for this purpose, and some are too fine. Experiment with brands until you find the right one.

Most often the visible Luos are very superficial. They need be barely nicked with the point of the lancet to bleed. Sometimes the Luos will be much deeper; you can see them but they look blurred or buried. If you stretch the skin a little, the lancet tip will reach these Luo vessels. Sometimes the Luos give off a crunching sound or a feeling of crackling. This is common especially when the patient is taking sedating or tranquilizing drugs. Stubborn Luo points and vessels sometimes require a slight turn on the lancet to encourage bleeding.

An alternative method to lancing is plum-blossoming which I think is far more invasive but can be desirable when moving Blood in a diffusely discolored area. Lightly tap the area a few times until the color changes.

> *Needling a Luo point rather than bleeding it does not constitute a Luo treatment. For a Luo treatment to function, Blood must be expressed from the surface of the body at the Luo point, even if only a tiny speck. Likewise, bleeding visible Luo vessels without first bleeding the Luo point of the affected trajectory does not constitute a Luo treatment.*

The 15 Luo Points and the 16 Luo Channels

There are 16 Luo Channels, 15 of which emanate from Luo points. The Great Luo of the Stomach—described in chapter 18 of the *Su Wen*—has no points and is described as a *pulsating Vessel* which can mean the heartbeat.

LU-7	*Lie Que*	Lightning Strike. To split from the center (the chest).
LI-6	*Pian Li*	Veering Passage
ST-40	*Feng Long*	Bountiful Earth
SP-4	*Gong Sun*	Grandfather Grandchild
HT-5	*Tong Li*	Breaking Through, Penetrating the Distance
SI-7	*Zheng Zhi*	The Upright Branch
BL-58	*Fei Yang*	Taking Flight
KI-4	*Da Zhong*	The Great Bell
PC-6	*Nei Guan*	The Inner Barrier
TH-5	*Wei Guan*	The Outer Barrier
GB-37	*Guang Ming*	Bright Illumination of Sight
LR-5	*Li Gou*	Insect Groove
CV-15	*Jiu Wei*	Turtledove Tail
GV-1	*Chang Qiang*	Long Endurance
SP-21	*Da Bao*	The Great Wrap, The Great Luo of the Spleen

Note: Located three cun below the axilla, not six. In the Ling Shu, *the Great Luo of the Spleen is located where we currently put GB-22.*

Great Luo of the Stomach *Xu Li* The Empty Mile*   **A Li is about a third of a mile.*

Locating Luo Points

Luo points are all in depressions in the body. They have a special feel to them, as though they are sitting within bands. When locating a Luo point, go to the textbook location of the point but don't press into the point. Glide your finger over the point and check that you feel an indentation or a crevice. If you don't find one, the textbook location has only brought you to the vicinity of the Luo point. The true anatomical location for this individual is likely to be close by. Gently feel around near the textbook location until you do find a slight depression. Often, Luo points are clearly visible, either because there is a Luo vessel or discoloration at the point, or because there is a visible depression.

Often the Luo points are found in locations with the following qualities:

LU-7* in a tight, narrow notch.

LI-6 in a wide, diagonal dish-like depression bound by bands.

ST-40 in a shallow dish like depression.

SP-4 in a bound depression.

HT-5 in a very deep depression.

SI-7 in a tiny dip which feels like an irregularity in the muscle.

BL-58* in a very large soft depression.

KI-4 in a moon-shaped depression against the tendon.

PC-6* level with the springiest part of the tendons.

TH-5 in a round depression. (Be sure to be radial to communis.)

GB-37 in a significant depression against (anterior to) peroneus.

LR-5* in a significant notch in the bone.

CV-15 in a depression immediately inferior to the base of the xyphoid.

GV-1 in a depression immediately inferior to the base of the coccyx.

SP-21* in a tight intercostal space, three cun (according to the *Ling Shu*) below the axilla.

*These points must be palpated with more pressure before they will reveal themselves.

Bleeding Luos Unilaterally

Chapter 26 of the *Nan Jing* says that the Primary Channels are on the same side of the body the pulse is found and the Luo Channels are found on the opposite side.

The *Nan Jing* says the Luo points are bled on the side opposite the pulse. This stipulation is made regardless of gender.

Therefore the following Luo points are bled on the right side: HT-5, SI-7, LR-5, GB-37, BL-58, KI-4.

The following Luo points are bled on the left side: LU-7, LI-6, SP-4, ST-40, TH-5, PC-6.

Longitudinal Luo Channel Trajectories

Longitudinal Luo	*Ling Shu* Trajectory	*Su Wen* Trajectory
Lung	LU-7, LU-10, PC-8.	
Large Intestine	LI-6, LI-11, LI-15, ST-5, splits into two branches, to ST-4 and to SI-19.	LI-6, LI-15, teeth, then splits to the ear and to the Large Intestine Primary Channel.

Longitudinal Luo	*Ling Shu* Trajectory	*Su Wen* Trajectory
Stomach	ST-40, ST-13, GV-20, ST-9 on the opposite side.	
Spleen	SP-4, intestines, Stomach at CV-12.	
Heart	HT-5, HT-1, LU-2, ST-11, BL-1. Two branches: from HT-1 to Heart organ, and from ST-1, through ST-5 to ST-11.	HT-5, CV-17, CV-14, CV-23.
Small Intestine	SI-7 to LI-15.	SI-7, SI-8, LI-15.
Bladder	BL-58, KI-4, then follows Kidney Longitudinal Luo, to GV-4.	
Kidney	KI-4, KI-21, CV-14, GV-4.	KI-4, genitalia, lumbar spine.
Pericardium	PC-6, HT-1, PC-1, Heart organ, the three Jiao's.	PC-6 to CV-17.
Triple Heater	TH-5, LI-15, LU-2, LU-1, CV-15, the three Jiao's.	TH-5, LI-15 or GB-21, ST-17, CV-17. In later editions CV-12 is added.
Gallbladder	GB-37 to ST-42.	
Liver	LR-5, CV-2.	LR-5 to the genitalia.
Ren	CV-15, spreads over abdomen.	
Du	GV-1, splits into two branches to follow along both sides of the spine. At BL-10 it splits again, one branch goes over the head to BL-1 and the other goes into the paravertebral muscles (the Bladder Sinew Channel).	
Great Luo of the Spleen		Begins three cun below the axilla and spreads to the breast and ribs.
Great Luo of the Stomach		Begins in the Stomach, penetrates the diaphragm, goes below the left breast and ends at the pulsating vessel (the heartbeat).

Points Beyond the Luo Point, Along the Longitudinal Trajectory

During a Luo treatment, points along the trajectory can be added if it is felt that their function will enhance the treatment. In my practice, I find that bleeding the Luo point and the visible vessels along the channel and using gua sha to release the obstructions along the channel is quite adequate. Below is a list of the Luo Channel trajectories. It should be noted that there are no points along the trajectory other than the Luo point itself. Rather, the Luos traverse areas, feathering out and dispersing along the way. ***The points listed in the trajectories below are intended merely to be markers for locating the pathway.*** Nonetheless the points can also be treated (by bleeding). It is not necessary to treat any points described below in order to have a successful Luo treatment.

Lung Luo Channel: Begins at LU-7, then travels through the areas around and including LU-10, PC-8.
LU-10: Heat in Lung and Stomach, sore throat, hunger, cough, fever, thirst, epistaxis, loss of voice, profuse sweat, reflux.
PC-8: Disturbed Shen, internal Wind, Damp-Heat, Blood Heat, halitosis.

Large Intestine Luo Channel: Begins at LI-6, then travels through the areas around and including LI-15, ST-5, ST-4, SI-19.
LI-15: Wind-Damp in the joints, especially shoulder and upper limbs, inflammation of the shoulders and arms.
ST-5: Lockjaw, toothache, TMD (temporomandibular joint disorder), inability to close mouth or eyes.
ST-4: Inability to eat, close eyes or speak.
SI-19: Opens ears and eyes. Treats madness.

Stomach Luo Channel: Begins at ST-40, then travels through the areas around and including ST-31, ST-13, ST-9.
ST-31: Atrophy of the lower limbs due to Wind-Cold, inability to extend the legs.
ST-13: Clears Heat and treats fullness and distention of the chest.
ST-9: Clears Heat, regulates Qi and Blood, treats dyspnea and ruddy complexion.

Spleen Luo Channel: Begins at SP-4, then travels to the area around and including CV-12.
CV-12: Regulates entire digestive system.

Heart Luo Channel: Begins at HT-5, then travels through the areas around and including (selected points): HT-1, LU-2, ST-11, BL-1.

HT-1: Opens chest, throat, treats thirst.

LU-2: Opens chest, clears Heat in chest and throat.

ST-11: Treats rebellious throat and Stomach Qi, goiters.

BL-1: Brings fluid to the eyes.

Small Intestine Luo Channel: Begins at SI-7, then travels through the area around and including LI-15.

LI-15: Wind-Damp Bi obstruction in the joints, Heat in the shoulders.

Bladder Luo Channel: Begins at BL-58, then travels to KI-4, then along Kidney Luo Channel.

KI-4: Constipation and blockage of urine. Harmonizes Blood. Treats coughing Blood, Blood in the sputum, stools, urine and vomit.

Kidney Luo Channel: Begins at KI-4, then travels through the areas around and including KI-21, GV-4.

KI-21: Harmonizes Spleen and Stomach, abdominal and diaphragmatic distention, vomiting, diarrhea, pain in the chest radiating to the lower back.

GV-4: Banks Essence, relaxes the sinews, harmonizes Blood, treats stiffness of the spine, impotence and seminal loss.

Pericardium Luo Channel: Begins at PC-6, then travels through the areas around and including PC-1, CV-17.

PC-1: Treats inability to move the limbs, oppression and pain in the chest, cough with copious Phlegm.

Triple Heater Luo Channel: Begins at TH-5, then travels through the area around and including CV-15, then to the three Jiao's.

CV-15: Transforms Wind-Phlegm, treats epilepsy, mania, fright palpitations, nourishes Yin.

Gallbladder Luo Channel: Begins at GB-37, then travels through the area around and including ST-42.

ST-42: Transforms Damp, supports digestion, stabilizes the Shen, treats swelling in the upper body, particularly the head.

Liver Luo Channel: Begins at LR-5, then travels to the area around and including CV-2.

CV-2: Warms the Yang, builds Kidneys, regulates menses, stops leakage in the Lower Jiao.

Ren Luo Channel: Begins at CV-15 and disperses over the abdomen.
No trajectory points.

Du Luo Channel: Begins at GV-1, then travels to the area around and including BL-10.

BL-10: Dissipates Wind-Cold, soothes the sinews, treats heavy headedness, stiff neck.

Great Luo of the Spleen Channel: Begins at SP-21 (3 cun below the axilla according to the *Ling Shu*) and disperses laterally over the chest.
No trajectory points.

Great Luo of the Stomach: Begins in the Stomach, penetrates the diaphragm, goes below the left breast and ends at the pulsating vessel (the heartbeat).

Lung Luo Channel

- Luo Point
- Longitudinal Luo
- Transverse First Segment
- Transverse Second Segment

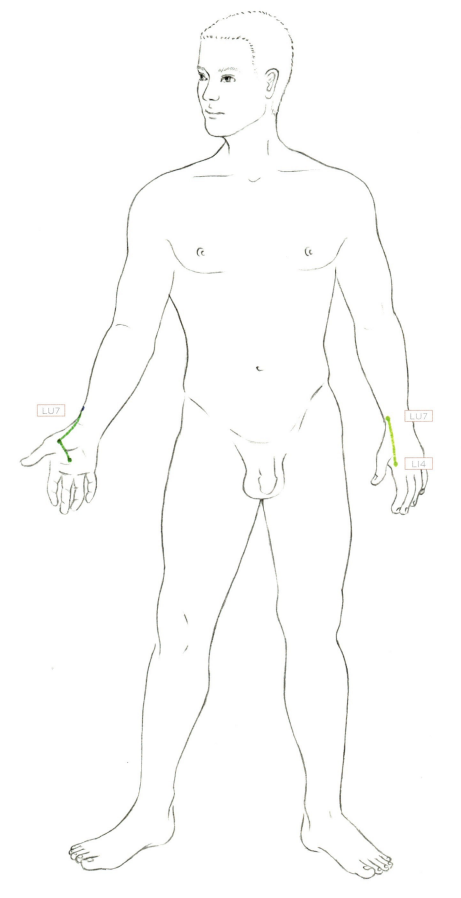
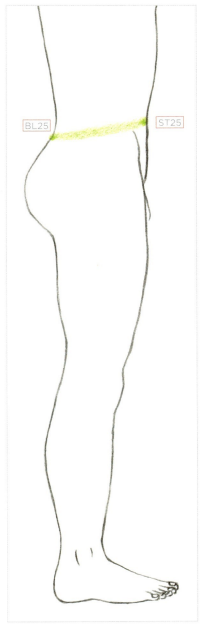

Large Intestine Luo Channel

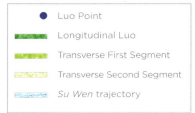
- Luo Point
- Longitudinal Luo
- Transverse First Segment
- Transverse Second Segment
- *Su Wen* trajectory

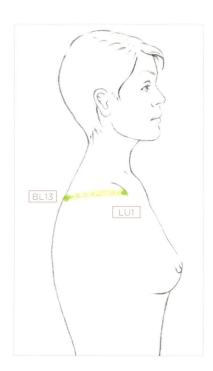

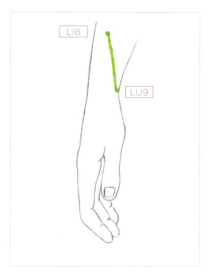

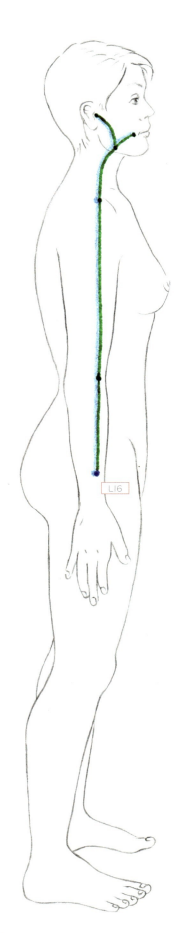

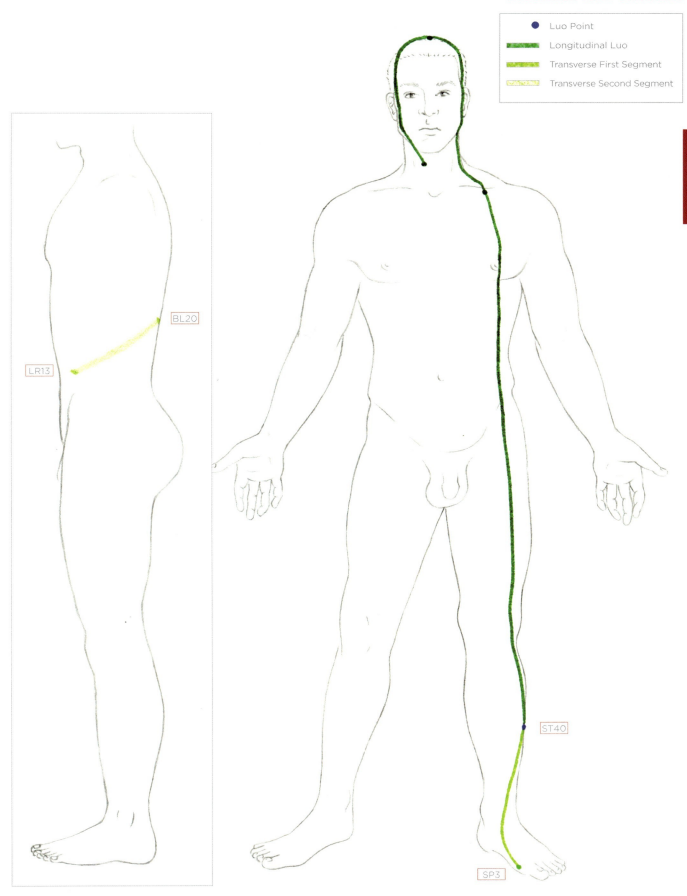

Spleen Luo Channel

- Luo Point
- Longitudinal Luo
- Transverse First Segment
- Transverse Second Segment

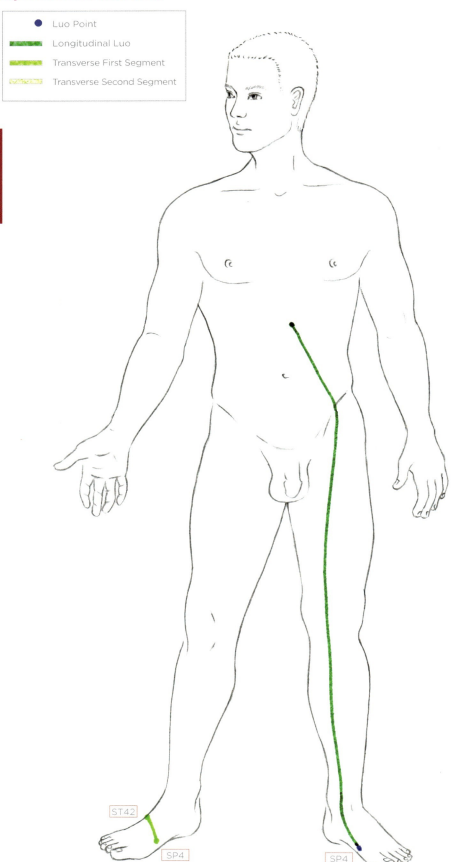
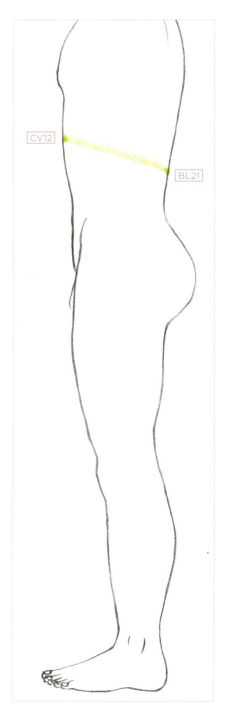

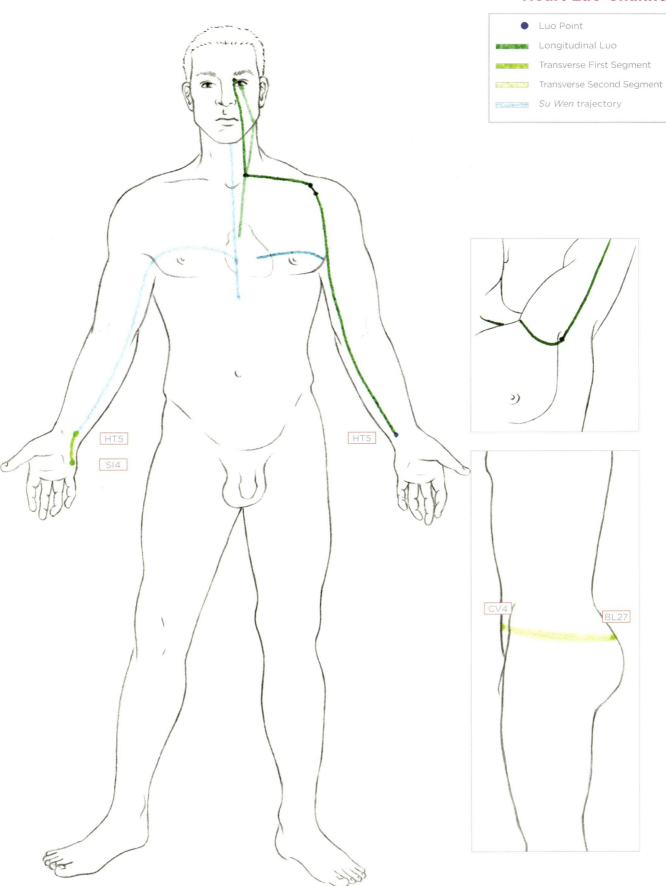

Small Intestine Luo Channel

●	Luo Point
▬	Longitudinal Luo
▬	Transverse First Segment
▬	Transverse Second Segment
▬	*Su Wen* trajectory

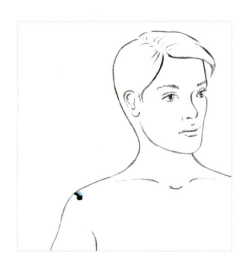

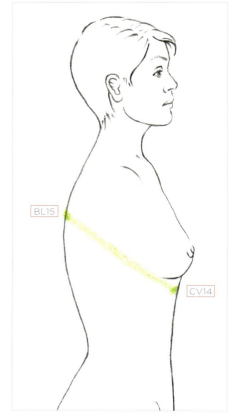

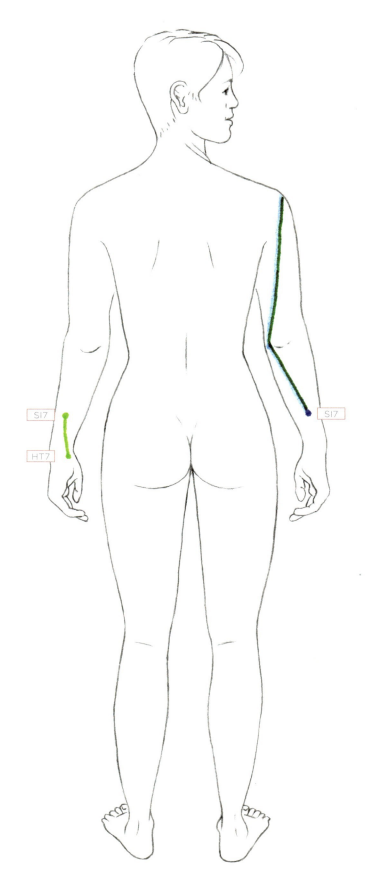

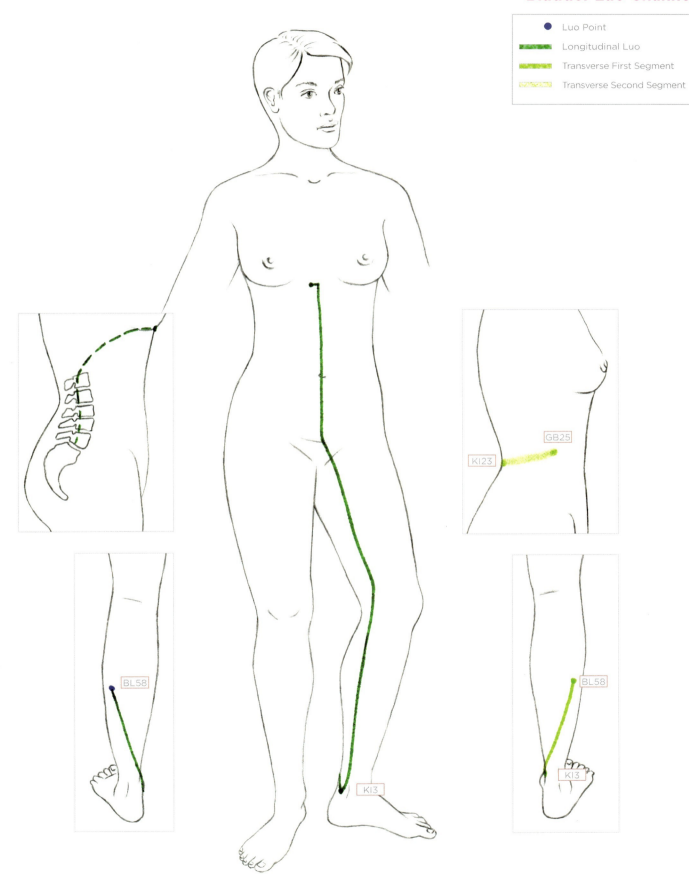

Kidney Luo Channel

- Luo Point
- Longitudinal Luo
- Transverse First Segment
- Transverse Second Segment
- *Su Wen* trajectory

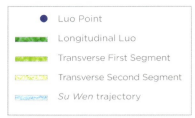
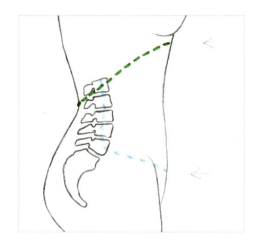
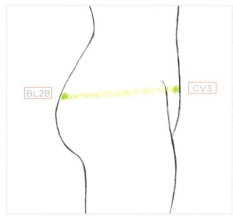
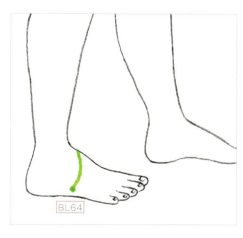
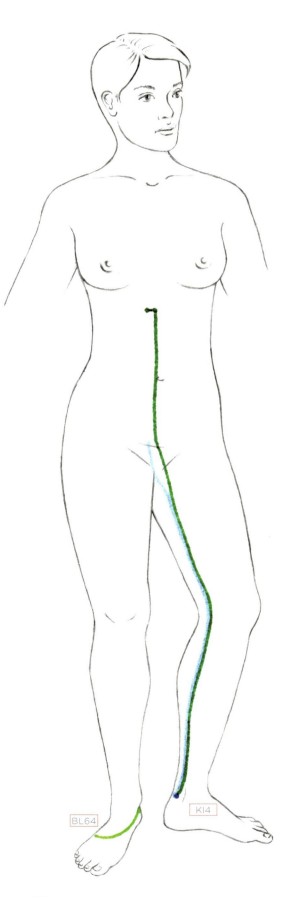

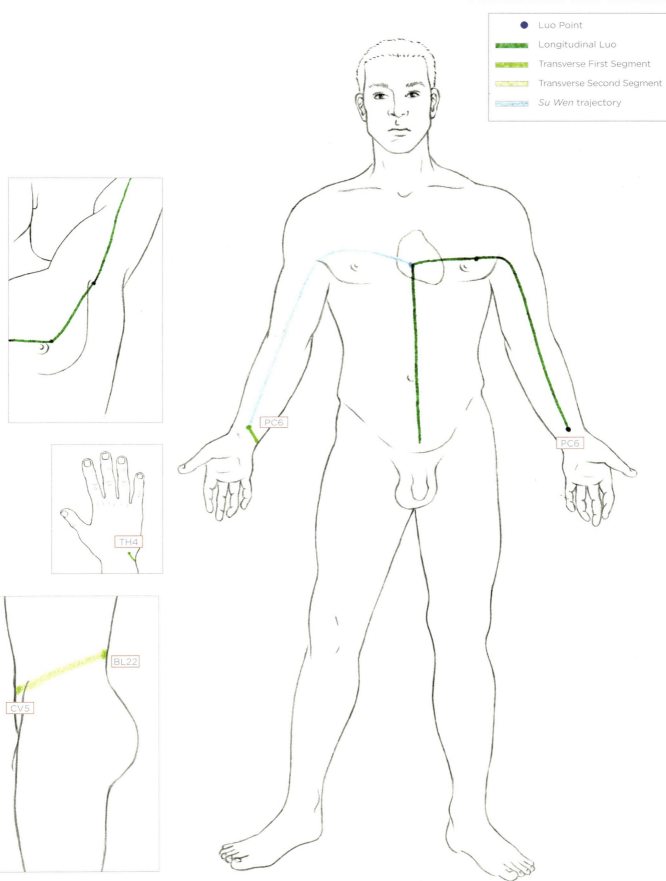

Triple Heater Luo Channel

●	Luo Point
▬	Longitudinal Luo
▬	Transverse First Segment
▬	Transverse Second Segment
▬	*Su Wen* trajectory

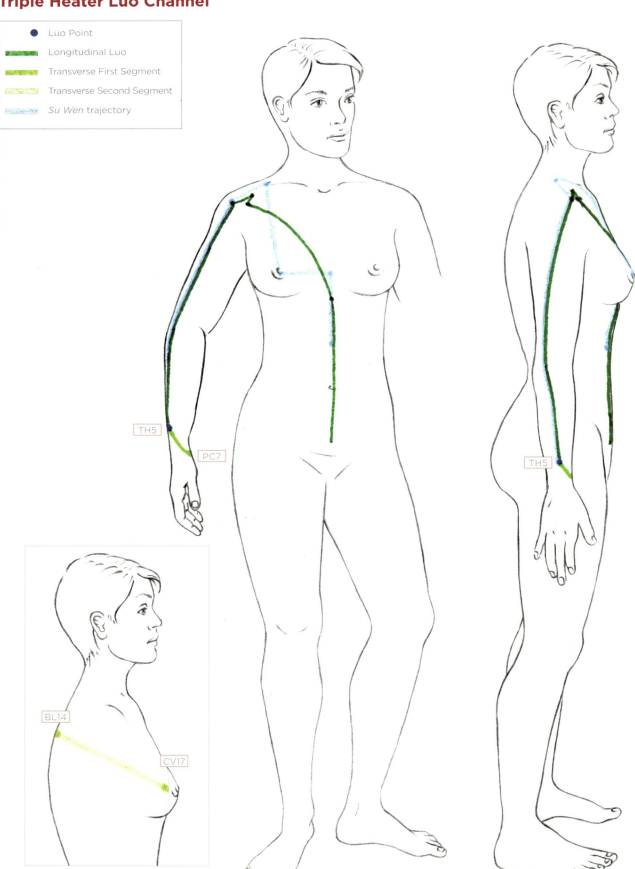

Gallbladder Luo Channel

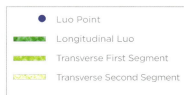
- Luo Point
- Longitudinal Luo
- Transverse First Segment
- Transverse Second Segment

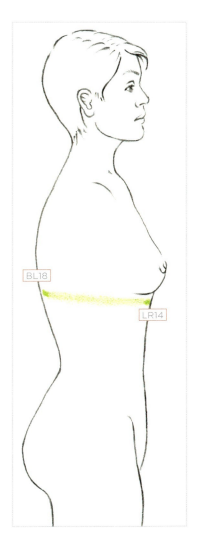
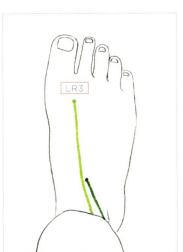
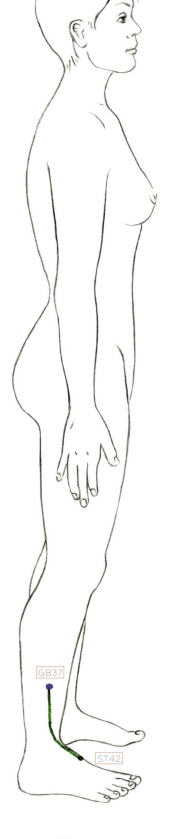
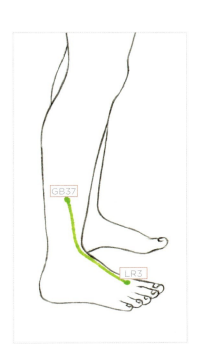

Liver Luo Channel

- Luo Point
- Longitudinal Luo
- Transverse First Segment
- Transverse Second Segment
- *Su Wen* trajectory

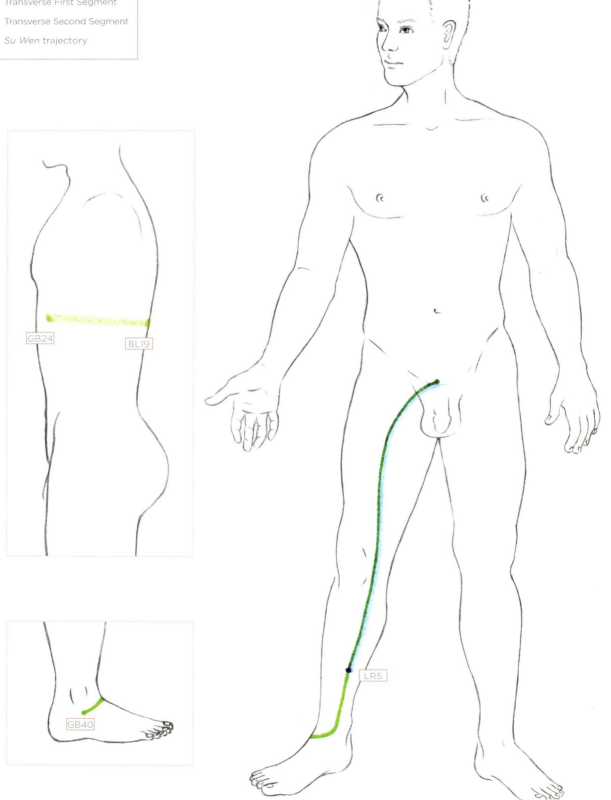

Ren Luo Channel

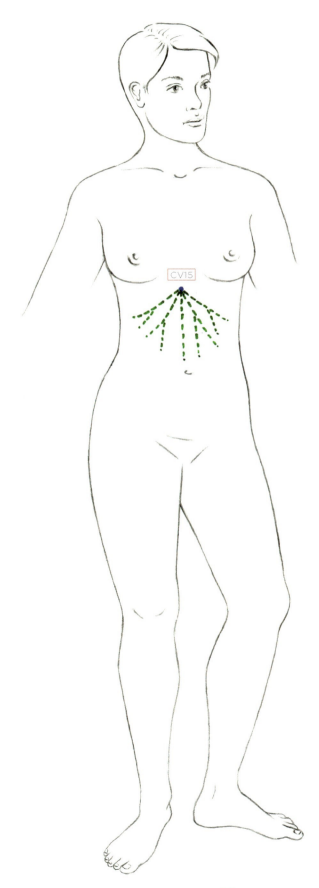

Du Luo Channel

- Luo Point
- Luo trajectory
- Branch 1
- Branch 2

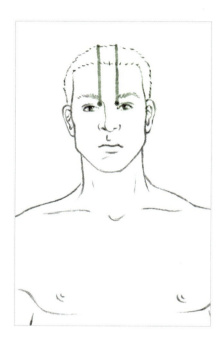
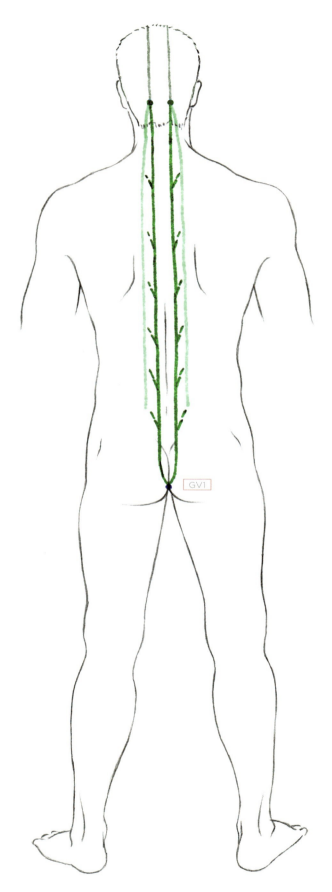

Great Luo of the Spleen

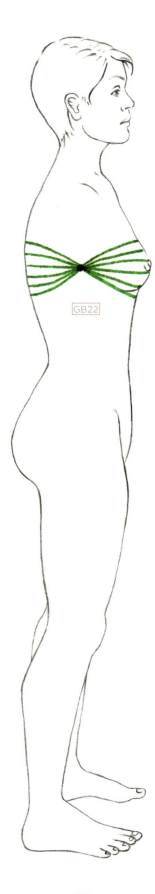

Great Luo of the Stomach

- Luo Point
- *Su Wen* trajectory

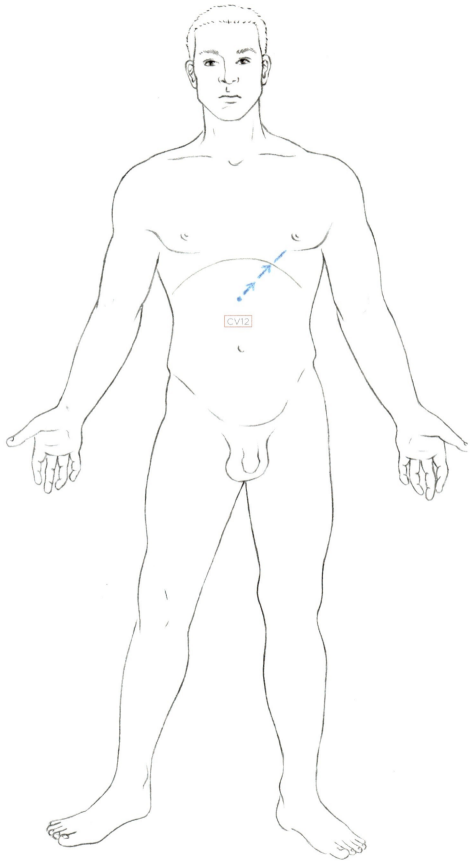

Luo Treatment Toolkit

1. *Luo points*

2. *Luo vessels*

    are where Blood is visible and includes capillaries, varicosities, and discolorations along the trajectory or at areas where the trajectory connects. It is not necessary to bleed all the visible Luos. Some practitioners start with the very fine ones, but my preference, after bleeding the Luo point, is to bleed in the following order:

    a. The darkest Luos
    b. Bulging Luos
    c. Intersections of Luos: places where two or more capillaries join.
    d. Ropey varicosities
    e. Fine spider veins

    Depending on the patient, the pulses, and the patient's tolerance of the treatment, I often stop after the very dark Luos, or the intersections. Tremendous healing can occur with the release of a single bulging Luo or a series of fine capillaries (spider veins). With practice, you'll know when to stop. Watch the patient's breathing and notice when there's a big release (a sigh or a deep breath). That's often a good place to stop.

3. *Yuan-Source points,* if required

4. *Harmonizing point*

    which is one point proximal to the He-Sea point.
    Harmonizing points normalize the circulation of Blood.
    LU-4, LI-12, ST-35, SP-10, HT-2, SI-9, BL-38, KI-11, PC-2, TH-11, GB-33, LR-9.

5. *Trajectory points*

    It is not necessary to needle any trajectory points in a Luo Channel treatment. However, if it is felt that the intention of the treatment is enhanced by doing so, the points should be needled with even technique.

6. *Indirect pole Moxa*

    is required in Emptied Luo treatments. If using smokeless moxa for practical reasons, make sure it is a solid pole and not hollow.

7. *Gua sha*

    can be useful in bringing Blood closer to the surface to facilitate bleeding. Gua sha is essential to remove obstructions (accumulations) in the Luo Channel if encountered along the channel.

Treatment Protocols

"If the Luo vessels around the point and along the channel are full and one can see Blood, then let Blood to end the illness. When the color of the Blood changes, stop." —Chapter 22, *Ling Shu*

Full Luo Protocol *(Protocols for each Luo Channel are given on pages 88-103)*

1. Assess which Luo is affected using the criteria for diagnosis above. (See Luo Channel Diagnosis on page 57 and signs and symptoms, pages 88-103.)
2. Bleed the Luo point. Wait for the color to change or brighten (2–5 drops).
3. Bleed any visible Luos vessels.
4. Palpate the channel. If obstructions and tensions are found, *gua-sa* to break them up. Free the entire channel.
5. Regulate the Blood by needling one point proximal to the He-Sea point on the related Primary Channel with even technique. When De Qi is obtained, remove the needle. The regulating point needs no retention.

"If the Luo Channel disease is emptied, harmonize it with moxa." —Chapter 27, *Ling Shu*

Emptied Luo Protocol *(Protocols for each Luo Channel are given on pages 88-103)*

1. Assess which Luo is affected using the criteria for diagnosis above. (See Luo Channel Diagnosis on page 57 and signs and symptoms, pages 88-103.)
2. Light a solid moxa pole and hold it in one hand.
3. Bleed the Luo point with your other hand.
4. Immediately moxa the point until the patient declares the point hot. Do this safely many times until you feel the point has taken a lot of heat. This may take several minutes.
5. WARNING: Sometimes the patient will not feel that the point is hot. After two seconds ask them can they feel the heat. After another two seconds ask them whether it's getting warmer. Repeat the question again and again. If they can feel it steadily getting warmer, it's likely they will tell you that it's hot when it's hot. If they can't really feel it, or if it seems that it should feel hotter than they report, stop the moxa when your "safety fingers" (fingers placed on either side of, and close to the moxa site) are very warm. It is possible to severely burn a patient without them feeling anything. Keep your patient safe.

6. Bleed and moxa nodules along the trajectory or break up the nodule with strong reduction technique. This can take a while. Traditionally, one would use the Tortoise Technique: surround the nodule with four needles, put one needle in the center of the nodule and strongly reduce all of them.
7. Gua sha any obstructions or tensions in the channel. Free the entire channel.
8. Harmonize Blood one point proximal to the He-Sea point using even technique. When De Qi is obtained, remove the needle. The regulating point needs no retention.

Treatment Course

> "Treat the Luo Channels every other day. Harmonize Blood after bleeding."
> —Chapter 10, *Ling Shu*

1. Treat the Luos every second day for 21 days (11 treatments).
2. If using essential oils to continue the Luo course, apply the oil to the Luo point every other day for 21 days.
3. If you cannot treat the Luos every second day, technically you are not performing a Luo treatment. The application of the appropriate essential oils *does* constitute a Luo treatment.
4. At the end of a Luo course, if there is no change in signs and symptoms, the person is said to be stubborn (don't announce it, of course). This indicates stagnation in all the Luos. (Also, your diagnosis may need reevaluating.)
5. If you want to do more Luo treatment, perform the following treatment (first) combined with your original treatment every second day for twenty-one days.
    a) Using only a lancet, no plum blossom, lance the Great Luo of the Spleen, SP-21, three cun below the axilla, (not six).
    b) Regulate SP-10 with even technique

Subjective Observations Associated with Luo Treatments

Patient experience on the table during Luo treatments occupies a broad spectrum. Some patients:

1. have major emotional releases on the table.
2. will not feel the use of the lancet at all.
3. feel extreme burning on insertion even though the insertion is very shallow.
4. enjoy the sensation of bleeding and feel immense relief immediately.
5. feel internal temperature changes.
6. feel nauseous as rebellious Qi is released.

7. feel a sensation of fluid streaming from the Luo point when only a tiny drop was let.
8. feel intense tingling for a short while after treatment.

It seems that all patients uniformly experience the sensation of relief soon after bleeding.

Healing Events

The following kinds of events are possible and are healing.

1. Emergence and processing of suppressed memories.
2. Intense dreaming.
3. Noticeable positive changes in the tenor of relationships.
4. Purges with or without a strong smell, such as vomiting, diarrhea, coughing, sneezing, sweating, increased defecation, dark urine. Purges can even include a desire to clean out closets, or to move.
5. If the patient is strong—if they have sufficient Yang Qi—the Luos might empty into the Sinew Channels. Sudden stiffness or reduced range of motion may arise. This is simply the pathogen coming up to the surface for release. Perform a Sinew treatment/s if this occurs.

The Psychosocial Luo Model

The Development of Luo Pathology

Luo theory could fill several books. Outlined below is a segment of Luo theory referred to in this book as the Psychosocial Luo Model. It conveys the detailed, highly sophisticated way Chinese medicine explains and treats the emotional issues that arise in the course of human development from the moment of birth to the moment of death, and the effects of the residency of that pathology in the Blood. It should be noted that while an emotional issue can progress and affect all the Luo Channels, it may also just remain latent in the channel associated with that development stage. What follows here is an introduction for easy clinic reference.

The Psychosocial Luo model follows the Primary Channel sequence because the Luo Channels are collaterals that come out of the Primary Channels. The sequence is divided here into three energetic levels.

1) Survival energetics: LU, LI, ST, SP
2) Interaction energetics: HT, SI, BL, KI
3) Differentiation energetics: PC, TH, GB, LR

While the Primary Channels carry out development, the Luo Channels are created to contain the emotion of the unresolved difficulties that occur along the way. These difficulties can arise anywhere in the sequence. They don't have to arise at the beginning. As these emotional holdings increase in quantity, the Luo Channels fill up. This can take days or decades.

Wei	LU, LI, ST, SP
Ying	HT, SI, BL, KI
Yuan	PC, TH, GB, LR

The Luos of the First Energetic Level

Emotions at the level of SURVIVAL
The Development of Perception, Sensation, Thought

The signs and symptoms apply equally to adults and children. All these signs and symptoms appear in Chapter 10 of the *Ling Shu*.

Here follows the progression of Luo pathology. The Lung Luo is explained in detail on this page as an introduction to the process. In the next section, you'll find all the progressions with full content but in fewer words. Not all signs and symptoms need be present to warrant the diagnoses. Even one sign presenting in the correct emotional context can justify a given diagnosis.

The Lung Luo Channel Progression

Lung Primary Channel functions normally. Free openness to the world through breath is experienced. There exists an easy readiness to encounter the outside world through the common medium, the breath. The Lung Channel is activated at birth.

Difficulty arises: The typical difficulty is the failure to bond. At birth, the bond with the maternal matrix is not made immediately; the reconnection to the mother through embracing and breastfeeding is delayed or compromised. This results in a heightened desire to bond and the child is often (much later) misdiagnosed as a "high needs" child. Also, the initial bond with the breast may have been weak, conditional, limited with scheduling, or absent and there remains the sense of profound missing intimacy, which affects interaction with the world.

Treatment: Establish the bond with the mother. Start process of relactation. Put baby in sling facing in, breastfeeding on demand until able to walk. If relactation is not possible, put the baby in a sling full-time, facing in, with maximum skin-to-skin contact.

Lung Luo formation and filling process: The pathology progresses if untreated and as a child or an adult the need to bond, to connect, becomes all-consuming. If that need is repeatedly denied, emotions of profound sadness and frustration arise. When the sadness and frustration become overwhelming, the body creates a reservoir, a Longitudinal Luo at the Luo point to contain the Blood that is containing those emotions so that they are in a reduced state of circulation. Over time, the Luo vessel becomes full and therefore visible.

Fullness of the Lung Luo Channel: The Longitudinal Luo fills up and fullness of the Luo signs occur: Luo vessels appear at or near the Luo point and/or along the Luo Channel.

Signs and Symptoms: Hot palms, looking for something to contact, needing constant stimulation, the inability to sit still.

Treatment: Full Luo treatment.
    i. Bleed LU-7.
    ii. Bleed Luo vessels along the Lung Longitudinal Luo trajectory.
    iii. Gua sha obstructions along the Lung Longitudinal Luo trajectory.
    iv. Harmonize Blood at the point which is one point proximal to the He-Sea point.

Lung Luo empties into the Lung Primary Channel: When the Luo vessel becomes very full, it begins to overflow back into the Primary Channel.

Emptied Lung Luo: Most or all of the varicosities fully or partially disappear because Blood is no longer able to keep pathology in latency. The neediness is in the process of internalizing. Nodules occur on the Lung Primary Channel trajectory as Yin is brought forward to prevent penetration of this emotional pathology into the Yuan-Source level now that the Primary Channel is trying to place the pathology elsewhere.

Emptied Lung Luo Signs and Symptoms: Disinterest in contact and stimulation, no sense of what in life is stimulating, no interest in life.
Treatment: Emptied Luo treatment.
    i. Bleed and moxa LU-7.

ii. Bleed and moxa nodules along the Lung Longitudinal Luo trajectory.
iii. Bleed and moxa nodules along the Lung Primary Channel.
iv. Harmonize Blood.

Note: When reading the following summaries, it's important to consider the information given here as being somewhere in a wide spectrum of possibilities within the nature of each of the Luos. In other words, these signs and symptoms may seem understated or overstated when compared with your patient's presentations. With practice, you'll learn the feel of a given Luo and won't feel the need to be very literal.

I'm using the word *literal* in the lists below, rather than *physical* to illustrate that these signs are intended as colloquial metaphors in the Classical texts (although these signs and symptoms do often appear in a physical sense). Likewise, one could view the signs and symptoms listed under "literal" as metaphors of the psyche.

The Significance of the Sequence of the Luos

In the following section I am using the sequence of the Luos used in the Psychosocial Model of the Luo Channels which follows the Primary Channels. However, the Longitudinal Luos are also described in chapter 10 of the *Ling Shu* as an anatomical progression: Yin arm channels to Yang arm channels to Yang leg channels to Yin leg channels to the constitutional Luos. In this order, the Luos are seen to return to the chest where Blood must return to be recirculated and refreshed. The order does not affect choices in diagnosis and is included here because it appears in the Classical texts. Anatomical order of the Luo Channels: LU, HT, PC, SI, LI, TH, BL, GB, ST, SP, KI, LR, CV, GV, Great Luo of the Spleen, Great Luo of Stomach.

The order of the Luo Channels given below has the Constitutional Luos (Ren and Du Luos) preceding those of the Great Luo of the Spleen and Stomach. Unresolved emotional issues are ultimately deposited in the Ren and the Du Luos for potential resolution in the following lifetime; LR-5 goes to Ren at CV-2, and GB-37 goes to Chong at ST-42. The Great Luo of the Spleen, however, controls all the Luos. This responsibility lasts as long as there is activity in the Great Luo of the Stomach (a heartbeat). Therefore the Great Luo of the Stomach is the last of the Luos.

Luo Channel Signs, Symptoms and Treatment Protocols

Lung Luo Channel Progression

1. **The Lung Primary Channel functions normally** and free openness to the world through breath is experienced.
2. **Difficulty is encountered and unresolved.** This is very often caused by the failure to bond. The initial bond with the breast was weak or absent and there remains the sense of profound missing intimacy, which affects interaction with the world.
3. **Lung Luo becomes full;** Luo vessels appear at or near the Luo point, LU-7 and/or along the Lung Longitudinal Luo Channel.
    - Psyche: Looking for something to contact, needing constant stimulation. Inability to sit still, restlessness, jumpiness, uneasiness.
    - Literal: Hot palms, Heat in the palms, itchy palms.
4. **Lung Luo becomes emptied**; nodules appear on the Lung Primary Channel.
    - Psyche: Disinterest in contact and stimulation. No sense of what in life is stimulating. Loss of interest in life.
    - Literal: Frequent yawning to help open the chest to free the pathogen from the interior. Frequent urination as Wei Qi–which is controlled by the Lungs–tries to move the pathogen out using Fluids.

Treatment

Treatment Protocol for Full Lung Longitudinal Luo
  i. Bleed LU-7.
  ii. Bleed visible Luos along the Lung Longitudinal Luo trajectory and as you proceed along the channel.
  iii. Gua sha obstructions along the Lung Longitudinal Luo trajectory.
  iv. Harmonize Blood at LU-4 with even technique.

Treatment Protocol for Emptied Lung Longitudinal Luo
  i. Bleed and immediately moxa LU-7.
  ii. Break up nodules and gua sha obstructions along the Lung Longitudinal Luo trajectory.
  iii. Break up nodules and gua sha obstructions along the Lung Primary Channel.
  iv. Harmonize Blood at LU-4 with even technique.

Large Intestine Luo Progression

1. **The Large Intestine Primary Channel functions normally** and the person is able to assimilate experience beyond that of the breath.

2. **Difficulty is encountered and unresolved:** The emotions of weaning early or too much stimulation, trying to assimilate too much. Food was introduced too early and the person had to very quickly grow teeth to be able to handle the excess stimulation to the gut. There were many bright colors in the child's room. The child has toys that make sounds on their own. There's a television in the child's room. The child plays with electronic screens, games, phones, and computers. Screens are overwhelming to a young child. There is too much to digest.

3. **Large Intestine Luo becomes full**; Luo vessels appear at or near the Luo point, LI-6 and/or along the Large Intestine Longitudinal Luo Channel.

    Psyche: Over-stimulation has led to the shutting down of response.

    Literal: Wanting to see something over and over again. Making repetitive actions. Toothaches as the teeth rebel against premature demands. Acute deafness or autism are possible as the child withdraws from the stimulation.

4. **Large Intestine Luo becomes emptied**; nodules appear on the Large Intestine Primary Channel.

    Psyche: Difficulty assimilating stimulus. Having difficulty sensing feelings in one's own Heart.

    Literal: Coldness of the teeth. Diaphragmatic numbness.

Treatment

Treatment Protocol for Full Large Intestine Longitudinal Luo

   i. Bleed LI-6.

   ii. Bleed visible Luos along the Large Intestine Longitudinal Luo trajectory.

   iii. Gua sha obstructions along the Large Intestine Longitudinal Luo trajectory.

   iv. Harmonize Blood at LI-12 with even technique.

Treatment Protocol for Emptied Large Intestine Longitudinal Luo

   i. Bleed and immediately moxa LI-6.

   ii. Break up nodules and gua sha obstructions along the Luo trajectory.

   iii. Break up nodules and gua sha obstructions along the Large Intestine Primary Channel.

   iv. Harmonize Blood at LI-12 with even technique.

Stomach Luo Channel Progression

1. **The Stomach Primary Channel functions normally** and governs preferences and the "gut feeling". The Stomach has no judgment.
2. **Difficulty is encountered and unresolved.** Feelings are regularly denied, undervalued or suppressed.
3. **Stomach Luo becomes full**; Luo vessels appear at or near the Luo point, ST-40, and/or along the Stomach Longitudinal Luo Channel.
    - **Psyche**: The rational mind cannot overcome the emotions. The patient acts without thinking, impulsively, "loses it". There is a feeling that there's too much stimulation. Acute madness, acute insanity.
    - **Literal**: Temper tantrums, hysteria, diaper rash, blemishes around oral cavity.
4. **Stomach Luo becomes emptied;** nodules appear on the Stomach Primary Channel.
    - **Psyche**: The desire to explore is harmed. Lack of feeling of destination in life. Feeling there are no conclusions along life's pathway. Stagefright. Lack of personal satisfaction.
    - **Literal**: Weakness or atrophy of the lower limbs, stiff feet, listlessness, lethargy, numbness of the throat with accompanying rebellious Qi signs and symptoms, sudden loss of voice.

Treatment

Treatment Protocol for Full Stomach Longitudinal Luo
  i. Bleed ST-40.
  ii. Bleed visible Luos along the Stomach Longitudinal Luo trajectory.
  iii. Gua sha obstructions along the Stomach Longitudinal Luo trajectory.
  iv. Harmonize Blood at ST-35 with even technique.

Treatment Protocol for Emptied Stomach Longitudinal Luo
  i. Bleed and immediately moxa ST-40.
  ii. Break up nodules and gua sha obstructions along the Stomach Longitudinal Luo trajectory.
  iii. Break up nodules and gua sha obstructions along the Stomach Primary Channel.
  iv. Harmonize Blood at ST-35 with even technique.

Spleen Luo Channel Progression

1. **The Spleen Primary Channel functions normally** and controls the Yi (thoughts), rationalization, habituation and skill.
2. **Difficulty is encountered and unresolved.** The patient overthinks and rationalizes too much.
3. **Spleen Luo becomes full**; Luo vessels appear at or near the Luo point, SP-4 and/or along the Spleen Longitudinal Luo Channel.
    - **Psyche**: Lack of control of emotions. Emotions seem to have no closure. Obsessiveness. Obsessive thinking.
    - **Literal:** Sharp pains in the middle of the gut, in the intestines.
4. **Spleen Luo becomes emptied**; nodules appear on the Spleen Primary Channel.
    - **Psyche**: Repetition of thoughts. Addictions. A nagging internal voice.
    - **Literal:** Drum-like distention in the abdomen, ascites.

Treatment

Treatment Protocol for Full Spleen Longitudinal Luo
   i. Bleed SP-4.
   ii. Bleed visible Luos along the Spleen Longitudinal Luo trajectory.
   iii. Gua sha obstructions along the Spleen Longitudinal Luo trajectory.
   iv. Harmonize Blood at SP-10 with even technique.

Treatment Protocol for Emptied Spleen Longitudinal Luo
   i. Bleed and immediately moxa SP-4.
   ii. Break up nodules and gua sha obstructions along the Spleen Longitudinal Luo trajectory.
   iii. Break up nodules and gua sha obstructions along the Spleen Primary Channel.
   iv. Harmonize Blood at SP-10 with even technique.

The Luos of the Second Energetic Level

Emotions at the level of INTERACTION
Emotions Governing the Capacity to Live a Coherent Life with Others

Heart Luo Channel Progression

1. **The Heart Primary Channel functions normally** and provides animation. It sets and then vocalizes goals. The Heart Primary Channel controls relationships.
2. **Difficulty is encountered and unresolved** resulting in Heartbreak. The Heart encounters the pain of not achieving what it wants. The patient feels betrayed because someone who imposed their morals and ethics denied them the right to express themselves.
3. **Heart Luo becomes full**; Luo vessels appear at or near the Luo point, HT-5 and/or along the Heart Longitudinal Luo Channel.
    - **Psyche:** Striving towards that which is no longer there. Heartbreak. A feeling of broken dreams.
    - **Literal:** Chest pains and chest oppression or heaviness. Heart pain. A feeling of suffocation.
4. **Heart Luo becomes emptied**; nodules appear on the Heart Primary Channel.
    - **Psyche:** Loss of speech due to having been stifled. Not knowing what to say. Not being able to express what's on the mind or in the Heart and being heavy-Hearted as a result. The inability to find the inner voice; the inability to be and express oneself fully.
    - **Literal:** Loss of speech, dyslexia, Tourette's syndrome, stuttering, language issues, a loss of engagement. A feeling that speaking one's thoughts makes no difference.

Treatment

Treatment Protocol for Full Heart Longitudinal Luo
i. Bleed HT-5.
ii. Bleed visible Luos along the Heart Longitudinal Luo trajectory.
iii. Gua sha obstructions along the Heart Longitudinal Luo trajectory.
iv. Harmonize Blood at HT-2 with even technique.

Treatment Protocol for Emptied Heart Longitudinal Luo
  i. Bleed and immediately moxa HT-5.
  ii. Break up nodules and gua sha obstructions along the Heart Longitudinal Luo trajectory.
  iii. Break up nodules and gua sha obstructions along the Heart Primary Channel.
  iv. Harmonize Blood at HT-2 with even technique.

Small Intestine Luo Channel Progression

1. **The Small Intestine Primary Channel functions normally** and separates the pure from the impure. Small Intestine creates one's feedback system, a personal system of checks and balances that enables a person to declare privately to oneself that they are doing okay. It produces dignity and criticism. Small Intestine has intelligence.

2. **Difficulty is encountered and unresolved**: A constant need to compare and self-check.

3. **Small Intestine Luo becomes full**; Luo vessels appear at or near the Luo point, SI-7 and/or along the Small Intestine Longitudinal Luo Channel.

    Psyche: A constant need for approval. Constant internal dialogue, annoyingly returning to the same thought. Trying to control people like an obsessive lover. Overwhelming obsessive thought. Looking for self-recognition through the feedback of others. Patient can become aggressive and violent.

Note: Small Intestine differs from Large Intestine because now intelligence is engaged.

    Literal: Easily dislocated loose joints, elbow atrophy. Atrophy of joints in general.

4. **Small Intestine Luo becomes emptied**; nodules appear on the Small Intestine Primary Channel.

    Psyche: Lost capacity to discern; the feedback system fails. Doubt and uncertainty about what to let go of. Looking at something over and over and having a lot of criticism and judgment. Having a dialogue with self: How did I do? Seeking constant feedback from the self. Uncertainty, doubt about decisions and about self. Brainstorming the possibilities.

Note: Spleen Luo does not have this dialogue – it just thinks in a straight line with no varying scenarios arising in the thoughts. Spleen Luo does not evaluate. Small Intestine Luo does evaluate actions.

    Literal: Lost capacity to separate pure from impure; pebbly stools. Small itchy or flaky swellings that scab (fungal infections).

Treatment

Treatment Protocol for Full Small Intestine Longitudinal Luo

i. Bleed SI-7.

ii. Bleed visible Luos along the Small Intestine Longitudinal Luo trajectory.

iii. Gua sha obstructions along the Small Intestine Longitudinal Luo trajectory.

iv. Harmonize Blood at SI-9 with even technique.

Treatment Protocol for Emptied Small Intestine Longitudinal Luo

i. Bleed and immediately moxa SI-7.

ii. Break up nodules and gua sha obstructions along the Small Intestine Longitudinal Luo trajectory.

iii. Break up nodules and gua sha obstructions along the Small Intestine Primary Channel.

iv. Harmonize Blood at SI-9 with even technique.

Bladder Luo Channel Progression

1. **The Bladder Primary Channel functions normally** and controls the exterior. It erects the boundary to exterior conditions.

2. **Difficulty is encountered and unresolved:** Too much feedback is received. The limits of the feedback system are exceeded.

3. **Bladder Luo becomes full**; Luo vessels appear at or near the Luo point, BL-58 and/or along the Bladder Longitudinal Luo Channel.

    Psyche: Panic. The alarm system is always activated; the body reacts to repel criticism. The patient sabotages relationships in order to return to the self. (This is why the Bladder Luo Channel goes to the Kidney Luo point; the Kidney contains the self.) The patient is constantly at the ready for the onslaught of a crisis. Constant crises ensue. The threshold between response and no response is very thin; reactivity is very high.

    Literal: Nasal congestion, allergies, sinusitis, headache and low back pain. Post-traumatic stress disorder (PTSD). The startle reflex is active.

4. **Bladder Luo becomes emptied**; nodules appear on the Bladder Primary Channel.

    Psyche: The threshold of tolerance for feedback disintegrates and the alarm system turns off through overstimulation. Addictive behavior is accompanied by the inability to set a limit to turn the behavior off. Lack of emotion, vulnerability, a constant need to feel loved. Fetishes emerge and are unstoppable. Not knowing enough is enough. The patient doesn't have emotions about, or place a value on, what they do.

Literal: Clear nasal discharge, nosebleeds.

Treatment

Treatment Protocol for Full Bladder Longitudinal Luo
i. Bleed BL-58.
ii. Bleed visible Luos along the Bladder Longitudinal Luo trajectory.
iii. Gua sha obstructions along the Bladder Longitudinal Luo trajectory.
iv. Harmonize Blood at BL-38 with even technique.

Treatment Protocol for Emptied Bladder Longitudinal Luo
i. Bleed and immediately moxa BL-58.
ii. Break up nodules and gua sha obstructions along the Bladder Longitudinal Luo trajectory.
iii. Break up nodules and gua sha obstructions along the Bladder Primary Channel.
iv. Harmonize Blood at BL-38 with even technique.

Kidney Luo Channel Progression

1. **The Kidney Primary Channel functions normally** and governs the Will (Zhi) effectively. (Will means the force of self-direction: one's drive.)
2. **Difficulty is encountered and unresolved.** The will is uncontrolled and misdirected.
3. **Kidney Luo becomes full**; Luo vessels appear at or near the Luo point, KI-4 and/or along the Kidney Longitudinal Luo Channel.
    Psyche: Obsessive, compulsive behavior emerges and the patient acts on it. The extreme of this is the death wish: constantly putting oneself in life-threatening situations. The inability to let anything go.
    Literal: Stagnation in the lower orifices, blockage of the lower orifices, constipation and/or anuria.
4. **Kidney Luo becomes emptied**; nodules appear on the Kidney Primary Channel.
    Psyche: Extreme paranoia. Being afraid of the self and afraid of loss. Fear of being left alone. Extreme fear, Fright. Depression. The patient constantly feels they are in a life-threatening situation and there's no way out. (Here the trigger is unknown, not to be confused with panic

or PTSD where the trigger is known.)

Literal: Pain in the Kidney region or pain in the genital region due to adrenal exhaustion.

Treatment

Treatment Protocol for Full Kidney Longitudinal Luo
i. Bleed KI-4.
ii. Bleed visible Luos along the Kidney Longitudinal Luo trajectory.
iii. Gua sha obstructions along the Kidney Longitudinal Luo trajectory.
iv. Harmonize Blood at KI-11 with even technique.

Treatment Protocol for Emptied Kidney Longitudinal Luo
i. Bleed and immediately moxa KI-4.
ii. Break up nodules and gua sha obstructions along the Kidney Longitudinal Luo trajectory.
iii. Break up nodules and gua sha obstructions along the Kidney Primary Channel.
iv. Harmonize Blood at KI-11 with even technique.

The Luos of the Third Energetic Level

Emotions at the level of DIFFERENTIATION
The Management of Emotions and the Development of the Ability to Deal with Stress

Pericardium Luo Channel Progression

1. **The Pericardium Primary Channel functions normally** and protects the Heart. The Pericardium Channel functions as a coping mechanism. It manages stress, preserves sanity, generates empathy, manages emotions, uses intelligence to rationalize.

2. **Difficulty is encountered and unresolved.** Betrayal of, or trauma to the Spirit is perceived. Patient experiences failure in achieving goals.

3. **Pericardium Luo becomes full**; Luo vessels appear at or near the Luo point, PC-6 and/or along the Pericardium Longitudinal Luo Channel.

    Psyche: Heart "pain". The inability to control emotions which are then verbalized or somatized. Split personalities. A constant need to lie. The inability to feel remorseful.

    Literal: Palpitations, anxiety, Heart pain.

4. **Pericardium Luo becomes emptied**; nodules appear on the Pericardium Primary Channel.

> **Psyche**: Inability to interact because of the inability to control the emotions. Self-mutilation, the inability to see options, inability to experience the pain of another person, inability to experience guilt. Sociopathic behavior. Absence of empathy.
>
> **Literal:** Rigidity and pain in the neck and head.

Treatment

Treatment Protocol for Full Pericardium Longitudinal Luo
  i. Bleed PC-6.
  ii. Bleed visible Luos along the Pericardium Longitudinal Luo trajectory.
  iii. Gua sha obstructions along the Pericardium Longitudinal Luo trajectory.
  iv. Harmonize Blood at PC-2 with even technique.

Treatment Protocol for Emptied Pericardium Longitudinal Luo
  i. Bleed and immediately moxa PC-6.
  ii. Break up nodules and gua sha obstructions along the Pericardium Longitudinal Luo trajectory.
  iii. Break up nodules and gua sha obstructions along the Pericardium Primary Channel.
  iv. Harmonize Blood at PC-2 with even technique.

Triple Heater Luo Channel Progression

1. **The Triple Heater Primary Channel functions normally** and controls the temperament successfully. It takes charge of changing who we are; it self-examines, and creates acceptance of responsibility for our own actions. Triple Heater finds options, handles situations by examining various angles, and uses intuition and ingenuity to come up with new possibilities.
2. **Difficulty is encountered and unresolved.** Intuition and ingenuity is programmed out by over-helpful parents or by the overuse of screens (games on electronic screens, computers), by discouragement, or failure to support.
3. **Triple Heater Luo becomes full**; Luo vessels appear at or near the Luo point, TH-5 and/or along the Triple Heater Longitudinal Luo Channel.

   > **Psyche:** Rigidity, stubbornness, the inability to change one's reactivity.

Literal: Stiffness, spasms and cramping in elbows. Dislocation of the elbows.

4. **Triple Heater Luo becomes emptied**; nodules appear on the Triple Heater Primary Channel.

   Psyche: Refusal even to look at own temperament. Indifference, numbness, failure to react to oneself.

   Literal: Weakness, loss of tonus of elbows, difficulty bending the elbow when it's bearing weight. Flaccid muscles.

Treatment

Treatment Protocol for Full Triple Heater Longitudinal Luo
   i. Bleed TH-5.
   ii. Bleed visible Luos along the Triple Heater Longitudinal Luo trajectory.
   iii. Gua sha obstructions along the Triple Heater Longitudinal Luo trajectory.
   iv. Harmonize Blood at TH-11 with even technique.

Treatment Protocol for Emptied Triple Heater Longitudinal Luo
   i. Bleed and immediately moxa TH-5.
   ii. Break up nodules and gua sha obstructions along the Triple Heater Longitudinal Luo trajectory.
   iii. Break up nodules and gua sha obstructions along the Triple Heater Primary Channel.
   iv. Harmonize Blood at TH-11 with even technique.

Gallbladder Luo Channel Progression

1. **The Gallbladder Primary Channel functions normally** and effectively controls decisiveness.
2. **Difficulty is encountered and unresolved.** A loss of certainty emerges and decision-making becomes difficult.
3. **Gallbladder Luo becomes full**; Luo vessels appear at or near the Luo point, GB-37 and/or along the Gallbladder Longitudinal Luo Channel.

   Psyche: Inability to see any options. Despair, hopelessness, introversion, isolation. Lack of courage in facing adversity or in facing the self. Severe denial of a quality of personality. Feeling there's only one way everything can be. Frustration.

   Literal: Various deficiency signs arise from an underlying Yang deficiency, e.g., cold feet, Spleen Qi deficiency.

4. **Gallbladder Luo becomes emptied**; nodules appear on the Gallbladder Primary Channel.

    Psyche: Feeling there's no place to go, so the patient doesn't even try walking. Severe introversion, a catatonic state, loss of motivation, severe depression, indifference to severe illness, loneliness, the "wandering corpse" (the Shen is apparently absent), suicidal tendencies.
    (These signs and symptoms are similar to, but more severe than "full".)

    Literal: Weakness or paralysis of the lower limbs. Inability to rise from a sitting position. Frozen limbs.

Treatment

Treatment Protocol for Full Gallbladder Longitudinal Luo
   i. Bleed GB-37.
   ii. Bleed visible Luos along the Gallbladder Longitudinal Luo trajectory.
   iii. Gua sha obstructions along the Gallbladder Longitudinal Luo trajectory.
   iv. Harmonize Blood at GB-33 with even technique.

Treatment Protocol for Emptied Gallbladder Longitudinal Luo
   i. Bleed and immediately moxa GB-37.
   ii. Break up nodules and gua sha obstructions along the Gallbladder Longitudinal Luo trajectory.
   iii. Break up nodules and gua sha obstructions along the Gallbladder Primary Channel.
   iv. Harmonize Blood at GB-33 with even technique.

Liver Luo Channel Progression

1. **The Liver Primary Channel functions normally** and effectively generates creativity, goal setting, and interest in the outside world.
2. **Difficulty is encountered and unresolved.** Disinterest emerges. The patient loses interest in achievement.
3. **Liver Luo becomes full**; Luo vessels appear at or near the Luo point, LR-5 and/or along the Liver Longitudinal Luo Channel.

    Psyche: Breaking from reality. Wanting to be somebody else. Hearing voices, seeing things, talking to oneself. Schizophrenia with multiple personalities. *Mild form:* daydreaming.

Literal: Abnormal sexual arousal or inappropriate erections. Testicular swelling as the body tries to create something, but is frustrated.

4. **Liver Luo emptied**; nodules appear on the Liver Primary Channel.

Psyche: Multiple personalities of a destructive nature. E.g., "I was possessed and instructed to kill." The extreme is suicide. Intolerance of self.

Literal: Cruel genital itch due to the inability to create what is wanted. Genital swellings, testicular, vaginal and scrotal swelling, uterine swelling. STDs including herpes. The extreme is stroke.

Treatment

Treatment Protocol for Full Liver Longitudinal Luo

i. Bleed LR-5.

ii. Bleed visible Luos along the Liver Longitudinal Luo trajectory.

iii. Gua sha obstructions along the Liver Longitudinal Luo trajectory.

iv. Harmonize Blood at LR-9 with even technique.

Treatment Protocol for Emptied Liver Longitudinal Luo

i. Bleed and immediately moxa LR-5.

ii. Break up nodules and gua sha obstructions along the Liver Longitudinal Luo trajectory.

iii. Break up nodules and gua sha obstructions along the Liver Primary Channel.

iv. Harmonize Blood at LR-9 with even technique.

Ren Luo Channel

Ren Luo full: Luo vessels appear at or near the Luo point, CV-15, and/or along the Longitudinal Luo Channel. Abdominal pain.

Ren Luo emptied; nodules appear on the Ren Channel. Abdominal itch.

The Ren Luo contains the accumulation of karma from the Yin Luos.

Unresolved emotions are deposited by the Luos into the Jing for processing in the next lifetime. This is the physicality of inherited karma. In other words, resistance to life stagnates the Blood and at the same time, the Blood is the residence of the Shen, the Spirit. So the Spirit, too becomes tainted by the experience of life. Every subsequent lifetime, therefore, is the opportunity to liberate oneself from all previous lives.

Treatment

Treatment Protocol for Full Ren Luo
  i. Bleed CV-15.
  ii. Bleed visible Luos along the Ren Luo trajectory (which disperses over the abdomen).
  iii. Gua sha obstructions along the Ren Luo trajectory.
  iv. Harmonize Blood at SP-10 with even technique. (SP-10 is used as a Blood regulator in the absence of a Blood regulating point on the Ren Channel.)

Treatment Protocol for Emptied Ren Luo
  i. Bleed and immediately moxa CV-15.
  ii. Break up nodules and gua sha obstructions along the Ren Luo trajectory.
  iii. Harmonize Blood at SP-10 with even technique.

Du Luo Channel

Du Luo full; Luo vessels appear at or near the Luo point, GV-1, and/or along the Luo Channel. Stiffness of the spine. Luo vessels appear at or near the Luo point and/or along the Luo Channel.

Du Luo emptied; nodules appear on the Du Channel. Heaviness of the head with shaking.

Du Luo contains the accumulation of karma from the Yang Luos. Unresolved emotions are deposited by the Luos into the Jing for processing in the next lifetime. The Ren and Du Channels communicate with the Chong. The Chong modifies the blueprint for the next incarnation and the next generation with the unresolved Luo pathology given it by the Ren and Du Luos. Hence, what we have not dealt with at the time we give our Jing to create conception, is transmitted to the next generation.

Treatment

Treatment Protocol for Full Du Luo
  i. Bleed GV-1.
  ii. Bleed visible Luos along the Du Luo trajectory.
  iii. Gua sha obstructions along the Du Luo trajectory.
  iv. Harmonize Blood at SP-10 with even technique. (SP-10 is used as a Blood regulator in the absence of a Blood regulating point on the Du Channel.)

Treatment Protocol for Emptied Du Luo

i. Bleed and immediately moxa GV-1 with care to part the buttocks.

Note: If you are worried about the proximity of heat to skin here, bleed GV-1, then insert a 2 inch needle half an inch or so until the needle can stand, part the buttocks at GV-1 and heat the needle with pole moxa.

ii. Break up nodules along the Du Luo trajectory.

iii. Gua sha obstructions along the Du Luo trajectory.

iv. Harmonize Blood at SP-10 with even technique.

Great Luo of the Spleen

1. **The Great Luo of Spleen functions normally** and controls all the sinews.
2. **Difficulty is encountered and unresolved.** A feeling of overwhelming suffering arises.
3. **Great Luo of the Spleen becomes full**; Luo vessels appear at or near the Luo point, GB-22 and/or along the Great Luo of the Spleen Channel.
    - **Psyche**: Wanting to hurt the self in a way that can be seen. The patient wants to hurt who they are. Being overwhelmed by the challenges of life to the point of incapacity. Feeling beaten, victimized. Severe depression. The feeling of martyrdom. The mind totally loses control. Schizophrenia, self-hatred. Defacing the self, cutting or slashing the throat or eyes.
    - **Literal**: Pain diffused all over the body. Fibromyalgia, Chronic Fatigue Syndrome.
4. **Great Luo of the Spleen becomes emptied**; nodules appear on the Great Luo of the Spleen Channel–the ring around the chest.
    - **Psyche**: Lack of will to live. Suicidal.
    - **Literal**: Looseness of all joints as pathology moves to the joints. The body holds it there by breaking down Marrow. A lack of integrity and strength in the structure.

Treatment

Treatment Protocol for Full Great Luo of the Spleen Longitudinal Luo

i. Bleed GB-22 (located three cun below the axilla).

ii. Bleed visible Luos along the Great Luo of the Spleen trajectory.

iii. Gua sha obstructions along the Great Luo of the Spleen trajectory.

iv. Harmonize Blood at SP-10 with even technique.

Treatment Protocol for Emptied Great Luo of the Spleen Longitudinal Luo
  i. Bleed and immediately moxa GB-22 (3 cun below the axilla).
  ii. Break up nodules and gua sha obstructions along the Great Luo of the Spleen trajectory.
  iii. Harmonize Blood at SP-10 with even technique.

Great Luo of the Stomach

The Great Luo of the Stomach is also known as the *Heartbeat*, the Qi that drives the flow of Blood. It begins in the Stomach and ends in the Lungs. The Great Luo of the Stomach empties directly into the Chong. The *Ling Shu* refers to the Great Luo of the Stomach as the *Empty Mile*, meaning that if one doesn't have enough Blood, one is running on empty. The *Ling Shu* says it begins "at the diaphragm, in the area of the left breast, where a pulsating vessel can be felt".

Great Luo of Stomach Full: Rapid, irregular breathing. Chest congestion, congestive Heart failure.

Great Luo of Stomach Emptied: Palpitations, fibrillations, tachycardia.

Treatment of the Great Luo of the Stomach

The Great Luo of the Stomach has no points and is treated with the Eight Extra Channels, usually Chong or Yin Wei Mai.

Longitudinal Luo Essential Oil Treatments

Essential oils can be used effectively in conjunction with acupuncture treatments. The oil treatments do not require needles and are topical (applied on the skin). Because there is no insertion, patients can learn to apply an oil at home. The acupuncturist selects the oil and the points, in accordance with Chinese medical theory, then instructs the patient on using the oil at home between treatments. The practitioner monitors progress through pulse reading and the patient's report at the next appointment.

The most important thing to know about the application of essential oils is that "less is more". It is critically important that the amount of oil applied to the point is extremely tiny, as the receptors in the body quickly become saturated when overwhelmed with oil and switch off, hindering the treatment. Essential oil therapy is one of the most misused and misunderstood modes of alternative therapy, mainly because the quantities of oil required to produce a therapeutic effect are not generally understood. Properly used, it is extremely potent medicine.

In Luo Channel treatments, the oil is applied only to the Luo point.[1] Choose the oil that resonates with the channel. Instruct the patient that every other day they should dip a toothpick into the oil and touch it to the Luo point which you might mark (if requested) with a fine surgeon's pen using a penny-sized circle, not a dot because the oil will dissolve the ink. Regulation of Blood is achieved by the patient through acupressure massage on the point which is one point proximal to the He-Sea point. These points could also be marked on the patient.

If the patient is having weekly treatments, try scheduling the acupuncture so that it is always on an odd numbered day, maintaining a day of rest between treatments (on the even numbered days).

A typical schedule might look like this:

Day 1, acupuncture; Day 3, 5, 7, essential oils applied at home.

Day 9, acupuncture; Days 11, 13, 15, essential oils applied at home.

Day 17, acupuncture; Days 19 and 21, essential oils applied at home.

---

[1] Blends that can be used on visible Luo vessels are beyond the scope of this book.

Essential Oil Application Method

Caution should be taken with essential oils. They can be caustic and must not come in contact with the eyes.

a. Dip the 'toothpick' in the oil.
b. If there is a visible drop of oil on the toothpick, let the drop fall back into the vial.
c. Touch the toothpick to the point/s to be treated.
d. Do not use a finger to apply the essential oil. It's extremely potent medicine and will affect the joints of the person applying the oil if overused.
e. The patient would put their toothpick back in a tiny ziploc bag and reuse it.
f. Wait 48 hours for the next treatment.

Essential Oils for Application on Luo Points

The Luos of the Emotions related to Survival
The Development of Perception, Sensation, Thought

Lung full	Ravensare, Myrtle
Lung emptied	Pine
Large Intestine full	Orange, Ti (Tea) Tree
Large Intestine emptied	Clove
Stomach full	Mimosa
Stomach emptied	Cedarwood
Spleen full	Rosewood[2], Ho Wood/Leaf, Camphor
Spleen emptied	Coriander, Patchouli

The Luos of the Emotions Related to Interaction
The Development of Social Skills and Living a Cohesive Life with Others

Heart full	Lemon Verbena
Heart emptied	Violet
Small Intestine full	Onion
Small Intestine emptied	Cumin
Bladder full	Styrax
Bladder emptied	Basil
Kidney full	Niaouli/MQV
Kidney emptied	Anise

---

[2] Rosewood is endangered. Use Ho Leaf as a substitute.

The Luos of the Emotions Related to Differentiation
Self-Preservation and the Management of Emotions

Pericardium full	Melissa
Pericardium emptied	Clary Sage
Triple Heater full	Petitgrain
Triple Heater emptied	Thyme
Gallbladder full	Rosemary
Gallbladder emptied	Vetiver
Liver full	German/Blue Chamomile
Liver emptied	Carrot Seed
Ren full	Sandalwood
Ren emptied	Niaouli/MQV
Du full	Fennel
Du emptied	Spikenard
Great Luo of the Spleen full	Rose
Great Luo of the Spleen emptied	Garlic

The Great Luo of the Stomach can be treated with oils prescribed for the Eight Extra Channels, on their Opening points, especially Yin Wei Mai and Chong. See page 230.

TRANSVERSE LUO TREATMENTS

Definition

A Transverse Luo is theoretically the pathway from a Luo point to an organ as it taps into the elemental Source energetics. They are not visible or palpable. A Transverse Luo is depicted as a connection from the Luo point of one channel to the Source point of its Yin-Yang pair, e.g., ST-40 to SP-3. However, the actual terrain of a Transverse Luo is much more extensive.

Importance of the Transverse Luo

The Transverse Luos are important because their treatment releases excess Heat, frees Yuan-Source Qi, and restores strength to the Primary Channels.

The Arising of the Transverse Luos

The Transverse Luos become active if the Longitudinal Luo empties into the Primary Channel *and* the Primary Channel is unable to contain the pathology through the use of swellings, cysts, nodules and other pathological Yin. When the Primary Channel begins to fail to control the pathology, the organ begins to be affected. Transverse Luo signs and symptoms then arise. It should be noted that the emergence of Transverse Luo signs and symptoms do not indicate that the pathology has gone to the Transverse Luos; they are warning signs that the organ is in danger of being reached by pathology, and indicate that the body is considering moving the pathology into the Transverse aspect of the Luo Channel, or that such movement is imminent.

If untreated, the body then begins to move the pathology to the Transverse Luo, the first segment of which extends from the Luo point of the failing channel to the Source point of the Yin-Yang related pair. Ideally, that Source point would keep the pathology still until the Luo Channel it came from regained some space (during treatment) and was able to receive the pathology back. Or, the body might create a connection from the Source point where the pathology arrived, to the Luo point on that same channel and hold it there. But if the pathology remains at that Source point and is not moved, or if it moves to the Luo and then makes a Luo-Source connection back to the Source point of the original channel by completing a figure eight type pathway (see diagram p. 117), the pathology moves deeper into the body, into the second segment of a Transverse Luo.

At that point it can enter Triple Heater,³ or the internal pathways of the Primary Channel and then access the organs. This is why Transverse Luo signs are the same as those of the internal branches of the Primary Channels. (If these various progressions to the Source are not intercepted by another channel, likely the Divergent Channels but possibly the Eight Extraordinary Channels, the pathology becomes fatal.)

For example, in the event of the failure of the Spleen Longitudinal Luo and then the Spleen Primary Channel, the pathogen goes from SP-4 to ST-42. This connection is called a *Transverse Luo*. I refer to that connection as the *first segment of the Transverse Luo*. The body is seeking to put the pathology in the Source point of the Yin-Yang related pair because when one member of a Yin-Yang pair is weakened, it's likely that its pair is considerably stronger. The Qi of Source points is dense and slow and the pathogen has a good chance of staying quiet there. Also, Source points are relatively distal and when the body has acquired the resources to push the pathogen out, the pathogen is not too far from the exterior. Pathology might reside in this part of the Transverse Luo for a period ranging from hours to decades.

When the pathology moves into the Transverse Luo, a tremendous amount of heat combined with the pathology moves from the Longitudinal Luo into the Transverse Luo. This is because long-term Longitudinal Luo pathology creates much stagnation. As Blood stagnates, the body mobilizes Yang to create heat to try to move it.

Ideally, a Transverse Luo treatment is given to make room for the pathology to return to the Luo point. If untreated, the next phase of pathology arises when the Yuan-Source point of the Yin-Yang related pair cannot move the pathology it is holding, or cannot contain more pathology. At that point, the pathology progresses from the first segment of the Transverse Luo to what I call the *second segment of the Transverse Luo*. The second segment occurs when the pathology overflows from the Source point of that Yin-Yang paired channel. The pathology would likely then move to the Luo point of that channel. When that Luo fills and empties (which could take any length of time), it moves back to the Source point of the original channel via the Source-Luo connection. Since that channel was weakened earlier, the pathology moves from there to the organ. (The pathology might stay in the Source of the second channel, however, and move further inward from *that* Source point.)

---

³ The Triple Heater mechanism originates at Ming Men and travels up the Hua To points adjacent to the spine, distributing Yuan Qi to each organ. If Triple Heater is affected by pathology, that pathology has ready access to the organs.

From the Source point, the pathology either moves into the internal branches of the Primary Channels which connect to the organs, or it moves into Triple Heater which connects to the Bladder Shu points and then to the organs. (The organs are represented in the drawings as the Mu points.) When the Transverse Luo overflows with pathology, the buffer between the pathogenic factor and the organ has been fully exhausted. Inflammatory conditions prevail because Heat has internalized. This becomes chronic inflammation, first of the membrane around the organ, and finally progressing to inflammation of the organ itself. Therefore any Zang Fu inflammatory condition will point you to the Transverse Luo. In Western terms, these conditions include infections of the organs: pleurisy, gastritis, colitis, enteritis, cholecystitis, cystitis, pancreatitis, hepatitis, pericarditis, pyelonephritis and myocarditis, and all organ Heat conditions. In terms of pulses, these conditions manifest as rapid pulses in the Yuan level. A patient might present with chronic infections that intermittently affect the organs. The disease at this point is terminal if untreated.

It is important to note that most likely, between the first and second segments of the Transverse Luos, the Divergent or Eight Extraordinary Channels intercept the pathology and move it into latency using their mechanisms. The pathology can also be shifted to the "terminations"[4] in an attempt to eradicate the pathology through the sensory orifices, the head, the chest, the abdomen and the Yang Jing-Well points of the feet. Even the zones can eradicate the pathogen; once Heat has reached the interior, the Yang Ming zone can make attempts to move the Heat out via Shao Yang and then Tai Yang. The body is always focussed on keeping pathology away from the organs and will exhaust all possible avenues to protect the internal organs.

The Transverse Luos can take several possible paths

The Transverse Luos extend from the Luo points to the Yin-Yang paired Source points and then terminate in the organs. They are not visible or palpable. They are repositories of the Longitudinal Luo Channels. The Ren and Du Luo Channels are sometimes referred to as Transverse Luo Channels because pathology is being held at the Yuan-Source level.

---

[4] The roots and terminations are beyond the scope of this book. SP-1 terminates at CV-12; LR-1 terminates at CV-18 and then CV-17; KI-1 terminates at CV-22 and CV-23, ST-45 terminates at ST-8; GB-44 terminates at GB-8; BL-67 terminates at BL-1.

The first segment of the Transverse Luos extends from the Luo point to the Source point of the Yin-Yang related pair.

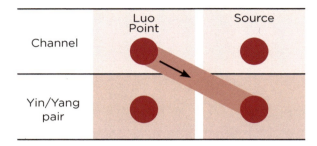

The second segment of the Transverse Luo can be any pathway from the Source point to the original organ.

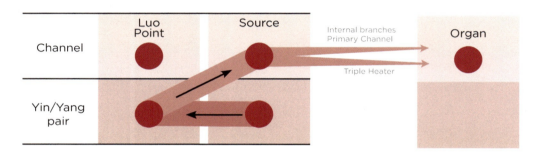

1. The second segment is often a loop from that paired Source point, to the Luo point on that paired channel and then back to the original Source point whereupon it moves:
   a. into the internal branches of the Primary Channels which connect to the organs, OR
   b. into Triple Heater which connects to the Bladder Shu points and then to the organs (represented in the drawings as the Mu points).

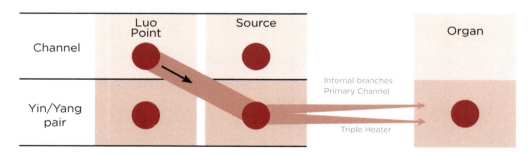

2. The pathology might move to a. or b. directly from the paired Source point in which case the signs and symptoms would be of the Transverse Luo of the Yin-Yang paired organ instead.

The Effect of Transverse Luo treatments

Transverse Luo treatments withdraw pathology from the Source level when signs and symptoms emerge indicating the Source is being challenged and pull it back to the Longitudinal Luo Channels. The treatments create space in the channel and generate Qi to enable the pathology to move. This is why the treatment principle is "to clear the Luos". After Transverse and empty Luo treatments, the pathology can move backwards into the Longitudinal Luos again. This is welcome.

Acute versus Chronic

The Transverse Luos can be used for any internal Heat pathology, acute or chronic. Luo pathology can develop very quickly or might take decades to evolve, depending on the status of Ying and Yuan Qi. The Transverse Luos can be used to clear pestilent pathology which has affected the organs directly and/or acutely. Hepatitis virus would be an example. The Transverse Luo can invite the pathology from the organ (the Source level) up to the Luo level which would be bled to release Heat from the organ. Point choices would be made according to the symptoms presented. Using Luo Channels to treat Heat affecting the organs requires Transverse Luos because the Longitudinal Luos do not reach the organs (with the exception of Heart and Pericardium).

The Luos and Psychology and Psychiatry

In any state of health, the dissemination of Yuan-Source Qi enables the organs to express their respective emotions. Since the Blood contains the emotions, once blood-borne pathology enters Yuan-Source level, the emotions expressed by that organ can become pathological, too. If this goes on in the long term, the pathology becomes part of the personality, and eventually, if not resolved, part of the constitution. This is why the Luo vessels are my first choice for psychological and psychiatric conditions, both acute and chronic.

Transverse Luo Signs and Symptoms

Symptoms include pain along the pathway of the Primary Channel, along both its internal and external pathways. Abdominal pain could be a symptom of the Transverse Luo of many of the organs. The Lung's internal pathway, for example, extends from CV-12 to ST-25 to CV-13 before going to LU-1. The Transverse Luos are not visible, because the pathology has gone to the interior.

Here is a chronological list of Transverse Luo symptoms which occurs if pathology is transmitted across the zones. If the Lung Source point fails, the pathology moves further inward. At that point, by definition, it affects *Yang Ming* which is the first level of the interior. Then, if unresolved outward through the Yang zones, it progresses inward to the organs. The following order is theoretical. Transmission order will change according to the unique weaknesses and strengths of the individual.

Transverse Luo Physical Signs and Symptoms, Theoretical Sequence Based on the Internal Pathways of the Primary Channels

Lung Transverse Luo: Chest fullness, cough, wheezing.

Stomach Transverse Luo: Fever with sweat, epigastric distention and burning, Phlegm, pain along the pathway, The Four Great Signs of Yang Ming: high fever, sweat, thirst, a flooding pulse; restlessness, irritability. Heat then rises above to affect the other Luo Channels:

Large Intestine Transverse Luo: Dry lips, mouth, damage to Fluids showing on tongue, dry throat.

Triple Heater Transverse Luo: Sweating, fever, pain along the pathway.

Small Intestine Transverse Luo: Ear issues, tinnitus, deafness, submaxillary swelling, long-term TMD, swollen salivary glands.

Gallbladder Transverse Luo: Sweating, fever, pain and achiness of the joints.

Bladder Transverse Luo: Eye symptoms, yellowing, glaucoma, watery eyes, eye discharge. Chronic inflammation, occipital headache, chronic neck pain, hemorrhoids, chronic bowel issues.

Spleen Transverse Luo: Heart pain, tongue pain, speech issues, stiffness of the body, diarrhea, chest oppression, depression.

Liver Transverse Luo: Nausea, vomiting, loss of appetite, diaphragmatic constriction, incontinence, anuria, chest pain, depression, an uneasiness with life, lack of desire to eat, lack of appetite, fatigue, loose stools, tightness in the sub-

	sternal area, Spleen Qi deficiency.
Pericardium Transverse Luo:	Heart pain, depression, hot palms, circulatory problems, cold limbs.
Kidney Transverse Luo:	Cold and numbness along the legs, neuropathy, diarrhea (cockcrow with undigested food), depression-introversion, lethargy, withdrawal, fainting easily, *Running Piglet Qi*, cold hands.
Heart Transverse Luo:	Yellow eyes, pain along the pathway, Shen disturbance, lost sparkle in the eyes, terminal illness.

The pathology can be arrested and turned around, and full healing can be achieved starting at any point along the progression. Transverse Luo treatments are particularly valuable because you are treating the internal branch of the Primary Channel and restoring strength to the Primary Channel by allocating the Yuan-Source Qi properly.

Treatment of Transverse Luos

To begin reversing the pathology, perform a Transverse Luo treatment when Transverse Luo signs and symptoms are evident. The patient must be exhibiting Transverse Luo signs for a treatment to be applicable, unless you want to promote a healing crisis, because a Transverse Luo treatment will move pathology which is latent, from the Yuan-Source level.

Transverse Luo Treatment Intention

The intention of a Transverse Luo treatment is to protect or tonify Yuan-Source Qi and to clear the Luo point by bleeding to pull the pathology away from the Yuan-Source level and back up into the Ying level (to the Luo point) where it is not imminently endangering the organs. If the origin of the pathology was the Source level, the Source point is reduced to free the pathology back to the Ying level for clearance by bleeding and moxaing the Yin-Yang paired Luo point.

Transverse Luo Diagnosis and Treatment

From the observation of signs and symptoms, determine which Transverse Luo is affected. The pulse will be rapid in the position of the organ affected at the Yuan level of the pulse. There may be some nodules remaining in the Primary Channel related to the affected organ from the time the body was trying to hold latency in the Primary Channel. When both Yin-Yang related channels are affected, determine the origin of the pathology and identify whether that channel is in excess or deficiency. If the channel of origin of pathology is in excess, reduce the Source of the channel of origin and tonify the Luo of the Yin-Yang related pair by bleeding and then moxaing. If the channel of origin is in a state of deficiency, tonify the Source of the channel of origin with moxa, and bleed the Luo point of the Yin-Yang related pair. This is an energy transfer treatment, allowing the return of the pathology to the channel of origin. Whatever treatment you do to the Luo (reduction by bleeding or tonification with moxa), you do the opposite to the Source.

In advanced cases, it's sometimes very difficult to determine the Luo Channel of the origin of pathology. If this happens, take the pulses of both members of the Yin-Yang pair, for example, the Lung and Large Intestine and determine which of the two is deficient. Moxa the Yuan-Source point of the channel of deficiency and bleed the Luo of the paired channel. Moxa LI-4, bleed LU-7 and harmonize Blood at LU-4. Or moxa LU-9, bleed LI-6 and harmonize Blood at LI-12. The treatments listed for each Transverse Luo are of this type.

Examples

A patient has a long history of gas and bloating. The patient presents with fever and sweating, epigastric distention and burning, and irritability. The Spleen pulse is weak. Tonify or moxa SP-3 and bleed ST-40.

A patient contracted a common cold and soon after developed a toothache. The Lung pulse is weak. This is a Source-Luo scenario of the Lung and Large Intestine. LU-9 was the origin (the Lungs failed to ward off the pathogen) and LI-6 would be the Luo (the Large Intestine Luo travels to the teeth). Tonify or moxa LU-9 and bleed LI-6.

A patient has an unresolved pathogenic factor and has developed body aches (Gallbladder) and a headache (Bladder). Moxa the Yuan-Source points of the Yin-Yang related pair: LR-3 and KI-3 and then bleed the Luo points on the affected channels, GB-37 and BL-58. Note that the Yuan-Source point is tonified because the Yuan-Source point of one or the other of the Yin-Yang pair must have failed for the progression to the interior to have taken place.

Transverse Luo Treatment Protocols

Moxa the Yuan-Source point of the channel of deficiency (Lung or Large Intestine). Bleed the Luo of the paired channel.

Lung Transverse Luo
Either moxa LI-4, bleed LU-7 and harmonize Blood at LU-4,
or moxa LU-9, bleed LI-6 and harmonize Blood at LI-12.

Large Intestine Transverse Luo
Either moxa LI-4, bleed LU-7 and harmonize Blood at LU-4,
or moxa LU-9, bleed LI-6 and harmonize Blood at LI-12.

Stomach Transverse Luo
Either moxa SP-3, bleed ST-40 and harmonize Blood at ST-35,
or moxa ST-42, bleed SP-4 and harmonize Blood at SP-10.

Spleen Transverse Luo
Either moxa ST-42, bleed SP-4 and harmonize Blood at SP-10,
or moxa SP-3, bleed ST-40 and harmonize Blood at ST-35.

Heart Transverse Luo
Either moxa SI-4, bleed HT-5 and harmonize Blood at HT-2,
or moxa HT-7, bleed SI-7 and harmonize Blood at SI-9.

Small Intestine Transverse Luo
Either moxa HT-7, bleed SI-7 and harmonize Blood at SI-10,
or moxa SI-4, bleed HT-5 and harmonize Blood at HT-2.

Bladder Transverse Luo
Either moxa KI-3, bleed BL-58 and harmonize Blood at BL-38,
or moxa BL-64, bleed KI-4 and harmonize Blood at KI-11.

Kidney Transverse Luo
Either moxa BL-64, bleed KI-4 and harmonize Blood at KI-11,
or moxa KI-3, bleed BL-58 and harmonize Blood at BL-38.

Pericardium Transverse Luo
Either moxa TH-4, bleed PC-6 and harmonize Blood at PC-2,
or moxa PC-7, bleed TH-5 and harmonize Blood at TH-11.

Triple Heater Transverse Luo
Either moxa PC-7, bleed TH-5 and harmonize Blood at TH-11,
or moxa TH-4, bleed PC-6 and harmonize Blood at PC-2.

Gallbladder Transverse Luo
Either moxa LR-3, bleed GB-37 and harmonize Blood at GB-33,
or moxa GB-40, bleed LR-5 and harmonize Blood at LR-9.

Liver Transverse Luo
Either moxa GB-40, bleed LR-5 and harmonize Blood at LR-9,
or moxa LR-3, bleed GB-37 and harmonize Blood at GB-33.

Permutations of the Progression of Luo Latency

- The pathology might not make the initial leap across to the Yin-Yang related channel but instead settle into the Source point of the first channel, especially if Yuan-Source Qi is weak.

- After going to the Source point of the Yin-Yang pair, it's possible that the pathology is pushed out partially to occupy the Luo point of that second channel, creating another Longitudinal Luo. For example, from the origin of SP-4 it moves into the Yin-Yang related pair at ST-42 and then into ST-40 on that same channel, creating fullness of that Luo. Then, after exhausting the Luo point of the Yin-Yang related pair, a Transverse Luo can be created from ST-42 to SP-3 which by now is greatly weakened.

- If there is not enough Blood to create a substantial Luo vessel, the Luo vessel might not fill, and the pathology might go to the Source point of the Yin-Yang related pair without ever filling the Luo vessel of the original channel.

- If the pathology arrives at a Yuan-Source point and saturates the point and the body cannot move the pathology it creates a Transverse Luo.

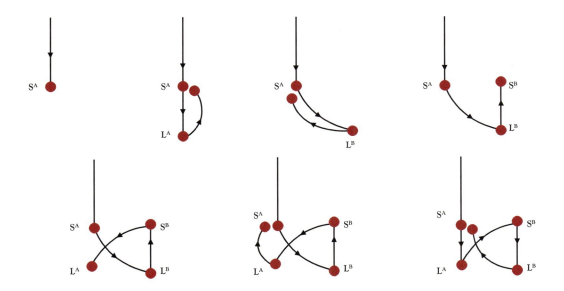

Some possible routes of Luo pathology to the Yuan-Source point.

Constitutional Acquisition of Pathology

When the pathology rests in a Source point, whether within a Transverse Luo scenario or not:

1. The pathology can drain into the Constitution because once it has entered the Yuan-Source level at the Yuan-Source point, it is in the terrain of the Eight Extraordinary Channels.

    a. It can drain into the Luos of Ren and Du. According to the *Ling Shu*, the Ren and Du Luos are the summation of all the Luo pathologies. The Ren and Du Channels communicate with the Chong. The Chong modifies the blueprint for the next incarnation and the next generation with the unresolved Luo pathology given it by the Ren and Du Luos. Hence, what we have not dealt with at the time we give our Jing to create conception is transmitted to the next generation. Likewise, what we do not deal with in this entire lifetime is again encountered in our next incarnation.

    b. It can drain into the Qiaos (according to the *Nan Jing, Chapter 26*). Pathology from the Yin Luos drains into Yin Qiao Mai and pathology from the Yang Luos drains into Yang Qiao Mai. The Qiao Channels control structure. This is why our emotional history is revealed in our posture and gait. (That could be the subject of a vast tome.)

2. When the pathology moves to the organ, the Divergent Channels may become active and move the pathology away from the organ to the joints in order to protect the organ.

Other Transverse Luo Applications

In the sections above, the discussion is about the Transverse Luos Channels being used for serious disease and for the release of Heat in an organ. In these treatments Luo points are bled. But Luo points can be used in their simple guise as connecting points that can be used to balance energy in two elementally related channels via the Luo to Source "gateway". In these cases, the Luo point is needled rather than bled because we are looking to tip the excess Qi from either of the related pairs into the one with deficiency. A simple example would be when the Stomach has fire and the Spleen has become deficient as a result. Needling SP-3 and ST-40 would function like balancing a scale, tipping the excess Qi into where it is needed.

Four different kinds of Transverse Luo treatments, each from a different tradition, are listed below in brief.

1. The Yin-Yang deficiency Transverse Luo treatment. A given deficiency is said to affect the Source of that channel and the Yin-Yang paired Luo counterpart. E.g., Deficient Heart Qi affects HT-7 and SI-7. Both are tonified.

2. The Energy Transfer Transverse Luo treatment. The cause of a Luo issue is observed to be an underlying deficiency. E.g., Stagnant Qi affecting the Liver with an underlying deficiency manifesting in the Spleen. Reduce LR-3, tonify GB-37 AND tonify SP-3 and Reduce ST-40. All needles.

3. The Narrative Model where chronology is important. The Source represents the Origin of the pathology and is reduced, and the Luo represents the Guest and is tonified. If both are excess, both are reduced. If both are deficient, both are tonified. In this model, the pairs do not have to be Yin-Yang related.

4. The Internal-External Connection: The Transverse Luo Model. If the pathology was allowed to enter the interior (via the Source), it means that the condition is in Yang Ming and internal Heat signs prevail. In this model the Luo is bled and the Source is tonified.

Narrative Model Examples

Example 1

A patient went out on Friday night, ate a "ton" of fried chicken and woke with intense pain on the right side of the abdomen and a thick yellow coat on the tongue. The fried food overworked the Gallbladder, requiring it to produce a lot of bile, so we would call Gallbladder the origin. Reduce GB-40, and tonify LR-5.

Example 2

A patient was in a fight with her boss and was very angry. She was so angry that she went out and ate too much fried chicken. She woke up the next morning with intense pain on the right side of the abdomen and a thick yellow coat on the tongue. Liver would be the origin, because the emotion of anger precipitated the illness. Reduce LR-3 and tonify GB-37.

Other Uses of the Luo Channels

The following treatments are simple but just as profoundly effective as a seemingly complicated Luo treatment.

"When there is counterflow Qi, examine the Luo Channels and bleed them."
—Chapter 21, *Ling Shu*

You might choose to treat the Luos if you see these rebellious Qi signs. Simply bleed the Luo point of the channel, any visible Luo vessels, and regulate the Blood.

LU-7	frequent yawning, frequent urination
LI-6	frequent bowel movements, flatulence, gas
SP-4	intestinal pain, bloating
ST-40	nausea, vomiting
HT-5	palpitations, tachycardia, arrhythmia
SI-7	cardiac reflux
BL-58	lack of urination
KI-4	wheezing
PC-6	palpitations
TH-5	alternating hot and cold
GB-37	alternating above and below, e.g., nausea above, diarrhea below, Sudden Turmoil Disorder
LR-5	dizziness, headaches

The Simple Three Level Emotional Luo Model

These are the simplest form of emotional Luo treatments because they don't encompass the concept of fullness or emptiness. They are nonetheless quite potent. In this model, ascertain whether the emotion to be treated is merely a mood (gan), an emotion (qing), or a product of the temperament, a constitutionally-derived emotion (xing).

A mood is seen as the result of the energy in the environment having penetrated the Wei level, leading to a feeling that is stuck in the Wei level (the level of Qi that senses the environment). The patient might be aware of the mood, but will not attribute a definite reason to it. Moods are acute and have no target. E.g., "I just feel angry; I can't explain why." Even if the patient is aware of the mood, he or she feels no control over it.

An emotion is seen as a feeling that has penetrated the Blood which enables that emotion to be explained or expressed. Emotions, in this sense, have a target. E.g., "I feel angry at my boss."

The temperament, or constitutional personality, is seen as a product of the way in which Yuan-Source Qi was distributed in the individual via the Triple Heater mechanism at birth. Because the temperament is an innate part of the patient, these feelings are often denied by the patient because he or she has no purchase on the perception of those emotions. The temperament also includes inborn tendencies and alterations made to the temperament through experiences during the first cycle of seven and eight.

The emotions being treated are pathological, obsessive, unresolved emotions the patient is trying to keep latent. These emotions may be latent and yet visible, that is, obvious to the practitioner. They may be deeply latent or repressed, causing the patient to act on patterns of grief or anger, for example, without acknowledging it to themselves.

An emotion becomes pathological if it is not experienced and let go, if it remains with the patient and controls or motivates them. It may be nurtured or harbored by the patient or, conversely, it may be suppressed in an attempt to avoid unpleasant issues.

The Levels of the Pathological Emotions

A pathological **mood** is a vague feeling that haunts us without reason.

A pathological **emotion** is one which can be expressed by the patient yet lingers and is undesired. The patient suppresses the emotion.

A pathological **constitutionally-derived** emotion is a repressed feeling the patient often denies having but is observed in the patient by the practitioner. It can also be a feeling the patient determines could possibly be there but is unable to interpret or raise to the level of conscious expression.

On all levels we are treating pathological emotions which are preventing the fullest expression of life in the patient. In these treatments, we are not trying to change the temperament, but to free the patient to be who they truly are.

Moods occur on the Wei level
Emotions occur on the Ying level
Temperament-derived emotions occur on the Yuan level

The **Wei level** is controlled by the Lungs which control the quantity of Wei being distributed to the exterior and by the Liver which is in charge of the smooth flow or the quality of Wei Qi.

The **Ying level** is controlled by the Spleen which holds Blood in its banks and the Heart which circulates Blood.

The **Yuan level** is controlled by the Kidneys which store Yuan-Source Qi and by Triple Heater which is responsible for its distribution.

Diagnosis in the Simple Three Level Emotional Luo Model

1. Choose the level at which the emotion resides.

Wei level	Mood
Ying level	Emotion (patient acknowledges and expresses the emotion)
Yuan level	Constitutional emotion (patient is unaware of or denies the presence of the emotion)

2. Label the prevailing emotion in a basic sense:
    Sadness
    Pensiveness
    Anxiety, over-excitement
    Fear
    Anger

Protocol for the Simple Three Level Emotional Luo Model

1. Bleed the two Luo points related to the level of your diagnosis on the side opposite the pulse:

Wei level	LU-7 and LR-5	Mood
Ying level	SP-4 and PC-6	Emotion
Yuan level	KI-4 and TH-5	Constitutional emotion/Temperament

2. Bleed one of the five Yang Luo points in the list below on the side opposite the pulse. E.g., LI-6 is bled on the left side, SI-7 on the right:

LI-6	Sadness
ST-40	Pensiveness
SI-7	Anxiety, over-excitement
BL-58	Fear
GB-37	Anger

3. Tonify the Source point of the related Yin pair. E.g., if you bled LI-6, tonify LU-9 with moxa or by lifting and thrusting.

Musculoskeletal Luo or Injury Luo Treatment

The musculoskeletal Luo protocol treats injury where there is bruising and Bi-Obstruction (pain caused by Qi and Blood stagnation in the sinews). The treatment brings Blood to nourish the sinews.

WARNING: Cold packs and ice packs force Wei Qi into the bones. This develops into what is known in Western terms as arthritis or even rheumatism as the body tries to move the Wei back to the surface and break up the Cold by generating heat in the bone. The body creates swelling to bring Qi and Blood to the area in order to heal it, and to immobilize the area so that it cannot be used. Swelling is an essential part of healing. To ice the swelling of an injury is to declare the body's natural response incorrect. The response is correct. The use of cold packs will greatly impede the efficacy of treatment.

Etiologies

1. Traumatic or non-traumatic injury. The injury allowed climatic factors to enter the injury site. Injury is due to an underlying Wei Qi deficiency. The injury responds to a climatic factor.
2. Emotional origin. The injury is unexplained. The patient cannot recall being injured.

The injury does not respond to a climatic factor. Qi and Blood stagnation is usually due to internal Pathogenic Factors. When the patient cannot remember being injured, the injury is said to be of emotional origin. This is also known as emotional armoring; the body holds and freezes emotions. If muscular pain is not affected by temperature changes (application of heat or cold) the injury has an emotional origin.

Principles of Diagnosis	Techniques of Treatment
Wind moves.	Needle and remove immediately.
Cold Manifests as sharp pain.	Moxa.
Damp manifests as heaviness.	Needle and moxa.

Musculoskeletal Luo Treatment Protocol

Day A:

1. Plum blossom the Luo of the injured Sinew with a scooping action (the hand will make circles perpendicular to the skin) towards the site of the injury, and then moxa it.
2. Needle to tonify Blood at the point proximal to the He-Sea point.
3. Do a movement assessment using the diagnostic protocols in the Sinew chapter. You might end up with a diagnosis of the channel that is exhibiting the injury, but the diagnosis could end up being that of any Sinew Channel.
4. Perform a full Sinew treatment of that Sinew Channel. That will include the Confluent point, the ah shi points along the channel and the Jing-Well point of that Sinew.
5. Moxa the Jing-Well of that Sinew to restore Wei Qi.

Note: There is no treatment on the even numbered days to allow the body to assimilate the treatment.

Day B:

6. Two days later, plum blossom the Luo of the injured Sinew away from the site of injury to move Blood.
7. Needle with even technique, the point one point proximal to the He-Sea point. This will bring fresh Blood in to replace the stagnated Blood.
8. If the injury persists, alternate the treatment for days one and three until it is relieved. Treatment could go on for 21 days if necessary. Day A's would be done on days 1, 5, 9, 13, 17, 21. Day B's would be done on days 3, 7, 11, 15, 19.

Example:
The patient was injured in a car accident and has a large hematoma near GB-34.

Day A:

1. Plum blossom GB-37 towards GB-34. Moxa GB-37.
2. Tonify GB-33.
3. Do a movement assessment. The patient reports that walking is the most difficult action. Therefore the Bladder Sinew is affected.
4. Needle SI-18, the ah shi points on the entire Bladder Sinew Channel. Needle and withdraw BL-67.
5. Moxa BL-67 to restore Wei Qi.

Day B:

6. Two days later, plum blossom GB-37 away from GB-34.
7. Needle GB-33 with even technique.
8. If the injury persists, alternate Days A and B until it is relieved. Treatment is performed every second day.

Frequently Asked Luo Questions and Troubleshooting

1. *Can't I simply needle the Luo point?* If the Luo point is not bled, a Luo Channel treatment has not been performed. It is essential to bleed the Luo point. There need only be a tiny amount of Blood visible at the Luo point after withdrawing the lancet. It doesn't have to release whole drops. Needling the Luo point will not treat emotional or Blood-engaged pathology because the pathology is held in the Blood.

2. *I can't get any Blood to come out!* Sometimes in an empty Luo treatment, and occasionally in a full Luo treatment, the Blood will not come to the surface when the Luo point is lanced. Cup or gua sha the point and try again. If it still won't come out, stimulate SP-10. If it still won't come out, the patient is either extremely Blood deficient or not yet ready for a major emotional shift.

3. *Can a Luo be half emptied?* Yes, a Luo can be emptied and full at the same time. Treat using the emptied Luo protocol.

4. *The Blood that's coming out is thick, sticky and looks almost black. What should I do?* Let the point bleed until the color changes and red Blood shows, this could be 3 to 5 drops.

5. **Help! I bled a Luo and the Blood isn't coming out but is pooling under the skin.** Immediately apply strong pressure to the area. Hold the pressure firmly for a few minutes. When you release it, the hematoma will be flat and the skin will be bruised. Apply a small amount of 2% dilution of myrrh[5] to the area and regulate the Blood one point proximal to the He-Sea point. This occurs when the patient has insufficient Lung Qi to move Blood to the surface, or if the patient is not yet ready to release the pathology.

6. **Sometimes I bleed a Luo and nothing happens but after a while I return to the point and it's running. Why?** This is a sign of Qi stagnation, probably of the Lungs.

7. **I bled the Luo point and instead of a drop coming out, it sprayed. What does this mean?** It means that there was tremendous pressure in the vessel. The treatment may have averted a heart attack.

8. **Sometimes on the table my patients say that they feel Blood is gushing out of the Luo point long after it is bled and even if the Luo point only yielded a tiny dot of Blood. Is this normal?** This happens quite often. It's the feeling of the Qi moving out after the movement of Blood. Qi follows Blood and Blood follows Qi.

9. **What would happen if I didn't harmonize Blood after a Luo treatment?** If the harmonizing point is omitted, the patient might not be able to make sense of the emotions that are being released. There might also be bruising.

10. **ST-35 is the harmonizing point for the Stomach Luo but I feel it has a different quality to the other regulators. Why?** ST-35 is the only regulating point distal to the major joint.

11. **Why is BL-38 the harmonizing point for the Bladder Luo and not BL-39?** BL-39 is the lower He-Sea point for Triple Heater. Also, it's not proximal to BL-40.

12. **Why is the Great Luo of the Spleen three cun below the axilla and not six?** The *Ling Shu* places the Great Luo of the Spleen "three inches below the axilla". The *Nan Jing* places the Great Luo of the Spleen three inches below GB-22, making the point SP-21. The *Nan Jing* and the *Ling Shu* do not agree with each other. Three inches below

---

[5] Make a preparation of 1 drop of myrrh in 50 drops of sweet almond oil.

the axilla is a key point for the Divergent Channels whose job it is to keep pathology away from the Source if the Luos have failed. In the Luo treatments described in this chapter, the Great Luo of the Spleen is understood to be three cun below the axilla.

13. **Why is the Great Luo of the Spleen after the Ren and the Du in the order of the Luos?** Because the Great Luo controls all the Luos. If you found multiple Luos were affected, you might choose to treat using the Great Luo.

14. **What point do I bleed to treat the Great Luo of the Stomach?** Great Luo of the Stomach is treated with the Eight Extra Channels.

15. **I did a Luo treatment and now the Liver pulse is very thin at the moderate level. What should I do?** Nourish Blood if there is a Blood deficiency showing in the pulses after the treatment. For example: LR-3, LR-8, LR-13, BL-17, -18, -20, etc. The Blood Mansion will build Blood (SP-21, HT-1, LR-13).

16. **My patient is extremely Blood deficient. Can I do any Luo treatments at all?** Yes, you can perform Luo treatments in cases of Blood deficiency, even a severe deficiency, but regulation of the Blood is absolutely essential. Taking the pulses after the treatment is also essential to see whether more Blood building treatment is required. Luo treatments help tremendously in cases of Blood deficiency because to stimulate the manufacture of Blood, Blood must move.

17. **Can Luo treatments treat Blood deficiency?** Yes, a Luo treatment can alleviate a Blood deficiency because to build Blood you must move it.

18. **My patient is taking Blood thinners. Can I do a Luo treatment?** If performing a Luo treatment on a patient taking a Blood thinning drug, bleed one point at a time, apply pressure to that point or Luo vessel, and wait until you are certain that the point has stopped bleeding before proceeding. Treat very few points. The treatment will help relieve the pathology which is being suppressed by the drugs.

19. **Do I always have to build Blood after a Luo treatment?** No. But if patient is pregnant, elderly, Yin deficient, menopausal, menstruating, dizzy or faint, Blood must be both regulated and built after the Luo treatment, not just regulated.

20. *My patient is pregnant. Can I perform a Luo treatment?* Yes, if strongly indicated. Do not bleed the Middle or Lower Jiaos.

21. *Is a varicose vein a kind of Luo vessel?* Yes. The term "Luo vessel" applies to discolorations, spider veins, visible veins and varicose veins of any description—yes, even the big, thick, ropey, knotted ones!

22. *My patient has so many Luo vessels all over the place that my diagnosis is fullness of all the Luo vessels that travel on the legs. Should I bleed all of them?* You can, but you might consider bleeding the Qiaos. Bleed the points belonging to the Qiao trajectory because when all the Luos become saturated they spill into the Qiaos. Yin Luos empty to Yin Qiao and Yang Luos to Yang Qiao. This is a grand version of the Luos emptying to the Source. Bleeding the Qiaos will take pressure off the Luos. In later treatments you could go back to the Luos and bleed them.

23. *My patient has dozens of spider veins along the channel. How many of them should I bleed?* You can bleed as many as you think is appropriate as long as you stop the flow of Blood after the color has changed (usually one to three drops) and regulate the Blood.

24. *When the pathology reaches the organs, what does it do to them?* Initially, the pathogen affects the organs by causing inflammation of the membranes surrounding them (the gao huang) so you'll see organ inflammation or infection, or lots of Heat signs. As the pathology progresses beyond the membrane, the organ degenerates.

25. *My Pericardium empty Luo treatment didn't work. Why?* The chest is not open. Do a Sinew treatment of the Lung Sinew Channel to enable the Lung to carry the pathology to the exterior.

26. *Is there a limit to the number of Luo Channels I can treat in one session?* No, as long as you can justify a diagnosis through signs and symptoms or through visibility.

27. *If I use a Luo point outside the context of the Luo Channels, must it be bled?* No.

28. **My patient is feeling overwhelmed by the emotions being released. What should I do?** Needle the first trajectory of the Chong vessel, or GB-42, to ground the patient.

29. **When diagnosing an empty Luo, should I take into account cysts, nodules or tumors on the organs?** No, you're interested in masses on the palpable Primary Channel.

30. **Are nodules and swellings Luo vessels?** No, in the context of the Luo Channels, these are a response to the failure of the Longitudinal Luos.

31. **When I palpate the channel I feel many tiny grainy nodules along sections of the channel. Can these constitute the nodules of an emptied Luo condition?** Yes.

32. **I can palpate some nodules along the Primary Channel, but my patient doesn't recall there ever being spider veins in that area. Does that mean that these are not indicative of an empty Luo condition?** Luo vessels are formed in the moderate level of the flesh and then float upward. If there's insufficient Qi to raise them to a state of visibility, they can fill at a level beneath the surface and then progress to being empty without becoming visible. This is uncommon, however.

33. **Are there unilateral bleeding recommendations pertaining to gender in Luo Channel theory?** No.

34. **If I see organ Heat signs, how do I know that I must diagnose a Transverse Luo issue?** Internal Heat affecting the organs can be treated using Eight Extra or Divergent Channels, also. Any condition can be treated using various Complement Channels. Organ Heat signs would lead you to diagnosing Transverse Luos if you had corroborating information to indicate such a treatment.

35. **Some of the signs and symptoms listed for the Transverse Luos seem as though they could belong to other channels. Are the symptoms listed unique to the Transverse Luos?** No, there is no sign or symptom that uniquely belongs to a category of Complement Channel. The choice of which channel to use is made after the various diagnostic data has been collected.

The Divergent Channels

DIVERGENT CHANNEL TREATMENTS

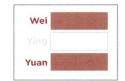

A Discussion of Chapter 11 of the *Ling Shu* and Chapter 63 of the *Su Wen*

Historical References to the Divergent Channels

Chapter 11 of the *Ling Shu* introduces the Divergent Channels in written form and describes all their pathways. Chapter 1 of Scroll 2 of the *Jia Yi Jing* also discusses the Divergent Channels (sometimes translated as Separate or Distinct Channels). In both the *Ling Shu* and the *Jia Yi Jing*, the Divergent Channels are described as branches of the Primary Channels. Chapter 63 of the *Ling Shu* does not specifically use the word "Divergent" but says the Channels mobilize pathogenic factors away from the Zang Fu (viscera) to the joints so that disease cannot manifest in the Zang Fu.

The *Ling Shu* says, in dialogue form, that one should:

"Study the Divergents first and work it out to the finish. The inexperienced clinician will think they are easy to understand, while the superior one knows their difficulty. The skilled pass right by them while they are the very breath of the superior physician. Please listen to these words." —*Ling Shu*, **Chapter 11**

Long before the *Ling Shu* was written down, the superior physicians had begun an oral tradition that includes extensive teachings on the Divergent Channels, their theory and their clinical applications. The material that follows constitutes a detailed introduction to the enormously complex study of the Divergent Channels, which could easily comprise several volumes. It is my hope that this may serve your cultivation as a practitioner and the health of your patients.

Description of the Divergent Channels

Divergent channels can successfully be used to treat a wide variety of chronic degenerative diseases. It is a natural response of the body to create a slow-progressing disease or milder chronic disease in order to prevent a more serious one. We know this as Disease Nemesis Theory. Divergent Channels are key players in this process. The Divergent Channels exist only in the presence of pathology. In the absence of pathology, there is no call for them.

The function of the Divergent Channels (also translated as "Distinct" or "Separate" Channels) is to divert the pathogen away from the Zang Fu organs, where it could be fatal, and send it to the joints (the deepest layer of the external anatomy) to be held latent (hidden). Therefore, Divergent Channels communicate between the Wei and Yuan levels, the Wei level being the level at which the pathogen entered and the Yuan level being the level at which the body contains the pathogen and keeps it quiet. The pathogenic factor remains in latency until the body seeks to clear it, or until latency is lost.

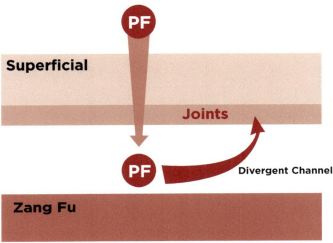

Case Study: A 46 year-old woman who described herself as "overworked and sleep-deprived" came to the clinic complaining of severe joint pain especially in the left hip, left elbow and left thumb. She reported gradually worsening digestive issues including reflux and gastritis. She said she'd been developing arthritis for years. Upon questioning she reported that about ten years earlier she was in bed for days with what she called a "Stomach flu," during which time she was vomiting and defecating greenish fluids. The pulses showed a marked thin quality in the moderate level of the guan position on both sides. None of her pulses were floating; her tongue was dry with a midline crack. The diagnosis was "deficient Stomach Fluids, and Wei Qi trapped in the joints leading to Bi-Obstruction." The etiology most likely was as follows: the viral infection which affected the Stomach was intercepted at that organ by the Divergent Channel and moved to the major articulations, the hips and shoulders. The patient recovered from the Stomach flu, but did not completely rid the pathogen. For ten years afterward, the body was able to keep the pathogen in latency in the major joints, while the patient's resources gradually became depleted due to lifestyle choices (overwork and lack of sleep.) At that point the Divergent Channel could no longer hold, allowing the pathogen to come out of latency and return to the organs from which it was diverted, causing her gastric problems. The treatment strategy was to build resources and return the pathogen to latency until the body had enough resources to finally be able to eradicate it. (In this case, the ST/SP confluence was used DSD.) The patient was treated three days in a row, rested and ate hearty soups, and although she was tired, she was without the described signs and symptoms on the fourth day. This meant the pathogen had been directed back to the joints. On the fourth day she developed low back pain and a sinus infection, indicating the pathogen had moved into the first confluence. BL/KI Divergents completed the eradication of the pathogen. Outcome: The patient has no arthritis or gastric issues.

A pathogenic factor is defined as a challenge to the body's defense. It can be a climatic factor (Wind, Cold, Damp), a dietary factor, an ecological factor (pollution, virus, bacteria, fungus, parasite), a toxin (e.g., asbestos, heavy metals) or an emotion.

Once the Divergent Channels have diverted the pathogenic factor (PF) to the joints, the maintenance of latency is entirely dependent on Jing-Essence to hold it there. As Jing-Essence becomes overly taxed, the body calls upon other Fluids and resources to assist the Jing-Essence in the following order: Blood, Jin-Thin (exocrine) Fluids, Ye-Thick (endocrine) Fluids, Qi and Yang. The art of using the Divergent Channels begins with the assessment of the depletion of these resources, the identification of the location of the pathogen, and the careful building of resources to either maintain latency or empower the body's eradication of the pathogenic factor.

The Divergents are referred to in the classics as Sun Luo, Grandchildren Luos, because they are two steps away from the Sinews. When pathology enters the Wei level and is not handled by the Sinews, the next level of the body that attempts to deal with it is the level of the Luo Channels. If the Luo Channels do not contain the pathogen, it can progress via the transverse Luos to the Source level (the Yuan level). Therefore the Yuan level latency is two generations of pathological encounters away from the Wei level where the pathogen entered. We could also think in terms of there having been two transitions (two generations, so to speak) of the pathogen after it encounters the Luos, one from Luo to Yuan, and another from Yuan to the joints. However, there are times when a pathogenic factor is diverted directly from the Wei level to the Yuan level, without engaging the Luo level at all. This scenario would occur in situations of Blood and fluid deficiency; in other words, the body does not have the Blood or fluid resources to finance latency in the Ying level.

Another way to think about the creation of the Divergent Channels is that the Primary Channels failed to deal with the pathogenic factor. Classically, the Primary Channels are thought of as waterways. Their Yang function, upon encountering a pathogenic factor, is to create a sweat to expel it. If a Divergent Channel is created, it means the Primary Channels were overwhelmed and unable to create a sweat to expel a pathogen.

For example: if the (Tai Yang) Bladder Channel fails to expel a pathogen with sweat, the pathogenic factor—if unchallenged at the Luo point—will travel along the channel and enter the He-Sea point (BL-40). Here the pathogen has access to Yuan-Source Qi so the body employs its strategy of putting the pathogen into latency. This is to keep the pathogen from progressing further along the channel and reaching the organs. And we find that BL-40 is the first point of the Divergent Channel continuum.

Another way a Divergent Channel moves a pathogen into latency is to make use of its zonal pair. Zonal Divergents connect zonally related Divergent pairs. For example, the Tai Yang Divergents, Bladder and Small Intestine connect to each other. Zonal treatments involve the cutaneous regions, which are areas of the surface anatomy that connect the paired zones. The cutaneous regions (pictured) are released (by gua sha) because the pathogen used them to cross into the zonally paired Divergent Channel, causing a musculoskeletal condition to worsen. For example, a patient with a tight sacrum (Leg Tai Yang) might report that suddenly the shoulder has the same kind of pain. This is an example of a pathogen being transferred to the paired zone (Arm Tai Yang).

The Six Divergent Confluences

There are twelve Divergent Channels arranged in six pairs or confluences, so named because the two member channels of each confluent pair have four important points in common (the confluent or meeting points). The order of these pairs is that of disease progression. When reversed, the order is that of disease resolution.

1st confluence:	Bladder and Kidney Divergent Channels
2nd confluence	Gallbladder and Liver Divergent Channels
3rd confluence:	Stomach and Spleen Divergent Channels
4th confluence:	Small Intestine and Heart Divergent Channels
5th confluence:	Triple Heater and Pericardium Divergent Channels
6th confluence:	Large Intestine and Lung Divergent Channels

Divergent Channel Needling Technique and Intention

Divergent treatments require the practitioner to choose how to direct the body in its management of the pathogenic factor, that is, to direct the body to eradicate the pathogen or to find latency for the pathogen. Once this choice is made, the Wei Qi and Yuan Qi are directed to support the intention of eradication of the pathogen, or the intention to re-establish latency of the pathogen. Divergent treatments involve engaging Wei Qi either at the Wei level or at the Yuan level and dragging it to the polar opposite level and back again. This needling technique is called "deep-superficial-deep" (DSD) or "superficial-deep-superficial" (SDS).

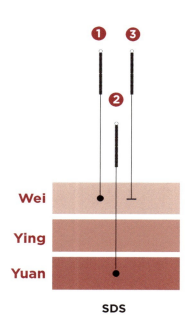

SDS

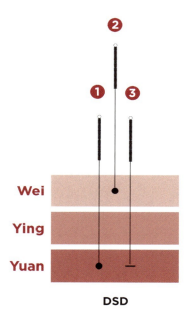

DSD

In SDS treatments, the **Wei Qi** level is stimulated to open the surface, then the needle is inserted deeply to engage **Wei Qi** which is trapped in the Yuan level with the pathogen. Then the needle is brought back to the surface where the **Wei Qi** level is engaged again so that the trapped **Wei Qi** and the pathogen are ready for release. SDS treatments are for the release of a pathogen trapped by **Wei Qi**.

In DSD treatments, the Yuan level is stimulated to make it receptive, then the needle is brought up to the surface where **Wei Qi** is engaged, then the needle is returned to the Yuan level where **Wei Qi** returns to its origin of Yang Qi. DSD treatments are consolidating: Yang is returned to the interior to hold a pathogen in latency. You're going up to the Wei level, lassoing the PF and escorting it to the Yuan level. Because DSD treatments also build the mediumship, the PF is "bricked in" at the Yuan level.

If needled DSD, the aim is to move the pathology to the densest, most Yin region of the body, the joints. DSD Divergent treatments accomplish this by increasing the mediumship at that confluence (that level or pair of Divergent Channels) in order to support Jing-Essence. This will enable the body to prolong latency of the pathology. DSD also gives the pathogenic factor the message to stay at the deep level (in latency). The joints affected in Divergent pathology are principally the major articulations: the hips and shoulders. As pathology progresses, more joints become involved.

To Perform the Deep-Superficial-Deep technique
a. Insert the needle deeply into the point (relative to the specific point).
b. Lift and thrust with very small movements within that deep (Yuan) level. If preferred, vibrating technique can be used in the Yuan level.
c. Drag the needle up to the Wei level and lift and thrust within that level. If preferred, circular technique can be used in the Wei level.
d. Push the needle back down and lift and thrust again within the Yuan level. If preferred, vibrating technique can be used in the Yuan level.

If needling SDS, the aim is to move the pathogenic factor from the Yuan level back to the exterior in order to be expelled.

To Perform the Superficial-Deep-Superficial technique
a. Insert the needle into the Wei level with a tube. That means it's tapped into the point the depth the tube allows and not inserted further. (BL-1 and GB-1 are always inserted freehand with a half inch needle. For these points, the Wei level is relative to the depth of the point: very shallow.)
b. Lift and thrust within the Wei level to engage Qi. This means the tip of the needle is moving up and down with very small movements. If preferred, circular technique can be used in the Wei level.
c. Push the needle in deeply, relative to the point and lift and thrust at the Yuan level to engage the Qi. If preferred, vibrating technique can be used in the Yuan level.
d. While the Qi is engaged, drag the needle back up to the Wei level and lift and thrust at the Wei level. Leave the needle inserted. It should be so shallow that it's almost dangling. If preferred, circular technique can be used in the Wei level.

If the vibrating and circular techniques are used, in SDS treatments the actions are fast. In DSD treatments, the actions are slow. Qi must be engaged at each level. If you lose the Qi on the way up or down, go back to the point where you lost the Qi, lift and thrust to re-engage the Qi and continue with the larger movement of the needle. The clinician's focus is essential in maintaining the engagement of Qi throughout the work with each needle.

In the simplest scenario you might choose to do all the trajectory points you have selected in an SDS treatment with SDS technique, and all the points you have selected in a DSD treatment with DSD technique. But as you get more experienced at the Divergents it's likely you'll want to do some points in either kind of treatment with the opposite technique to the one you used on the Confluent points, depending on your intention for that individual point. You might even decide to do a given point simply superficial or simply deep.

Indications of the Divergent Channels

The Divergent Channels are indicated for chronic, intermittent, one-sided signs and symptoms, and signs and symptoms that alternate sides.

CLINICAL APPLICATION OF DIVERGENTS

The Divergent Channel Toolkit

1. *The Confluent Points*[1]

(also known as "meeting points") function as transporting points. As such, their function is to move Wei Qi. Each pair of Divergent Channels shares a set of four Confluent points. When needled as a group they signal to the body that a Divergent treatment is underway. They also indicate the confluence. The Confluent points must be needled in any and all Divergent treatments, elemental or zonal. They are always needled with SDS or DSD technique. A rare exception could arise if a Confluent point is obscured by an obstruction, e.g., if a goiter is located at LI-18, use the remaining three Confluent points.

Divergent Confluent Points and their Classical Names

BL/KI	BL-10 *Tian Zhu*, Celestial Pillar	BL-40 *Wei Zhong*, Center of Bend
GB/LR	GB-1 *Tong Zi Liao*, Virgin Child's Bone Hole	CV-2 *Qu Gu*, Curved Bone

---

[1] The functions of the Divergent Confluent points are discussed in appendix II, page 366.

ST/SP	BL-1 *Jing Ming*, Eye's Clarity	ST-30	*Qi Chong*, Qi Thoroughfare
SI/HT	BL-1 *Jing Ming*, Eye's Clarity	GB-22	*Yuan Ye*, Armpit Abyss
TH/PC	SJ-16 *Tian You*, Celestial Orbit	CV-12	*Zhong Wan*, Central Vessel
LI/LU	LI-18 *Fu Tu*, Support the Chimney	ST-12	*Que Pen*, Broken Dish[2]

Note: Divergent Channel points are common to the Primary Channels. When speaking of Divergent Channels by point number, the Primary Channel numbers are used, but it would be equally valid to number the points for the Divergent Channels specifically. For example, BL-40 could be called Bladder Divergent point number 1, BLDC-1.

2. The Crossing Point

A single acupuncture point on the midline, used in SDS treatments only. They encourage the Wei Qi to cross to the side of the body that has the Jing-Well point. They are not on the trajectory. The crossing point is inserted superficially with no manipulation, pointed to the side of the body that has the Jing-Well. The most common crossing point chosen is GV-20.

3. Opening Points

Used to differentiate between the two Divergents in each confluence. In the cases of the Bladder and Stomach Divergent Channels, the Opening points are the same as the lower confluence.

Opening Points:			
BL DC	BL-40	KI DC	KI-10
GB DC	GB-30	LR DC	LR-5
ST DC	ST-30	SP DC	SP-12
SI DC	SI-10	HT DC	HT-1
TH DC	GV-20	PC DC	GB-22
LI DC	LI-15	LU DC	LU-1

4. Trajectory Points

are points on the Divergent Channel that are neither confluent nor Opening points. They enhance and fine-tune the intention of a Divergent treatment. It's usually unnecessary to use all the trajectory points in a Divergent treatment. In fact it is quite inadvisable to needle all the trajectory points, except in cases where the trajectory points are few, e.g., Heart Divergent Channel. Choose which points are appropriate from the trajectory by correlating point function with the patient's signs and symptoms. Choose points which elucidate the broad intention of the treatment.

---

[2] ST-12 is called "Broken Dish" because by the sixth confluence, mediumship is exhausted.

The effectiveness of a treatment is greater when fewer needles are used. The trajectory points can be inserted unilaterally according to the pulse or the organ. For example the Spleen and Stomach points could be needled on the right, Liver points on the left. To needle more than a few trajectory points, or more than is necessary, gives too many messages for a treatment to be fully potent.

5. Local Points (ah shi)

can certainly be added to Divergent treatments. Gua sha the painful area before needling, insert all the Divergent needles, then palpate the ah shi again. Very often the pain will not be present because it has already shifted down the channel and there is no reason to treat the former ah shi further. If the ah shi are still present, needle them in Divergent fashion. If an SDS treatment, the ah shi needle has no retention. If a DSD treatment, the needle remains in deep.

6. Jing-Well Points

are not on the trajectory of the Divergent Channels but they are added in an SDS treatment to activate the related Sinew Channel in order to provide a delineated exit route for the pathogen once it has been freed for release. Failure to needle the Jing-Well point in an SDS Divergent Channel treatment may result in an uncomfortable and apparent worsening of the condition because the pathogen is raised to the Wei level. There it can be felt more strongly, but without an exit offered, it may back up in the channel, resulting in discomfort or pain.

7. The Cutaneous Regions

These regions can be gua sha'd in any Divergent treatment whether elemental or zonal (explained later) and whether SDS or DSD. Gua sha on the cutaneous regions frees Wei Qi so that it can be directed inward (for DSD treatments) or outward (for SDS treatments).

8. Points that Can be Added to a Divergent Treatment

Yuan level points can be added to a Divergent treatment. These include:
    a. Bladder and Kidney Shu points
    b. Yuan-Source points (often used to protect the organ if there's concern about the pathogen beginning to affect the organ)
    c. He-Sea points
    d. Influential points
    e. Mu points
    f. Xi-Cleft points (these are not Yuan level, but they can be used in cases of Qi and mediumship leakage, or lost latency)

Unblocking Wei Energetics

Ensuring the Routes of Elimination are Open

It's important to check with a patient about their elimination patterns. If they are constipated or have pebbly stools, Wei Qi is not moving well in the bowels and so if the body were to choose that route, the pathogen would not be evacuated. Adding ST-25 to any Divergent treatment when the bowels are compromised is very important.

Ensuring Scars are Freed

Even if a scar is very fine, it can be blocking the flow of Wei Qi. Scar treatments are important in preparation for Divergent treatments. They can be done on the same day. See my "Advanced Acupuncture Scar Treatment" video on the web and see the Scar Treatment section on page 18.

Clinical Notes

Divergent Treatment Duration

DSD: 40 minutes from the time the meeting points were all inserted.

SDS: 20 minutes from the time the Jing-Well was inserted. If much De Qi was elicited during the needling, the needles can be withdrawn after the last needle is inserted.

The treatment can also be said to be complete when the pulses reveal that the change you are looking for has occurred, whether it be SDS or DSD.

Divergent Course Duration

Divergent treatments generally require a frequency and rhythm unusual by today's standard. Treat for 18 days: Three cycles of three days on and three days off. That is: 3 days of treatment, 3 days off, 3 days of treatment, 3 days off, 3 days of treatment, 3 days off, then evaluate. If more treatment is needed, keep going by performing another cycle of treatment.[3] Any Wei level treatment must be consistent in order for the Wei Qi to learn its new instruction. If the patient can only come once a week, get them to massage the Confluent points. (In the old days, the patient would moxa the Confluent points to keep the treatment going.)

If the three days on and off schedule is not followed, it cannot be said that Divergent Channel protocols are being fully performed. Practically speaking, strictly fol-

---

[3] These treatments might end up being quite different to those of the previous course.

lowing the three days on and off protocol is often not feasible. If weekly treatments are the most frequent possible, rely on cultivation and strong intention to fill the gap. If the treatments are less frequent than classically prescribed, they can also be reinforced by the patient using specific essential oils on the Confluent points. See the Essential Oils section at the end of this chapter, on page 212.

Clarity of Treatment

The most important aspect of any acupuncture treatment is clarity of treatment principle. Some say that any point on the channels of confluences adjacent to that being treated can be added if it is a point that aligns powerfully with the treatment principle. It is also possible to treat more than one Divergent Channel at the same time (not described in this book). However, these variations are best explored after fluency is gained with the Divergents in their theoretically individual form. That way the unique personality of each Divergent Channel is experienced by the practitioner.

BASIC TREATMENT PRINCIPLES

What is happening when the Divergent Channels are needled DSD or SDS?

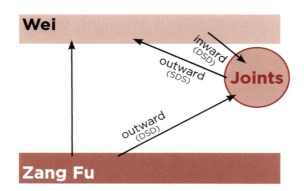

Whether needling the Divergent Channels SDS or DSD, the pathogen is moved away from the organs.

The First Confluence

When BL/KI Divergent Channels are needled DSD, the pathogen is being brought TO the joints, either inward to the joints from the Wei level, or outward to the joints from the Bladder or the Kidney organ. At the joints, the pathogen will be held latent in the medium of Jing-Essence.

When BL/KI Divergent Channels are needled SDS, the pathogen is being brought TO the Wei level, either outward FROM the joints or outward FROM the Bladder or the

Kidney organ. At the Wei level the pathogen is then expelled from the body via the Bladder and/or Kidney Sinew Channels which are activated by the Jing-Well point.

The Second Confluence

When GB/LR Divergent Channels are needled DSD, the pathogen is being brought TO the joints, either inwards to the joints from the Wei level, or outward to the joints from the Gallbladder or the Liver organ. At the joints, the pathogen will be held latent in the Jing-Essence with the assistance of the Blood. Blood is supporting the function of the Jing-Essence here.

When GB/LR Divergent Channels are needled SDS, the pathogen is being brought TO the Wei level either outward FROM the joints or outward FROM the Gallbladder or the Liver organ, using the medium of Blood for its conveyance. At the Wei level the pathogen is then expelled via Gallbladder and/or Liver Sinew Channels which are activated by the Jing-Well point.

Note: The second confluence connects to the eyes and ears.

The Third Confluence

When ST/SP Divergent Channels are needled DSD, the pathogen is being brought TO the joints, either inwards to the joints from the Wei level or outward to the joints from the Stomach or the Spleen organ. At the joints, the pathogen will be held latent in the Jing-Essence with the assistance of the Jin-Thin Fluids. Jin-Thin Fluids are supporting the function of Jing-Essence here.

When ST/SP Divergent Channels are needled SDS, the pathogen is being brought TO the Wei level, either outward FROM the joints, or outward FROM the Stomach or the Spleen organ, using the medium of Jin-Thin Fluids for its conveyance. At the Wei level the pathogen is then expelled via the Stomach and/or Spleen Sinew Channels which are activated by the Jing-Well point.

Note: The third confluence connects to all the sensory orifices.

The Fourth Confluence

When HT/SI Divergent Channels are needled DSD, the pathogen is being brought TO the joints, either inward to the joints from the Wei level or outward to the joints from the Heart or the Small Intestine organ. At the joints, the pathogen will be held latent in the Jing-Essence with the assistance of the Ye-Thick Fluids. Ye-Thick Fluids are supporting the function of Jing-Essence here.

When HT/SI Divergent Channels are needled SDS, the pathogen is being brought TO the Wei level, either outward FROM the joints or outward FROM the Heart or the Small Intestine organ, using the medium of Ye-Thick Fluids for its conveyance. At the Wei level the pathogen is then expelled via the Heart and/or Small Intestine Sinew Channels which are activated by the Jing-Well point.

From this point onward, all Fluids (Blood, Thin Fluids and Thick Fluids) have been used up and the release of the pathogen is not possible because there is no mediumship for conveyance. The fifth and sixth confluences therefore, are generally used for the attainment of latency at the expense of Qi (5th) and Yang (6th).

The Fifth Confluence

When TH/PC Divergent Channels are needled DSD, the pathogen is being brought TO the joints, either inward to the joints from the Wei level or outward to the joints from the Triple Heater or the Pericardium organ. At the joints, the pathogen will be held latent in the Jing-Essence with the assistance of Qi. Qi is supporting the function of Jing-Essence here.

When TH/PC Divergent Channels are needled SDS, it is for Wind that has entered the Triple Heater or Pericardium Sinew Channels and is affecting those Sinew Channels chronically, unilaterally and intermittently. This treatment would also be applicable when bringing out an acute infection of the Pericardium if there were sufficient Fluids to enable that to happen.

The Sixth Confluence

When LU/LI Divergent Channels are needled DSD, the pathogen is being brought TO the joints, either inward to the joints from the Wei level or outward to the joints from the Lung or the Large Intestine organ. At the joints the pathogen will be held latent in the Jing-Essence with the assistance of Yang. Yang Qi is supporting the function of Jing-Essence here.

When LU/LI Divergent Channels are needled SDS, it is for Wind that has entered the Lung or Large Intestine Sinew Channels and is affecting those Sinew Channels chronically, unilaterally and intermittently. This treatment would also be applicable in bringing out an acute infection of the Lungs or the Large Intestine if there were sufficient Fluids to enable that to happen.

Preparation for Diagnosis

Views of the Divergent Confluent Sequence

There are many different ways to view the six confluences of the Divergent Channels and a number of ways for practitioners to orient themselves when using Divergents.

1. The Mobilization of Mediumship

BL/KI	GB/LR	ST/SP	HT/SI	TH/PC	LU/LI
Jing	Blood	Thin Fluids (Jin)	Thick Fluids (Ye)	Qi	Yang

Divergents can be viewed as a progression of the mobilization of mediumship to contain a pathogenic factor in the Yuan level. This mobilization results in a gradual depletion of Fluids. In this view, there is mild disease at the first level (Bladder and Kidney) and severe disease at the sixth level (Large Intestine and Lung). When used in this way, the practitioner's intention is to build mediumship in order to contain the pathogen or to build mediumship to allow the movement of the pathogenic factor to the exterior for expulsion.

This view of the Divergents can be seen as an opportunity to back out the pathogen. The release of the pathogen can be brought out with SDS or DSD treatments; SDS because the pathogen is being instructed to go to the Wei level for release; DSD because inherent in a DSD treatment is an instruction to the body to gather mediumship for the conveyance (or latency) of the pathogen. The practitioner chooses the level at which the pathogen is present and treats that level either DSD or SDS depending on the status of Fluids (determined by pulse assessment), until the pathogen moves to an earlier confluence. The diagnosis is then changed as the pulses and signs and symptoms change, and the newly indicated confluence is needled until the pathogen backs up into an even earlier confluence. Near the conclusion of the treatment there is often a release of the pathogen which looks like the beginning of the disease (healing event). These symptoms, which often resemble a common cold with copious Phlegm, clear after a few days and the disease is resolved.

2. Non-Sequential Model.

Each confluence can also be viewed on its own without reference to a progression. This is a common point of view in the context of musculoskeletal conditions, for treatment of chronic conditions where the choice of treatment is determined by the pathway of the channel, and for acute organ infections.

3. Constitutional Predisposition.

The non-sequential framework can also be used when the patient consistently presents with the symptoms of one confluence, perhaps due to a constitutional issue.

4. Metaphorical Time-Clock

The Divergents can also be seen as a metaphorical time-clock. Briefly, the chaos/water from which life sprouts (BL/KI) gives birth (GB/LR) to form (ST/SP) which in time decays (HT/SI) as we are consumed by our desires (TH/PC). These desires are in conflict with the world (LI/LU). The Divergent Channels reflect the capacity of ourselves (Yuan Qi) to accept the world as it is (Wei Qi). This relates not only to the idea of disease progression, which is the process by which the body slowly sacrifices its resources in order to keep the pathogen away from the viscera, but also to the primary cause of all illness: a failure to accept the world in which we live as it is.

Diagnosis

Divergent Pulse Diagnosis

The thorough study of classical pulse taking would require a few volumes on its own and is beyond the scope of this book. (Traditionally, classical pulse taking is learned at the teacher's side.) However, this book would not be complete without at least an introduction to the Divergent pulses and how to take them.

Both Eight Extra and Divergent Channels are reflected in Fu Mai - Hidden Pulses. The difference is that the Eight Extra have a hidden vibrating quality, and the Divergents often have a floating element discernible alongside their hidden quality. Hidden does not mean difficult to find—it means you must occlude the flow of Blood through the radial artery to get it to emerge. In brief: apply pressure to the bone to occlude the flow of Blood in the radial artery (15 "Mung beans" of pressure). Release very slightly (14 "Mung beans" of pressure). Notice which pulse is pushing against the finger. Return to the bone (15 beans) and notice whether that pulse you felt at 14 beans is still there at 15 beans. If it's NOT there–it's a Divergent pulse. That means the

Divergent Channel of that position does have the ability to hold latency. In other words, your manipulation of the pulse stimulated a reading on the presence of the pathology in the Yuan level but when you pressed it back, it went back into latency.

Pulse Positions of the Divergents

Left Cun:	SI/ HT	Right Cun:	LI/LU
Left Guan:	GB/LR	Right Guan:	ST/SP
Left Chi:	BL/KI	Right Chi:	TH/PC

> **WARNING: Choose SDS or DSD based on the presence of mediumship at the Divergent confluence you have diagnosed. Choosing SDS when the patient has insufficient mediumship at that confluence is dangerous and can cause autointoxication as the pathogen is mobilized within the body while the body does not have the mediumship or Qi to expel it. Do not use Divergent Channels SDS if the pulses are thin or choppy. If in doubt use DSD and build mediumship for latency which will finance the expulsion via SDS at a later date. DSD will also secure the exterior.**
>
> **Note: The body might try to evacuate the pathogen on its own without the assistance of an SDS treatment. That is to say, if you treat DSD and the body acquires or musters sufficient resources, the pathogen may be evacuated.**

Choose which Divergent to use according to the following criteria. Not all need be met, but ideally all are considered:

1. *The status of resources*

The width of the pulse at the moderate level indicates the status of resources. In Divergent pulse diagnosis, the width of the pulse is more important than the strength of the pulse because Divergent Channels are dependent on Fluids. When finding a wide pulse at the moderate level in either the Kidney, Liver, Spleen or Heart, we know that the respective Divergent Channel is likely capable of dealing with the pathogen. If all the mediumship appears lost in the pulses, choose the fifth or sixth confluence.

Choosing the confluence based on resources available (for SDS or DSD)

    i. E.g., if all the Fluids are present, use the 1st confluence.

    ii. If there is an abundance of Blood, use the 2nd confluence.

    iii. If there is a good complement of Thin Fluids, and a deficiency of Blood, use the 3rd confluence.

    iv. If there is a good complement of Thick Fluids, and a deficiency of Thin Fluids and Blood, use the 4th confluence.

2. Superficial tight pulses

If the pulse in a given position is pushing up against your finger and is tight at superficial level of the pulse, this is considered evidence of an attempt by the body to push the pathology to the sinews. An SDS treatment of that confluence would be applicable.

3. The strength of an organ at a particular level

E.g., A patient is Blood deficient but Spleen is strong. Use Spleen Divergent Channel to shore up Liver Divergent Channel for use later.

4. The dearth of the mediumship at a given level resulting in the inability to maintain latency

E.g., A patient is very fluid deficient and the Spleen is weak. Use HT/SI Divergent Channel to build the previous Divergent level in the sequence (ST/SP) before going to the SP/ST Divergent Channels.

E.g., There is Blood deficiency. Use GB/LR with Source points added to consolidate Blood. Alternatively, use ST/SP DSD to support the Fluids to take pressure off the GB/Liver confluence by providing more mediumship for the production of Blood.

Try not to use confluences whose pulses are weak or thin. If you do decide to go ahead, use them DSD with Source points added.

If the pulses are floating and rapid in all positions there is insufficient Yin to use the first four confluences. Use Triple Heater and Pericardium Divergent.

5. The location of chronic, one sided, intermittent issues

E.g., A patient has chronic, intermittent pain at LI-15. Use Large Intestine Divergent Channel.

6. The progression of the condition

The order of the Divergent Channels illustrates the spectrum of humors and Qi, from Jing to Yang. (The signs and symptoms that would confirm the choice are listed with each confluence in detail later.)

- When Jing-Essence is over-taxed by having to chronically contain a pathogenic factor, BL/KI Divergent signs and symptoms occur, as the pathogen starts to escape.
- When Blood is over-mobilized and depleted, GB/LR Divergent signs and symptoms occur, as Blood is insufficient to support Jing-Essence in maintaining latency.
- When Thin Fluids are over-mobilized and depleted, ST/SP Divergent signs and symptoms occur, as Thin Fluids fail to finance Blood to support Jing-Essence to maintain latency.
- When Thick Fluids are over-mobilized and depleted, SI/HT Divergent signs and symptoms occur, as Thick Fluids are insufficient to support Thin Fluids to support

Blood to support Jing-Essence to maintain latency.
- When Qi is mobilized to try to hold Yin in place, TH/PC Divergent signs and symptoms occur.
- At the end of the Divergent Channel sequence, when Yang is mobilized in an effort to suppress the pathogen, LI/LU Divergent signs and symptoms occur.

7. Signs and symptoms

The appearance of signs and symptoms related to a given Divergent confluence indicates that the confluence is failing to maintain latency of the pathogen. They also signify that a particular confluence may have insufficient mediumship to be able to follow a request to support latency of the pathogen.

Signs and symptoms for each of the 12 single Divergent Channels can be categorized as:

a. Trajectory signs

These are signs that emerge along the pathway.

b. Wei Qi signs

These are signs that emerge due to the excess or deficiency of Wei Qi. Often they are heat signs because Wei Qi is a subset of Yang Qi. Often they involve inflammation because when Wei Qi is trapped, heat accumulates.

c. Mediumship mobilization signs in the Yang of the pair

These are signs that emerge as mediumship is called upon to move location to enable the pathogen to go into latency. As the medium (usually substance) is moved, deposits (lumps, masses) occur.

d. Mediumship depletion signs in the Yin of the pair

These are signs that emerge as a medium (Jing, Blood, Thin Fluids, Thick Fluids, Qi or Yang) is commandeered to enable the pathogen to go into latency. This leaves the body unable to perform functions requiring that medium. Also, the body may display heat signs as the medium—which was balancing the heat—is depleted. As the medium is depleted, the body attempts to accumulate pathological Yin which results in lumps, abscesses and swellings.

Notes: The category in which signs and symptoms (S&S) appear does not determine whether to needle SDS or DSD (this decision is based on the presence of mediumship at the confluence, as mentioned above). The S&S are listed here to identify which confluence might be chosen. The patient need not exhibit all or even many S&S to justify a diagnosis in that confluence. The number of S&S increases as the disease progresses in that confluence.

Divergent Channel Signs and Symptoms Listed in the Su Wen, Chapter 63

The superficial-deep-superficial and deep-superficial-deep needling technique is introduced in the first (the Bladder) Divergent description with the use of the term "three times."*

In the treatments explained below, we can see from the use of the Jing-Well points that the Sinew Channel is being used as a pathway for the exit of the pathology from the Divergent Channels.

BL DC: Neck and shoulder pain. Needle BL-67. If no result, needle BL-63 on the opposite side. For sudden spasm of the back and radiating pain from the back to the ribs, needle the Hua To points along the trajectory *three times.

KI DC: Heart pain, abdominal distention, diaphragmatic fullness. Bleed KI-2. For throat pain with difficulty in swallowing, anger for no reason and Running Piglet Qi, needle KI-1. Bleed KI-2 if the throat is swollen.

GB DC: Labored breathing, cough with spontaneous sweat, chest or rib pain. Needle GB-44 and withdraw needle when breathing improves or sweating stops. For hip pain with difficulty flexing the thigh, use a long needle at GB-30.

LR DC: Sudden pain in the genitals, e.g., hernia, conglomerations (fibroids and cysts). Needle LR-1.

ST DC: Sneezing, nasal discharge, nosebleed, coldness of the upper teeth. Needle ST-45. If no improvement, add ST-44.

SP DC: Low back pain, drum-like distention of the abdomen, labored breathing when looking upward (throat Bi).

SI DC: Lower abdominal pain that radiates to the lumbar region or genitalia, constipation (dry stools) and diarrhea.

HT DC: Chest and rib pain, palpitations, difficulty breathing especially when lying down, disturbed sleep, dizziness.

TH DC: Throat pain with soreness and constriction, dry mouth, restlessness, irritability, retracted (short) tongue, difficulty lifting head or arms. Needle TH-1. If no relief, needle TH-2 on the opposite side.

PC DC: Pain in the wrist (Carpal Tunnel Syndrome), hot palms. Needle around PC-1 and ah shi on the thenar eminence. Later versions of the *Su Wen* include chest fullness and oppression, palpitations, restlessness, delirium, stuttering and constant laughter.

LI DC: Chest and flank fullness, heat sensations on the chest, dyspnea, intermittent or long-term deafness. Needle LI-1 on the opposite side for deafness. If no improvement, add PC-9.

LU DC: Chest fullness and oppression, cough, wheeze, rapid breathing, restlessness, coughing of blood and phlegm, heat in the palms.

Note: Heart, Small Intestine, Lung and some Large Intestine Divergent signs and symptoms were not given in the original version of the *Su Wen*.

Key Phrases for the Divergent Channels

Remembering key phrases can help guide you in the selection of the appropriate Divergent Channel:

BL DC: "Finding latency for the pathogenic factor in the Yuan level of the exterior—the bone and joints—and revealing the pathogenic factor due to the decline in Jing-Essence."

KI DC: "Yang activity transformed from Yin. Kidney Divergent Channel is a buffer zone for Dai Mai (keeping the pathogenic factor from the Source)."

GB DC: "Moving Qi to put the pathogenic factor into latency. You need Blood to carry the Qi." If the Essence is used up, Blood is used to hold the pathogenic factor at the Mu points where Essence is stored. (That is what's meant by "Blood supports the Essence.") Gallbladder Divergent Channel, using Qi, makes this movement of Blood to the Mu points happen.

LR DC: "Uses Blood to support Essence." Liver Divergent Channel is generally needled DSD to build Blood. Gallbladder Divergent Channel moves while Liver Divergent Channel is a quiet, deep Blood builder.

ST DC: "Thin (exocrine) Fluids move to support Blood."

SP DC: "Wind stirs due to the depletion of Thin Fluids."

SI DC: "Thick Fluids (endocrine) are mobilized to support Thin Fluids and Wei Qi is internalized to the chest."

HT DC: "Loss of Thick Fluids results in loss of latency. Yang is unable to anchor to low back and Wei atrophy begins."

TH DC: "Loss of latency is complete. Qi is being lost."

PC DC: "Severe loss of Fluids and Blood."

LI DC: "End stage. Yang is nearly lost."

LU DC: "Brings Wei Qi to join the Primary Channels and the Zang Fu. The pathology enters the Zang Fu at the beginning of the Primary Channel sequence at LU-1."

> *Diagnostic Styles*
>
> Some Divergent practitioners choose the channels they will treat by focusing on the pulses and consider the signs and symptoms secondarily. Others are interested in the signs and symptoms primarily and then the pulses. Some practitioners will not treat the confluence pertaining to the signs and symptoms but choose another confluence to shore up resources. Others will only treat the confluence pertaining to the signs and symptoms. Some practitioners will only treat SDS and add Source and He-Sea points to support the resources that will facilitate the outward movement of the pathology. Others are very cautious about making that demand on the body until they're sure the resources are there, and treat DSD. The Divergent Channels are a vast study and there is a wide spectrum of subtle variations in their use. As you practice the Divergents you develop a style unique to you. There are no absolutes here as is the case throughout the practice of Chinese Medicine.

Single Divergent versus Complete Confluence (two Divergents).

It is not necessary to use both of the confluences in the pair chosen. The Yin and Yang Divergents of each pair do have a different feel about them, however. The Yang Channel of the pair provides the movement needed to move the pathogen and the Yin Channel of the pair provides the mediumship to hold the pathogen latent. The choice of whether or not to use both is a clinical decision of the practitioner.

Advanced Treatment Principles

After considering the broad treatment principles discussed above, more finely-tuned treatment principles can be applied.

While most often the treatment principle is adequately covered by the points in the Divergent Channel you have chosen, it is possible to choose points from adjacent confluences in order to enhance your intentions. A list of such point selections is below. In superscript you will see the name of the confluence of which the point is a member. Use the applicable point only if it belongs to the confluence that you are using or to an adjacent confluence. For example, if you are using Stomach Divergent, you can add points from Gallbladder and Liver and also from Heart and Small Intestine Divergent Channels. I do not often use these additional points in my practice because I prefer treatments to be very focused and simple.

I have left some points without superscript because:
- They are on implied parts of the trajectory and are not actual designated points on the trajectory;
- They are on the trajectory based on tradition; or
- They can be used based on the broader principle that, because Divergent Channels address the Wei and Yuan levels, it is okay to add Yuan level points to Divergent treatments.

Examining the list below can also help to deepen understanding of the mechanism of the Divergent Channels.

1. ***Soothe the sinews (Shu Jin):***
   BL-40 *Wei Zhong*$^{BL/KI}$, BL-36 *Cheng Fu*$^{BL/KI}$, BL-10 *Tian Shu*$^{BL/KI}$, GB-25 *Jing Men*$^{GB/LR}$, GB-22 *Yuan Ye*$^{SI/PC/LU}$, SI-10 *Nao Shu*^{SI}. Ancestral Sinew: ST-30 *Qi Chong*$^{ST/SP}$.

2. ***Secure the root (Gu Ben):***
   a. Secure the Essence (*Gu Jing*): CV-4 *Quan Yuan*$^{BL/KI}$, CV-3 *Zhong Ji*$^{BL/KI/GB/TH}$, GV-4 *Ming Men*$^{BL/KI}$, BL-28 *Pang Gang Shu*$^{BL/KI}$, BL-23 *Shen Shu*$^{BL/KI}$.
   b. Warm the Yang (*Wen Yang*): CV-2 *Qu Gu*$^{GB/LR/TH}$, GB-25 *Jing Men*$^{GB/LR}$.
   c. Strengthen the Yang (*Jian Yang*): GV-4 *Ming Men*$^{BL/KI}$, GV-14 *Da Zhui*^{LI}.
   d. Supplement the Spleen and Harmonize the Stomach (*Bu Pi He Wei*): KI-16 *Huang Shu*^{KI}, CV-12 *Zhong Wan*$^{ST/SP}$, ST-42 *Chong Yang*.

3. *Disinhibit the portals (Li Qiao):*
   a. Disinhibit the Lower Jiao: BL-36 *Cheng Fu*^(BL/KI), GV-1 *Po Men*^(BL/KI), CV-3 *Zhong Qi*^(BL/KI), BL-34 *Xia Liao*^(BL/KI), KI-10 *Yin Gu*^(KI), SP-15 *Heng Gu*^(KI).
   b. Disinhibit the Upper Jiao: BL-1 *Jing Ming*^(ST/SP, SI/HT), GB-1 *Tong Zi Liao*^(GB/LR).
      i. Brain: GB-13 *Wan Gu*
      ii. Head: BL-10 *Tian Shu*^(BL/KI)

4. *Regulate Qi (and Blood) (Tiao Qi):*
   ST-12 *Que Pen*^(GB/LR, LI/LU), ST-9 *Ren Ying*^(ST/SP), ST-30 *Qi Chong*^(ST/SP).
   a. Blood: LR-13 *Zhang Men*^(GB/LR), SI-10 *Nao Shu*^(SI)
   b. Regulate Qi: BL-15 *Xin Shu*^(BL), BL-17 *Ge Shu*
   c. Rectify Qi: BL-32 *Ci Liao*^(BL/KI), PC-1 *Tian Chi*^(GB/LR/PC), LR-13 *Zhang Men*^(GB/LR), LR-5 *Li Gou*^(LR), HT-1 *Ji Quan*^(SI/HT/LI), CV-14 *Ju Que*^(GB/LR, ST/SP)
   d. Normalize: GB-22 *Yuan Ye*^(SI/PC/LU)
   e. Course Qi: GB-24 *Rue Yue*^(GB/LR), LR-13 *Zhang Men*^(GB/LR), LU-1 *Zhong Fu*^(LI/LU)
   f. Relieve pain: BL-10 *Tian Shu*^(BL/KI), BL-32 *Ci Liao*^(BL/KI), GV-1 *Po Men*^(BL/KI), KI-16 *Huang Shu*^(KI), SI-18 *Quan Liao*^(SI), TH-16 *Tian You*^(TH/PC)
   g. Unbind the chest: GB-22 *Yuan Ye*^(SI/PC/LU), BL-15 *Xin Shu*^(BL/KI), PC-1 *Tian Chi*^(GB/LR/PC), HT-1 *Ji Quan*^(SI/HT/LI), CV-17 *Tan Zhong*^(BL, ST/SP, SI/HT, TH/PC).
      i. Unbind knotting/clumping: SI-10 *Nao Shu*^(SI)
   h. Diffuse Lung Qi: ST-12 *Que Pen*^(GB/LR, SI, TH/PC, LI/LU), PC-1 *Tian Chi*^(GB/LR, PC), CV-22 *Tian Tu*^(GB/LR, ST/SP, HT), LU-1 *Zhong Fu*^(LU)

5. *Clear Heat, Resolve Damp (Qing Re Jie Shi):*
   a. Wind-Damp: BL-40 *Wei Zhong*^(BL/KI), GB-30 *Huan Tiao*^(GB)
   b. Wind-Cold: BL-10 *Tian Shu*^(BL/KI)
   c. Expel Damp: KI-10 *Yin Gu*^(KI), TH-16 *Tian You*^(TH/PC)
   d. Disperse Water: SP-15 *Heng Gu*^(KI)
      i. Disperse Swelling: TH-16 *Tian You*^(TH/PC)
   e. Disinhibit Damp: GB-26 *Dai Mai*^(KI), CV-12 *Zhong Wan*^(ST/SP, TH/PC)
   f. Transform Damp: ST-25 *Tian Shu*^(KI), CV-14 *Ju Que*^(GB/LR, ST/SP), ST-42 *Chong Yang*
   g. Phlegm:
      i. Expel with CV-23 *Lian Quan*^(ST/SP), CV-17 *Tan Zhong*^(BL, ST/SP, SI/HT, TH/PC), CV-22 *Tian Tu*^(ST/SP)
      ii. Transform with LR-14 *Qi Men*^(GB/LR), LI-15 *Jian Yu*^(LI)
      iii. Disperse with CV-14 *Ju Que*^(ST/SP)
   h. Clear Heat: LI-20 *Ying Xiang*^(ST/SP), ST-9 *Ren Ying*^(ST/SP), CV-23 *Lian Quan*^(ST/SP),

GV-14 *Da Zhui*, LI-15 *Jian Yu*, CV-14 *Ju Que*$^{ST/SP}$, CV-17 *Tan Zhong*$^{BL/KI, ST/SP, SI/HT, TH/PC}$, BL-1 *Jing Ming*$^{ST/SP, SI/HT}$, LU-1 *Zhong Fu*^{LU}.

    i. Blood Heat: BL-40 *Wei Zhong*$^{BL/KI}$

    ii. Damp-Heat: Transform with GB-24 *Rue Yue*$^{GB/LR}$, Disinhibit with LR-5 *Li Gou*^{LR}

i. Wind:

    i. Course with ST-5 *Da Ying*$^{GB/LR}$, BL-1 *Jing Ming*$^{ST/SP, SI/HT}$

    ii. Expel with ST-4 *Di Cang*$^{ST/SP}$, TH-16 *Tian You*$^{TH/PC}$

    iii. Dissipate with GV-1 *Po Men*$^{BL/KI}$, GB-12 *Wan Gu*$^{TH/PC}$, LI-20 *Ying Xiang*$^{ST/SP}$

    iv. Extinguish with GV-20 *Bai Hui*TH

Note: Give the patient plain flat, room temperature water to drink prior to treatment. Divergent treatments are about the use of Fluids in pathology. Hydrating before treatment gives a message to the body that Fluids are and will be available for transformation. Advise the patient to hydrate well, especially first thing in the morning before food.

Deep-Superficial-Deep Divergent Treatment Protocol

Deep-Superficial-Deep Order of Insertion

1. Confluent
2. Opening
3. Trajectory points

1. Needle the Confluent points (Meeting points) usually from top to bottom depending on the confluence (each is spelled out in this manual) using no crossing point.
2. Needle the Opening Point either bilaterally (in the order of the sides needled in the loop if using looping) or unilaterally on the side of the first needle inserted.
3. Needle selected, appropriate Trajectory points.

Note: It's important not to needle the Jing-Well point in a DSD treatment because the aim of the treatment is to return the pathogen to latency and to build mediumship, not to release a pathogen.
Note: If there is tightness in the neck or upper back, it's very important to gua sha these areas before beginning needling, to allow Wei Qi to be free in order to be directed.

Order of Withdrawal of Needles in DSD Treatments

1. Yuan level points that were added to the standard protocol, if any.
2. Trajectory points
3. Opening point
4. Upper Confluent/Meeting points, lower Confluent/Meeting points

Superficial-Deep-Superficial Divergent Treatment Protocol

The Divergent Loop

The most important points in Divergent Channel treatments are the Confluent points. These four points (two points needled bilaterally) combined with the technique used to needle them signal the body that a Divergent treatment is being performed. This prepares the body to move Wei Qi. In an SDS treatment, especially in musculoskeletal conditions, these points are needled in a loop, meaning the lower confluent is needled on one side and then the upper point is needled on that same side, followed by the upper Confluent point and then the lower Confluent point on the opposite side. (In a DSD treatment the loop is not applicable.) In DSD treatments insert the two upper Confluent points first and the lower ones second.

When using SDS and looping to address a musculoskeletal condition, what is the direction of the loop? Decide which side to begin needling in an SDS treatment based on the origin of the injury. The basic rule of thumb is that the Jing-Well is needled on the side the injury originated.

Scenario 1: If the injury began on the left but pain is manifesting on the right, begin the loop on the right and put the Jing-Well on the left. The theory is that the body used up its capacity for latency on the left—the left-side "filled up"—and the injury "overflowed" to the right. Loop the injury back out to the left where it entered. For example, the patient reports right knee pain but does not remember it being injured. Upon questioning he reports that twenty years earlier he badly injured his left knee. This tells us the injury began on the left, went into latency, migrated to the right, exhausted the latency available for the right knee and then became apparent. In this case, you would begin the loop on the right and use the Jing-Well point on the left, the side of origin.

Scenario 2: If the injury is on the right and there is no history of it manifesting on the left, start the loop on the left and needle the Jing-Well point on the right. (The theory is that the right side has not yet "filled up" so the right side should still be strong enough to push it out.)

Scenario 3: If the injury is very long-term (chronic) and intermittent and is manifesting on one side, it probably did originate on the other side (the currently painless side) even if the patient has no memory of how it began. All the latency capacity of the left side was used up and the pathology then overflowed to the right side (the currently painful side) and used up the latency capacity of the right side, where it finally became apparent. If this is your assessment, begin the loop on the side of the pain, the right side in this scenario, and needle the Jing-Well point on the opposite side of the pain, the left side. In all cases, your intention is to facilitate the injury exiting on the side that it originally entered.

In SDS treatments the Confluent point needles do not have to be inserted at an angle to point along the pathway of the trajectory, although they can. Pointing GB-1 to delineate the trajectory is only a good idea if the needle is particularly superficial. Pointing GB-22 inferiorly or superiorly is only possible in people with plenty of padding, otherwise, it should be needled very obliquely in line with the ribs. BL-1, of course, should not be needled with directionality. Of course, intention must always be strongly in place so that the Qi does follow the trajectory.

Jing-Well Point Function and the Loop

Jing-Well points are not part of the trajectory of the Divergent Channels. In an SDS Divergent treatment the function of the Jing-Well point is to activate the Sinew Channel so that the pathology has a ready exit at the level of the exterior. (Jing-Well points are not used in DSD treatments unless a healing crisis emerges.)

Superficial-Deep-Superficial Order of Insertion

1. Gua sha cutaneous region or tight areas
2. Confluent (Meeting points)
3. Opening point
4. Trajectory points
5. Jing-Well

1. If treating a musculoskeletal condition or dermatological condition, gua sha or sliding cup the cutaneous region shown in the drawing or any areas of binding or tightness. If

not treating a musculoskeletal or dermatological condition, begin at step 2.

2. Needle the Confluent points in a loop using a crossing point on the midline. Either:

    Lower left, upper left, crossing point, upper right, lower right, or

    Lower right, upper right, crossing point, upper left, lower left.

    The crossing point is any appropriate point on Ren or Du. GV-20 works well. The function of the crossing point is to allow the pathology to shift to the other side of the body where there is more strength to push the pathogen all the way out of the body in an SDS treatment. The crossing point is not part of the trajectory but is used in all SDS treatments.

Note: Some practitioners when doing SDS needle both lower confluences followed by both upper confluences. I find this to be less powerful because the pathway for the pathogen does not feel strong and obvious.

3. Needle the Opening point either bilaterally (in the order of the sides needled in the loop if using looping), or unilaterally on the side of the first needle inserted.

Note: In Bladder and Stomach Divergents, the Opening point is the same as the lower Confluent point.

4. Needle selected, appropriate Trajectory points following the order of the trajectory. Begin with the most distal point on the side the first-inserted Confluent point, work up that side and then cross over and work downwards on the opposite side.

5. Needle the Jing-Well point on the same side as the last inserted Confluent point.

> In my practice I often add the Jing-Well point after the last Confluent point because often the Wei Qi accumulates at the last Meeting point and as it looks for an outlet it can become uncomfortable. The Jing-Well point if added then will release this pain entirely. Sometimes during the treatment, the patient will feel pressure against the Jing-Well point. This means the Wei Qi is "knocking" at the Jing-Well "door". Remove the needle immediately. The point will likely bleed.

Order of Withdrawal of Needles in SDS treatments

1. Yuan-Source level points that were added to the standard protocol, if any.
2. Trajectory points.
3. Opening point where applicable (where the Opening point is not a Confluent point).
4. Confluent points on the side that didn't have a Jing-Well, the crossing point, Confluent points on the side of the needled Jing-Well.
5. Jing-Well point(s).

Blockages

Divergent treatments are greatly enhanced when blockages are addressed first through cupping or gua sha. Often the success of a Divergent treatment depends on the release of blockages. This would be in addition to the treatments of the zones, where applicable (see information on Zonal Divergent Channel treatments below). Blockages stagnate Wei Qi and prevent it moving, thereby compromising Divergent treatments which require the movement of Wei Qi. Blockages are commonly found in the neck, pelvis, paravertebral muscles, scapulae, anywhere on the SCM, shoulders, trapezius, rectus abdominis, around the breast, at the floating ribs, on the ribcage, under the ribcage, in the gluteus, and in gastrocnemius (referred to as the Five Pillars in Wu Shu). I use a porcelain Chinese soup spoon or an animal horn gua sha tool on these areas in a scooping motion until sha appears and the area loosens. A water buffalo horn would be more traditional because horns, in herbal medicine, move Wind. Gua sha increases the efficacy of Divergent treatments enormously. This is true for both SDS and DSD treatments. Wei Qi must be freed from a blockage before you can move it.

Healing Events

Healing events are re-emergences of suppressed, unresolved or latent illnesses that sometimes arise after a healing acupuncture treatment. They are an important part of the peeling back of layers of energetic blockages that conceal natural good health.
See Healing Events Appendix, page 375.

Troubleshooting

Pain and stiffness remained after an SDS treatment.

Did you remember to gua sha the cutaneous region(s)?
Is the patient eating cold or raw foods or drinks, including salads, smoothies, refrigerated water, juices or ice cream?

Is the patient using an ice pack or seeing a well-meaning practitioner who is using ice packs? Ice is contraindicated in cases of pain and stiffness because it restricts the flow of Wei Qi. Ice slows the healing flow of Blood and Qi to the area and forces Wei Qi and inflammation into the joints. This often leads to joint bi (arthritis) in later years.

Patient suddenly experiences the emergence of pain during a DSD treatment.

Locate the pain, insert a needle into the Wei level, turn it 180 degrees away from the midline and immediately remove it. Leave the hole open. In nearly all cases, the pain will disappear. If it is still present, needle the Jing-Well point corresponding to the Sinew Channel on which the pain is felt, with no retention.

I can't get the Qi to stay engaged with the needle between the superficial and deep levels.

If you are having trouble getting the needle to "drag" between the levels, it is probably because it is made of the wrong kind of metal or has the wrong kind of handle. See Equipment appendix, page 379.

My treatment failed.

It's possible that latent pathology needs to be released by gua sha on muscular or accessible bony regions of latency: sternocleidomastoid, diaphragm, iliopsoas, abdominals, paravertebrals, gluteus, sternum, sacrum.

My patient is on steroids and it's slow-going. Do steroids affect Divergent treatments?

Yes, very much so. Steroids damage Yang Qi and result ultimately in a reduction of the capacity of the body to hold mediumship in place. The body displaces the steroids and when it gains enough strength to push the pathogen out again, it mounts another attempt which is in turn thwarted by the ongoing steroid use. This leads to the prescription of higher doses of steroids which damage Yang Qi even further.

My patient shows hyperactivity of the immune system in their blood test and yet there is no pathogen showing in the blood. Are Divergents applicable?

Yes, the Divergents are applicable in all immune system illnesses. The pathogen is not showing in the blood because the body is fighting an energetic state, for example, Cold, or the pathogen is being held nearly fully latent.

What is the purpose of treating the Divergents three days on and three days off?

Every day you are nagging the body, preventing the body from remaining in the habit of either keeping pathology in or trying unsuccessfully to push it out. During the three days off, the body is allowed to integrate this message. If the treatments were every day, the body could decide to ignore the message.

I find that the insertion of the last Confluent point in a looping treatment is painful. What should I do?

The last Meeting point can be painful if the body is very willing to raise the Wei Qi to the surface. The Wei comes up and looks for an outlet. If you feel that the Wei Qi is accumulating, add the Jing-Well point early to release the Wei Qi.

Frequently Asked Questions

If the pathogen is stuck in the body because the body failed to sweat, why can't I simply do a treatment to induce a sweat?

If the pathogen is in the Divergent Channels it means the Sinews which produce sweat have failed and the opportunity of this simple healing mechanism has been missed.

In any DSD treatment we are returning Yang to the interior to tonify the medium of latency, but then why is Yang said to be the last resort for holding latency?

Divergent treatments move Wei Qi. Wei Qi is derived from Yang Qi. When you needle DSD, you capture the Wei at the surface and return it to its origin, that of Yang Qi. In the sixth confluence you're using Yang Qi to hold the pathogen in latency as best you can. In the first, second, third and fourth confluences the body is holding the pathogen latent by also making use of Jing, Blood, Fluids, etc. Only when media of Blood, Thin Fluids, Thick Fluids and Yin have been exhausted does the body use Yang, and only Yang, as a last resort for maintaining latency.

Divergent Channels seek latency in the major joints but my patient has problems only in her knees. Is this Divergent pathology?

Yes, all joint pathology can be viewed in the context of the Divergent Channels. In this case, the hips and shoulders are likely successfully holding latency and are therefore asymptomatic.

How long should I keep a pathogen in latency?

A pathogen is kept in latency until the practitioner determines there are enough Fluids (and Qi) to expel it. This can take a few days, weeks, or even three months (more than one 18 day Divergent cycle), but sometimes, especially if the person will not change their diet or lifestyle, this is never achieved. In that case, acupuncture becomes a method of prolonging organ function by protecting the organs using DSD treatments. (Treatment frequency is determined by pulse status.)

DIVERGENT CHANNELS IN DETAIL
BLADDER DIVERGENT CHANNEL

Key Phrases

"Finds latency for the pathogenic factor in the deepest level of the exterior where Yuan is relatively superficially expressed, the bone and joints."

"The pathogenic factor has been revealed due to the decline in Jing."

"Pull the pathology from the Zang Fu via Shu points and Hua To points to the joints."

"Consolidates Essence."

"Pulls pathology out of the Shu points and displaces it to the joints via the Confluent points."

Trajectory Signs

Tumors at the knees and along spine, anus problems, urine issues, lumbar pain, stiff knees, tight psoas, scoliosis, occipital headaches.

Wei Signs

Pain along the trajectory, peristalsis signs (the gastrointestinal tract moves due to Wei Qi), Wei diarrhea (hot and frequent), urine issues, hypertension, prostatitis, acute meningitis.

The Bladder Shu Points

Bladder or Kidney Shu points in Divergent treatments are always 0.5 cun from the midline because that is the location at which latency is mediated. Divergent Bladder Shu points are in the Hua To positions.

Points

Confluent points: **BL-40, BL-10**

Trajectory points: **BL-36, GV-1, GV-4, BL-23** (Hua To), **CV-4, CV-3, BL-32, BL-28,** up the Hua To line to **BL-15** (as a Hua To point) and **GV-11, BL-15, BL-44** and **CV-17, BL-15,** (to **BL-10**).

If SDS: Jing-Well: **BL-67**

Entire Channel: **BL-40, BL-36, GV-1, GV-4, BL-23** (Hua To), **CV-4, CV-3, BL-32, BL-28,** up the Hua To line to **BL-15** (as a Hua To point) and **GV-11, BL-15, BL-44** and **CV-17, BL-15, BL-10**

Note: The trajectory points chosen here are a sample selection only. Every treatment will be different according to the finer points of the diagnosis.

Note: If there is tightness in the shoulders, neck, paravertebral muscles, scapulae, rhomboids, etc., gua sha these areas before commencing treatment so that trapped Wei can move.

Bladder Divergent DSD Treatment Protocol

Order of Insertion

1. Confluent points
2. Trajectory points

Note: If there is tightness in the shoulders, neck, paravertebral muscles, scapulae, rhomboids, etc., gua sha these areas before commencing treatment so that trapped Wei can move.

1. *Needle the Confluent points (Meeting points) with DSD technique.*

Needle the Confluent points from top to bottom:

BL-10 left and right

BL-40 left and right

2. *Needle selected, appropriate Trajectory points according to the unique diagnosis of the individual.*

E.g., (selected points): BL-36, GV-4, BL-23, BL-15, BL-15, BL-23, BL-36 with DSD technique or SDS technique or simply superficial or simply deep depending on your intention for each individual point.

Bladder Divergent SDS Treatment Protocol

Order of Insertion

1. Gua sha cutaneous region or tight areas
2. Confluent points with cross-over point
3. Trajectory points
4. Jing-Well

1. *If a musculoskeletal or dermatological condition, gua sha or sliding cup the Tai Yang cutaneous region:*

"The ring around the chest" shown in the drawing or any areas of binding or tightness.

If not treating a musculoskeletal or dermatological condition, begin at step 2.

2. *Needle the Confluent points (Meeting points) with SDS technique*

Needle the Confluent points in a loop. Either:

a. BL-40 (L), BL-10 (L), crossing point (e.g., GV-20), BL-10 (R), BL-40 (R) or

b. BL-40 (R), BL-10 (R), crossing point, BL-10 (L), BL-40 (L).

Bladder Divergent Channel

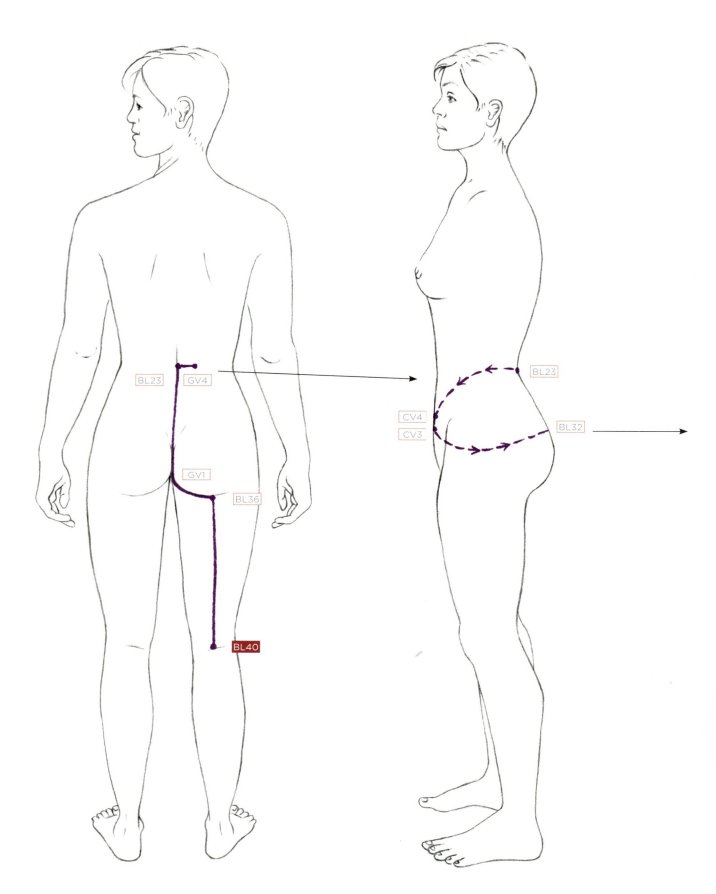

Bladder Divergent Channel

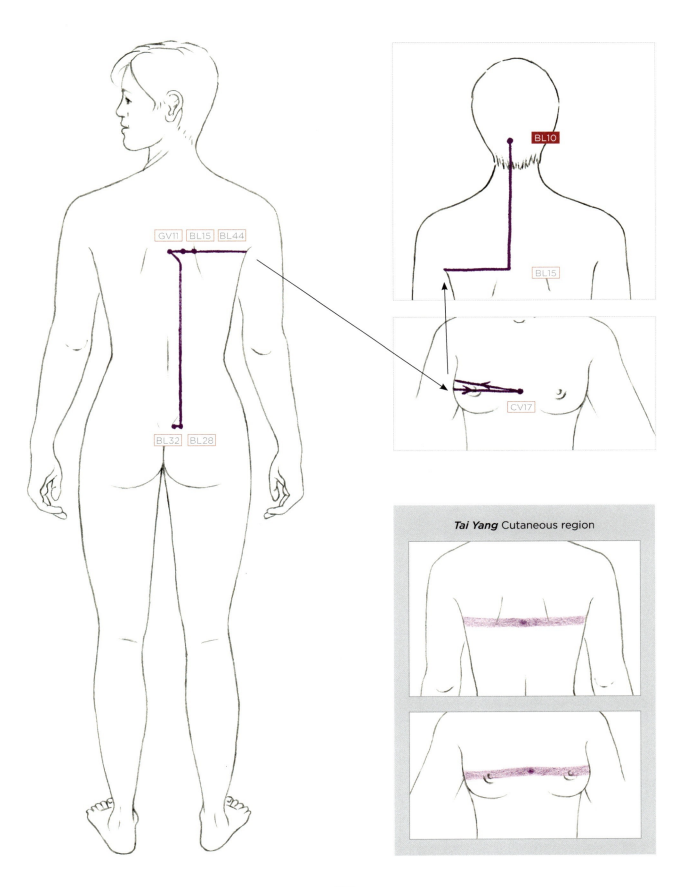

Tai Yang Cutaneous region

3. *Needle selected, appropriate Trajectory points according to the unique diagnosis of the individual, with SDS technique.*

    E.g., with selected points (if the Confluent points were started on the left): BL-36 (L), GV-4, BL-23 (L), BL-15 (L), BL-15 (R), BL-23 (R), BL-36 (R), with SDS technique or DSD technique or simply superficial or simply deep depending on your intention for each individual point. Note that the Bladder Shu points are all 0.5 from the midline, on the Hua To line.

4. *Needle the Jing-Well point, BL-67, on the same side as the last inserted Confluent point.*

Frequently Asked Questions Related to Bladder Divergent Channel

1. *Why are the Hua To points used instead of the Bladder Shu points?*

    The trajectory traverses the Hua To points and not the Bladder Shu points because the Hua To points control latency and the Shu points do the opposite, they transport. To put something into or out of latency it's necessary to use a point whose function includes capacity for latency. When you needle a Hua To point you are saying that you are:

    a. stopping the transference of the pathology to the Zang Fu and diverting that pathology to the joints (DSD), or you are

    b. pulling pathology from the reservoir of latency that features the Hua To points and sending it to the sinews (SDS), or you are

    c. pulling the pathology directly from the Zang Fu to the Bladder Shu points and then further to the Hua To points so that it can be brought to the sinews using SDS technique.

2. *Why do some patients have a bulge at BL-10?*

    BL-10 is a major site of latency, and Wind and Damp can accumulate at that site. It can be gua sha'd in an SDS treatment to instigate the movement of Blood. Moving Blood expels Wind.

3. *How can I needle CV3 and still needle the rest of the Bladder Divergent Channel trajectory if I have the patient lying supine on the table?*

    To include CV-3 in the treatment (necessary in chronic urinary tract infection cases, for example): If the treatment is SDS, needle the CV-3 SDS and tape the needle down flat to the skin with micropore surgical tape. Turn a corner of the tape onto itself so that you have something to pull to get the tape off again. Alternatively, needle SDS and remove. If the treatment is DSD, you might choose to tape the needle down, but if the patient finds it's very uncomfortable it's best to needle DSD and remove immediately.

4. If I am looping, should BL-10 be pointed in the direction of the loop?

In SDS, the first needled BL-10 can be pointed towards the other BL-10 and the second needled BL-10 can be pointed down towards BL-40 to delineate a loop.

5. How should BL-10 be needled for a DSD treatment? Perpendicularly.

Note: Never point BL-10 (or any point near the base of the skull) superior to the site of insertion, not even slightly. The cerebellum is close to these points.

6. How should BL-40 be needled?

BL-40 is either pointed:

    a. to the floor in DSD or SDS, or

    b. In SDS treatments, first inserted BL-40 is pointed very slightly superiorly to delineate a loop. The second BL-40 can be pointed very slightly inferiorly to delineate the loop. Loops can also be delineated by intention alone. This allows for deeper needling.

7. When can I not use BL/KI Divergent Channels? After all, when Jing has run out, life stops!

You can always use Bladder and Kidney Divergent Channels because everybody alive has Jing. The body will choose to stop using the first confluence (BL/KI Divergent Channels) long before Jing runs out, so you wouldn't say that the body moved to another confluence for the reason that Jing became overly depleted. The body uses the Jing as a temporary holding site while the body returns to the level of health needed to push the pathogen out. If we lived with the seasons, most often that would take a very short time. It moves to other confluences to preserve Jing.

8. My patient has crackling sounds in her knees, but no Divergent Channels signs per se. Should I still treat the Divergents?

Yes, these crackling sounds are a sign that the body has diverted pathology to the joints. Treat the BL/KI Divergent Channels.

9. Are there pulse determinations for BL/KI Divergent?

Yes, theoretically you would check the width of the chi pulse on the left side (Kidney). But BL/KI Divergent can be used any time because there is always Jing available. When Jing runs out, life is over. The reason the body switches out of the BL/KI confluence and asks for support from another medium is that it tries to preserve the Jing to prolong life.

KIDNEY DIVERGENT CHANNEL

Key Phrases

"Yang activity transformed from Yin. Kidney Divergent Channel is a buffer zone for Dai Mai. It keeps the pathogenic factor from Source and in so doing, maintains latency. Kidney Divergent Channel consolidates the Essence."

Trajectory Signs

Damp-Heat in the Lower Jiao (Jing stasis), ovarian cysts if ruptured (if not ruptured use Dai Mai), fibroids, chronic vaginitis, chronic cystitis.

Wei Signs

Pain along the trajectory, neck rigidity, throat issues, chronic sore throats and swollen glands, skull and jaw tension, dizziness and hypertension as Essence is relocated to maintain latency allowing Yang to rush up (empty heat).

Mediumship Depletion Signs

Sore throat, goiter, hyper- and hypothyroidism, impotence.

Points

Confluent points: **BL-40, BL-10**
Opening point: **KI-10**
Trajectory points: **BL-36, GV-1, GV-4, CV-4, CV-3, BL-32, BL-28**, then emerges at **BL-23, GB-26, SP-15, ST-25, KI-16, CV-8, KI-16, KI-27** at 0.5 cun lateral to the midline, **CV-23**, (to **BL-10**).
Entire Channel: **BL-40, KI-10, BL-36, GV-1, GV-4, CV-4, CV-3, BL-32, BL-28**, then emerges at **BL-23, GB-26, SP-15, ST-25, KI-16, CV-8, KI-16, KI-27** at 0.5 cun lateral to the midline, **CV-23, BL-10**

Kidney Divergent DSD Treatment Protocol

Order of Insertion

1. Confluent points
2. Opening
3. Trajectory points

Note: If there is tightness in the shoulders, neck, paravertebral muscles, scapulae, rhomboids, etc., gua sha these areas before commencing treatment so that trapped Wei can move.

Note: This is a side-lying treatment.

1. *Needle the Confluent points (Meeting points) with DSD technique.*

Needle the Confluent points from top to bottom:

BL-10 on both sides

BL-40 on both sides

2. *Needle the Opening point.*

KI-10 either bilaterally or unilaterally on the side of the first needle inserted, with DSD technique.

3. *Needle selected, appropriate Trajectory points.*

E.g., with selected points (if the Confluent points were started on the left): BL-36, GV-1, GV-4, CV-4, CV-3, BL-32, BL-28, BL-23, GB-26, SP-15, ST-25, KI-16, CV-8, KI-16, KI-27 at 0.5 cun lateral to the midline, CV-23, with DSD technique or SDS technique or simply superficial or simply deep depending on your intention for each individual point.

Note: The trajectory points chosen here are a sample selection only. Every treatment will be different according to the finer points of the diagnosis.

Kidney Divergent SDS Treatment Protocol

Order of Insertion

1. Gua sha cutaneous region or tight areas region
2. Confluent points with cross-over
3. Opening point
4. Trajectory points
5. Jing-Well

1. *Gua sha Cutaneous Regions.*

If a musculoskeletal or dermatological condition, gua sha or sliding-cup the *Shao Yin* cutaneous region: the CV-23 area shown in the drawing or any areas of binding or tightness. If not treating a musculoskeletal or dermatological condition, begin at step 2.

Kidney Divergent Channel

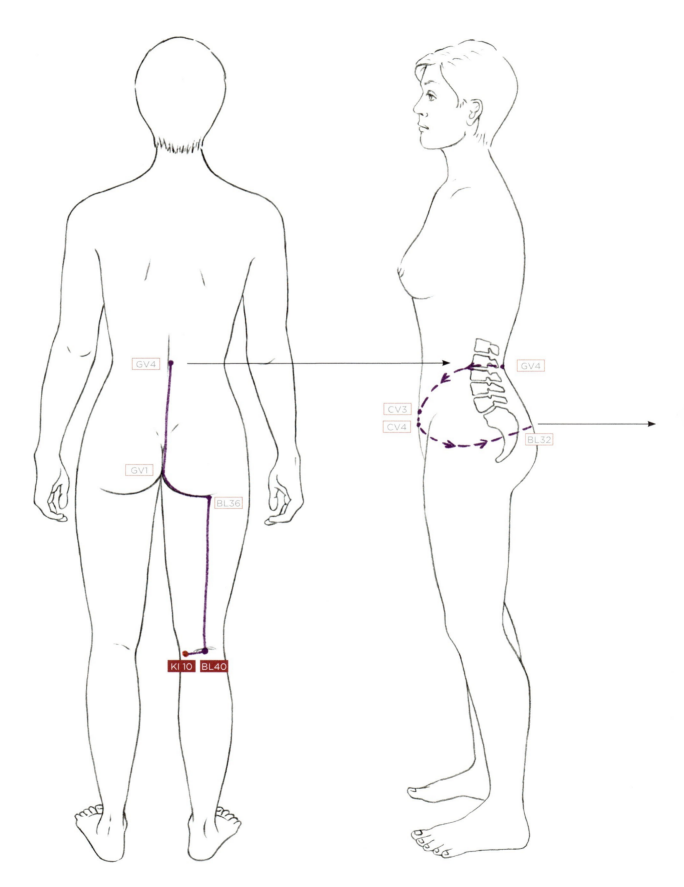

Kidney Divergent Channel

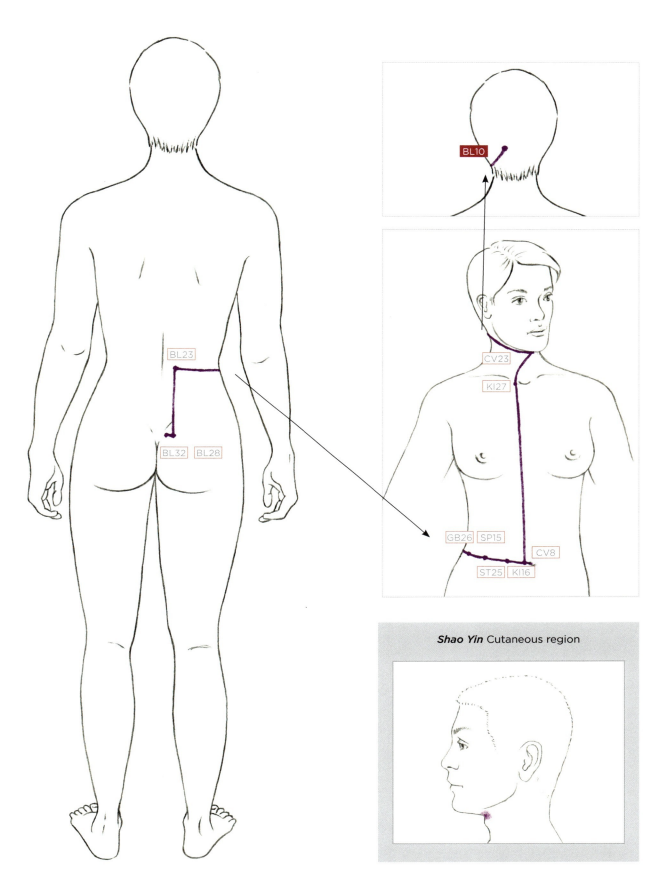

Shao Yin Cutaneous region

2. Needle the Confluent points (Meeting points) with SDS technique.

Needle the Confluent points in a loop. Either:

a. BL-40 (L), BL-10 (L), crossing point (e.g., GV-20), BL-10 (R), BL-40 R) or

b. BL-40 (R), BL-10 (R), crossing point, BL-10 (L), BL-40 (L).

3. Needle the Opening point with SDS technique.

KI-10 either bilaterally in the order of the sides needled in the loop, or unilaterally on the side of the first needle inserted.

4. Needle selected, appropriate Trajectory points

following the order of the trajectory with SDS technique or DSD technique or simply superficial or simply deep depending on your intention for each individual point.

5. Needle the Jing-Well point, KI-1 on the same side as the last inserted Confluent point.

Point Location and Clinical Tips

KI-10 is located between two tendons that are often very close together. Use the guide tube to gentle pry these apart so that the needle can be inserted in that gap. Sometimes the needle will want to point slightly superior in order to reach the deep level.

Kidney Divergent Channel uses the Kidney Shu points along the sternum as areas of latency but they also treat stagnation of Yin, Blood and Fluids. Palpate for sensitivity and needle sensitive points deeply and obliquely for DSD treatments or superficially for SDS treatments. Kidney Shu's are 0.5 lateral to the Ren line. They relate to specific organs: KI-22 (Kidney), KI-23 (Spleen), KI-24 (Liver), KI-25 (Heart), KI-26 (Lung), KI-27 (Master Kidney Shu).

Kidney Divergent Channel connects to the Chong, Ren and Du and brings postnatal Qi to nourish the Jing to support latency in the Jing.

Bladder Divergent Channel includes Da Bao and Kidney Divergent Channel includes Dai Mai. Therefore, as a pair, the first confluence affects communication between the Heart and Kidney.

Kidney Divergent Channel can divert Dai Mai excess upward. So you may see an accumulation which manifests as a fibroid in Dai Mai later manifesting as a goiter.

GALLBLADDER DIVERGENT CHANNEL

Pulses

Examine the width of the moderate level of the Liver position. This indicates the status of Blood. If the pulse is thin, choppy or very weak, Blood is inadequate to provide sufficient mediumship. Therefore, you might consider a different confluence. If you decide to go ahead, use the confluence DSD but begin the treatment with tonification of the Source point of the Liver, LR-3.

If the Liver pulse is tight, indicating constraint, the pathogen might not move. Begin the treatment with LR-3.

Key Phrases

"Moving Qi to put the pathogen into latency. You need Blood to carry the Qi. If the Essence is unwilling to hold the pathology any longer, Blood is used to hold the pathogen at the Mu points where Essence is stored. That's what is meant by 'Blood supports the Essence'. Gallbladder Divergent Channel makes this movement happen. Secures the Essence."

Trajectory Signs

Acute Blood stagnation, e.g., optic nerve issues, all eye issues, ear issues, vocal cord issues, laryngitis, Heart issues, chest and rib pain, pain with hip flexion, thigh, pelvis, hip arthritis.

Wei Signs

Pain along the trajectory, heaviness of the head or dizziness (Gallbladder Divergent Channel balances Yin and Yang in the head), chronic upper respiratory tract infections (URTI), acute allergies, asthma attack, skin conditions, psoriasis, eczema.

Mediumship Mobilization Signs

Irritated ears, nose, vocal cords, jaw, throat, laryngitis, rhinitis, spasms, stiff shooting pain, palpitations, cough with spontaneous sweat, cough with alternating chills and fever.

Mediumship Depletion Signs

Swollen liver organ and spleen organ, Alzheimer's disease, psychosomatic conditions.

Points

Confluent points: **GB-1, CV-2**

Opening point: **GB-30**

Trajectory points: **CV-2, CV-3, GB-25, LR-13, GB-24, LR-14, CV-14, PC-1, CV-22,** (**CV-23** often mentioned), **ST-12, ST-5, GB-1**.

Entire Channel: **GB-30, CV-2, CV-3, GB-25, LR-13, GB-24, LR-14, CV-14, PC-1, CV-22, (CV-23), ST-12, ST-5, GB-1**

Gallbladder DSD Treatment Protocol

Order of Insertion

1. Confluent points
2. Opening points
3. Trajectory points

Note: If there is tightness in the shoulders, neck, paravertebral muscles, scapulae, rhomboids, etc., gua sha these areas before commencing treatment so that trapped Wei can move.

1. Needle the Confluent points (Meeting points) with DSD technique.

GB-1 bilaterally, then CV-2

2. Needle the Opening point.

GB-30 either bilaterally or unilaterally on the side of the first needle inserted, with DSD technique.

3. Needle selected, appropriate Trajectory points.

For example: GB-25, LR-13, CV-14, ST-12, ST-5, PC-1, LR-14, GB-24, with DSD technique or SDS technique or simply superficial or simply deep depending on your intention for each individual point.

Note: The trajectory points chosen here are a sample selection only. Every treatment will be different according to the finer points of the diagnosis.

Gallbladder Divergent SDS Treatment Protocol

Order of Insertion

1. Gua sha Cutaneous region or tight areas
2. Confluent points with cross-over point
3. Opening point
4. Trajectory points
5. Jing-Well

Gallbladder Divergent Channel

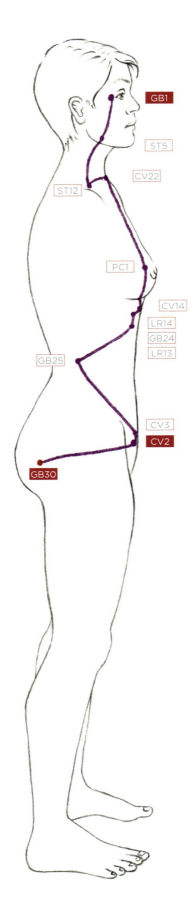

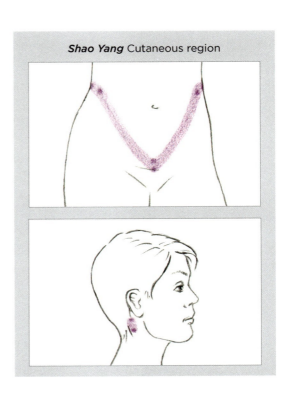

1. ***Gua sha Cutaneous Regions.***

    If a musculoskeletal or dermatological condition, gua sha or sliding-cup the three Shao Yang cutaneous regions shown in the drawing or any areas of binding or tightness. If not treating a musculoskeletal or dermatological condition, begin at step 2.

2. **Needle the Confluent points (Meeting points) with SDS technique.**

    Needle the Confluent points in a loop. Either:

    a. CV-2, GB-1 (L), GB-1 (R) or

    b. CV-2, GB-1 (R), GB-1 (L)

3. **Needle the Opening point with SDS technique.**

    GB-30 either bilaterally in the order of the sides needled in the loop, or unilaterally on the side of the first needle inserted.

4. **Needle selected, appropriate Trajectory points following the order of the trajectory.**

    For example: Here is a suggested order if the Confluent points were started on the right. I'm suggesting that the Mu points be needled according to the side the pulse of that organ is found: GB-25 (R), LR-13 (R), CV-14, ST-12 (R), ST-5 (R), PC-1 (L), LR-14 (L), GB-24 (L). Use SDS technique or DSD technique or simply superficial or simply deep depending on your intention for each individual point.

5. **Needle the Jing-Well point.**

    GB-44 on the same side as the last inserted Confluent point.

Point Location and Clinical Tips

GB-1 is in the hollow lateral to the corner of the eye and is needled freehand only, with a half-inch needle.

CV-2 is located immediately superior to the top of the pubic bone, on the midline.

Notes

The *Nei Jing* has an alternative trajectory for Gallbladder Divergent Channel. It says the trajectory moves internally along the sides, goes to GB-22 and then to CV-17, ST-12, then behind the ear to TH-16 and TH-17, then to "Tai Yang" point at the temple, then to GV-20 where it communicates with the brain. Then it emerges at GB-1. From GB-1 it crosses over to opposite side to LI-20. The application of this alternative trajectory includes treatment of chills and fever, migraines and earaches.

Questions

I can't lie my patient on his side for more than a few minutes. Is there a way of getting GB-30 inserted easily? I do this treatment a couple of different ways. Because I try to avoid side-lying treatments, occasionally I'll break a rule and needle GB-30 first, then ease the patient down onto their back. Sometimes, after insertion of the meeting points I bend the hip, push down on the table and needle diagonally upwards into GB-30.

LIVER DIVERGENT CHANNEL

Pulses

Examine the width of the moderate level of the Liver position. This gives the status of Blood volume. If the pulse is thin, choppy or very weak, you might consider a different confluence. If you decide to go with a DSD treatment, begin the treatment by tonifying the Source point, LR-3. If you decide to go ahead with an SDS treatment, tonify LR-3 first, check the width of the Liver pulse again, and then proceed when the pulse is stronger. If the Liver pulse is tight, the pathogen might not move and LR-3 should be reduced.

Key Phrase

"Uses Blood to support Essence."

Trajectory Signs

Pain along the trajectory, spotting, bleeding from genitals.

Wei Signs

Pain along the trajectory, dysmenorrhea, pelvic inflammatory conditions, vaginitis, endometriosis. Infertility due to Wei Qi over-acting on the uterus, making it unable to receive Essence, and infertility due to insufficient Blood moving to the uterus. Herpes and other sexually transmitted diseases, genital swellings as Jing stasis is moved, HPV, sudden genital pain, abnormal sexual arousal due to Wei Qi being active because there is not enough Blood to control Wei. Frequent uterine contractions due to insufficient Blood to subdue Wei Qi, cruel itching often in the genital area, genital swellings, testicular swellings, swellings of the uterus, vagina or scrotum. Fluid not properly regulated in the Lower Jiao. Blood toxins, e.g., genital herpes, toxins at Jing level.

Mediumship Depletion Signs

Chronic angry mood, "infertility" from fear of sex, hernia, fibroids, cysts, infertility, psychosomatic conditions, hypertension, rheumatoid conditions, thyroiditis, allergies, asthma, skin problems, psoriasis, eczema due to stress.

Points

Confluent points: **GB-1, CV-2**
Opening point: **LR-5**
Trajectory points: **GB-25, LR-13, GB-24, LR-14, CV-14, PC-1, CV-22, ST-12, ST-5**
Entire Channel: **LR-5, CV-2, GB-25, LR-13, GB-24, LR-14, CV-14, PC-1, CV-22, ST-12, ST-5, GB-1**

Liver Divergent DSD Treatment Protocol

Order of Insertion

1. Confluent points
2. Opening point
3. Trajectory points

Note: If there is tightness in the shoulders, neck, paravertebral muscles, scapulae, rhomboids, etc., gua sha these areas before commencing treatment so that trapped Wei can move.

1. Needle the Confluent points (Meeting points).

GB-1 bilaterally, then CV-2, with DSD technique.

2. Needle the Opening point.

LR-5 either bilaterally or unilaterally on the side of the first needle inserted, with DSD technique.

3. Needle selected, appropriate Trajectory points.

With DSD technique or SDS technique or simply superficial or simply deep depending on your intention for each individual point. E.g., GB-25, GB-24, LR-14, LR-13, CV-14, PC-1, CV-22, ST-12, ST-5.

Note: The trajectory points chosen will differ according to the finer points of the diagnosis.

Liver Divergent Channel

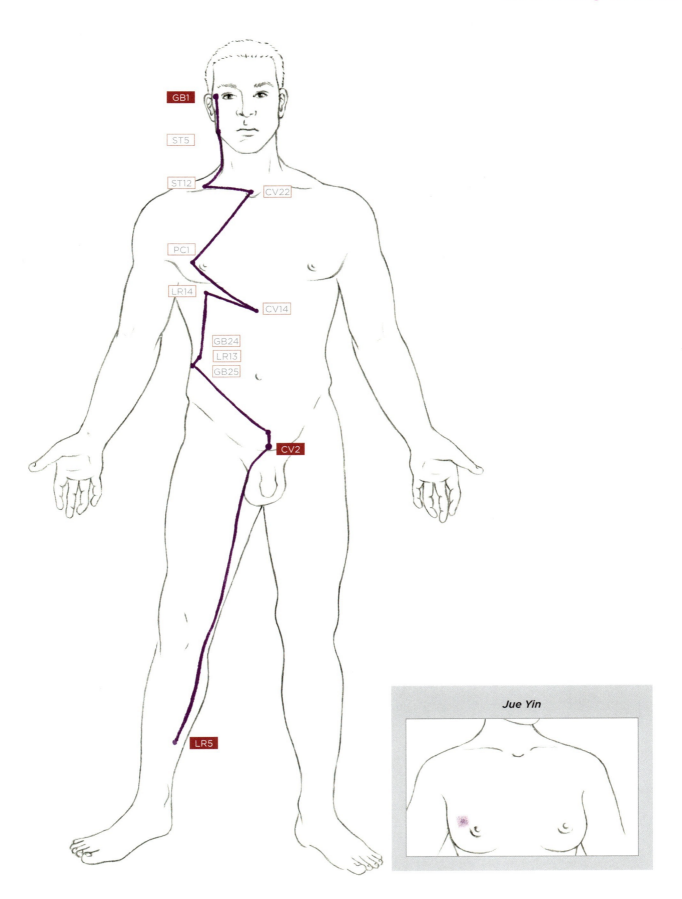

Jue Yin

Liver Divergent SDS Treatment Protocol

Order of Insertion

1. Gua sha Cutaneous Regions or tight areas
2. Confluent
3. Opening point
4. Trajectory points
5. Jing-Well

1. Gua sha Cutaneous Regions

If treating a musculoskeletal or dermatological condition, gua sha or sliding cup the Jue Yin cutaneous region, the PC-1 area shown in the drawing or any areas of binding or tightness. If not treating a musculoskeletal or dermatological condition, begin at step 2.

2. Needle the Confluent points (Meeting points) all with SDS technique.

Needle the Confluent points all SDS in a loop. Either:

    a. CV-2, GB-1 (L), GB-1 (R) or

    b. CV-2, GB-1 (R), GB-1 (L)

3. Needle the Opening point with SDS technique.

LR-5 either bilaterally in the order of the sides needled in the loop, or unilaterally on the side of the first needle inserted.

4. Needle selected, appropriate Trajectory points following the order of the trajectory.

E.g., with selected points (if the Confluent points were started on the right): GB-25 (R), LR-13 (R), CV-14, CV-22, ST-12 (R), ST-5 (R), PC-1 (L), LR-14 (L), GB-24 (L) with SDS technique or DSD technique or simply superficial or simply deep depending on your intention for each individual point.

5. Needle the Jing-Well point.

LR-1 on the same side as the last inserted Confluent point.

Point Location and Clinical Tips

LR-5 is inserted perpendicular to the flat face of the medial side of the tibia and needled towards the table so that it can almost penetrate the notch in the bone.

If uncomfortable doing gua sha on PC-1 on a female patient, gua sha GB-22 instead.

STOMACH DIVERGENT CHANNEL

Pulses

Examine the width of the moderate level of the Spleen position. This gives the status of Thin Fluids, the Jin. If the pulse is thin, choppy or very weak, you might consider a different confluence. If you decide to go ahead with a DSD treatment, begin the treatment with the Source point, ST-42. If you want to go ahead with an SDS treatment, give the patient water, tonify ST-42, check that the moderate Spleen pulse has widened at least somewhat, and then proceed.

Key Phrases

"Thin (exocrine) Fluids move to support Blood."

ST-30 is the Sea of Food and Drinks and affects peristalsis. The Divergents connect to Chong here; we can regulate Blood through that Chong connection.

BL-1 connects to Yin and Yang Qiao Channels and regulates our response to the external world.

BL-1 activates ST-42 which in turn ascends Pure Yang (moisture) to the face. Pure Yang is the moisture that goes to the sensory orifices. Stomach Divergent Channel opens the sensory orifices. ST-30 relaxes the ancestral sinews to treat chronic Wei Qi obstruction.

Trajectory Signs

Painful abdomen, inability to shift weight forward due to pain in the legs, thigh, or pelvis, inner thigh pain, ulcers, gastritis, ulcerative colitis, painful swallowing, pain of esophagus, tooth decay especially in the upper teeth, epistaxis, acute blindness.

Wei Signs

Pain along the trajectory, upper respiratory tract infections, acute and chronic allergies, rhinitis, sinusitis, signs and symptoms of all the sensory orifices: ears, eyes, nose, mouth and throat, including tinnitus, red swollen eyes with eye degeneration, cataracts, and glaucoma. Pelvic pain during ovulation, tight ancestral sinews causing Gastroesophageal Reflux Disease (GERD), colitis, cystitis, irregular menses.

Mediumship Mobilization Signs

Excess mucus, excess fluid accumulations such as edema, nasal discharge.

Mediumship Depletion Signs

Nasal and intestinal polyps, hyper- and hypothyroidism, ulcers, Lupus, Sjogren's Syndrome, chronic allergies, sinusitis, rhinitis, conjunctivitis, styes, tinnitus, ear lesions, chronic eczema, cold sores.

Points

Confluent points: **ST-30, BL-1**[4]

Trajectory points: **CV-12, CV-14, CV-17, ST-12** (often not mentioned) **CV-22, CV-23, ST-9, ST-4, LI-20**

Entire Channel: **ST-30, CV-12, CV-14, CV-17, ST-12, CV-22, CV-23, ST-9, ST-4, LI-20, BL-1**

> Note: Give the patient plain flat, room temperature water to drink prior to treatment. Because Stomach Divergent involves the assimilation of Thin Fluids you might find the patient will be quite thirsty during a ST/SP Divergent treatment. Many times I have experienced a patient drinking more than 64oz of water during the SDS or DSD treatment and they haven't needed to go to the bathroom at the conclusion of treatment. Use a bendy straw so they don't need to raise their head.

Note: BL-2 is not a replacement for BL-1. BL-2 and BL-1 have different functions. BL-1 gives access to pineal and pituitary function in the brain. If you or your patient is really afraid of it, needle BL-2 with great intention. To needle BL-1 safely, do not move the eye. The point is superior to the canthus, not medial and superior to the canthus.

Stomach Divergent DSD Treatment Protocol

Order of Insertion

1. Confluent points
2. Trajectory points

Note: If there is tightness in the shoulders, neck, paravertebral muscles, scapulae, rhomboids, etc., gua sha these areas before commencing treatment so that trapped Wei Qi can move.

1. Needle the Confluent points (Meeting points) with DSD technique.

BL-1 both sides, then ST-30 both sides, with DSD technique.

2. Needle selected, appropriate Trajectory points.

In the following order: CV-12, CV-14, CV-17, ST-12, CV-22, CV-23, ST-9, ST-4, LI-20, with DSD technique or SDS technique or simply superficial or simply deep depending on your intention for each individual point.

---

[4] ST-1 has been postulated as the Confluent point of Stomach Divergent Channel, but ST-1 has no capacity for latency.

Stomach Divergent Channel

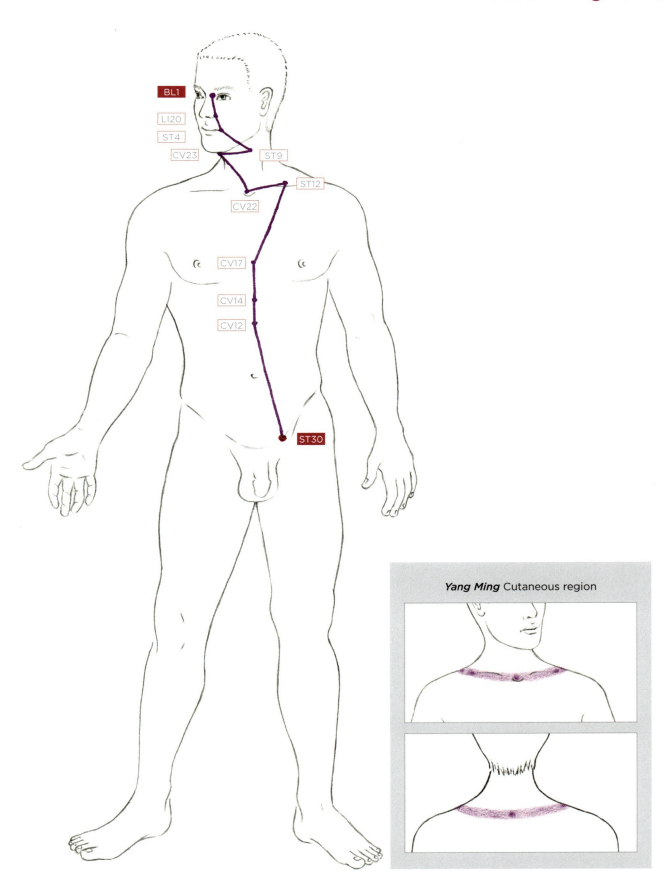

Yang Ming Cutaneous region

Note: The trajectory points chosen here are a sample selection only. Every treatment will be different according to the finer points of the diagnosis.

Stomach Divergent SDS Treatment Protocol

Order of Insertion
1. Gua sha cutaneous region or tight areas
2. Confluent points with cross-over
3. Trajectory points
4. Jing-Well point

1. Gua sha Cutaneous Regions

If a musculoskeletal or dermatological condition, gua sha or sliding cup the Yang Ming cutaneous region: "the ring around the collar" shown in the drawing or any areas of binding or tightness. If not treating a musculoskeletal or dermatological condition, begin at step 2.

2. Needle the Confluent points (Meeting points) with SDS technique.

Needle the Confluent points in a loop. Either:
    a. ST-30 (L), BL-1 (L), crossing point (e.g., GV-20), BL-1 (R) ST-30 (R), or
    b. ST-30 (R), BL-1 (R), crossing point, BL-1 (L), ST-30 (L).

3. Needle selected, appropriate Trajectory points.

With SDS technique or DSD technique or simply superficial or simply deep depending on your intention for each individual point, following the order of the trajectory with selected points: CV-12, CV-14, CV-17, ST-12, CV-22, CV-23, ST-9, ST-4, LI-20.

4. Needle the Jing-Well point.

ST-45 on the same side as the last inserted Confluent point.

SPLEEN DIVERGENT CHANNEL

Pulses
Examine the width of the moderate level of the Spleen position. This gives the status of Stomach Fluids. If the pulse is thin, choppy or very weak, you might consider a different confluence. If you decide to go ahead with a DSD treatment, begin the treatment with the Source point, ST-42 to provide Fluids. SP-3 can also be added. If you want to go ahead with an SDS treatment, give the patient water, tonify ST-42, check that the moderate Spleen pulse has widened at least somewhat, and then proceed.

Key Phrase
"Wind stirs due to the depletion of Thin Fluids."

Trajectory Signs
Hiatal hernia, esophageal pain, mouth pain, tongue pain, conjunctivitis.

Wei Signs
Pain along the trajectory, tight painful abdomen, food allergies, frequent spasm or cramping in jaw (TMD), poor digestion, diarrhea and constipation, heat in the Spleen causing rebellious Qi, varicosities, hemorrhoids, prolapse, pain during ovulation.

Mediumship Depletion Signs
Internal Wind, Wind signs and symptoms in the face due to deficient Fluids, eye tics, Bell's Palsy, facial tics, spasms, sensory motor tract issues, Parkinson's disease, strokes and the lesions associated with them, Multiple Sclerosis, dryness of Blood and Fluid complicated by Phlegm leading to neurological signs, Chong issues accompanied by Wind, Wind-Phlegm in the limbs, seizures, stuttering, Tourette's, autism, polycystic ovaries, acute food stasis, food poisoning, nasal polyps.

Points:
Confluent points: **ST-30, BL-1**
Opening point: **SP-12**
Trajectory points: **CV-12, CV-14, CV-17, ST12, CV-22, CV-23, ST-9**
Entire Channel: **SP-12, ST-30, CV-12, CV14, CV-17, ST12, CV-22, CV-23, ST-9, BL-1**

Spleen Divergent DSD Treatment Protocol

Order of Insertion

1. Confluent points
2. Opening point
3. Trajectory points

Note: If there is tightness in the shoulders, neck, paravertebral muscles, scapulae, rhomboids, etc., gua sha these areas before commencing treatment so that trapped Wei Qi can move.

1. Needle the Confluent points (Meeting points) all with DSD technique.

BL-1 both sides then ST-30 both sides with DSD technique.

2. Needle the Opening point with DSD technique.

SP-12 either bilaterally or unilaterally on the side of the first needle inserted with DSD technique.

3. Needle selected, appropriate Trajectory points.

Following the order of the trajectory CV-12, CV-14, CV-17, CV-22, ST-9, CV-23, with DSD technique or SDS technique or simply superficial or simply deep depending on your intention for each individual point.

Note: The trajectory points chosen here are a sample selection only. Every treatment will be different according to the finer points of the diagnosis.

Spleen Divergent SDS Treatment Protocol

Order of Insertion

1. Gua sha cutaneous region or tight areas
2. Confluent points with cross-over
3. Opening point
4. Trajectory points
5. Jing-Well

1. Gua sha Cutaneous Regions

If a musculoskeletal or dermatological condition, gua sha or sliding cup the Tai Yin cutaneous region: "the band at the throat" shown in the drawing or any areas of binding or tightness. If not treating a musculoskeletal or dermatological condition, begin at step 2.

Spleen Divergent Channel

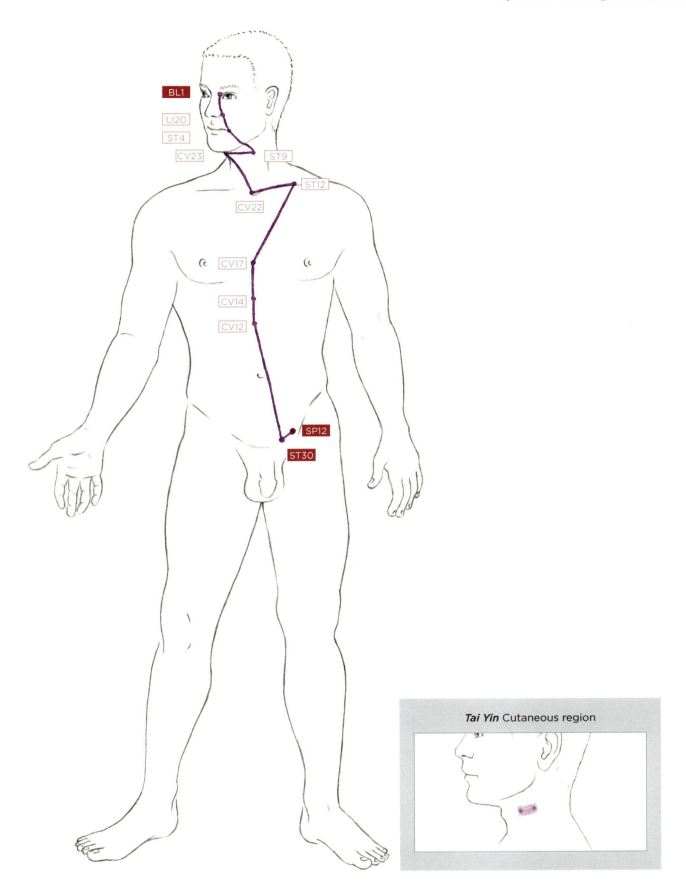

Tai Yin Cutaneous region

2. Needle the Confluent points (Meeting points) with SDS technique.

Needle the Confluent points in a loop. Either:

      a. ST-30 (L), BL-1 (L), crossing point (e.g., GV-20), BL-1 (R), ST-30 (R) or

      b. ST-30 (R), BL-1 (R), crossing point, BL-1 (L), ST-30 (L).

3. Needle the Opening point with SDS technique.

SP-12 either bilaterally in the order of the sides needled in the loop, or unilaterally on the side of the first needle inserted.

4. Needle selected, appropriate Trajectory points.

CV-12, CV-14, CV-17, CV-22, ST-9, CV-23 with SDS technique or DSD technique or simply superficial or simply deep depending on your intention for each individual point.

5. Needle the Jing-Well point.

SP-1 on the same side as the last inserted Confluent point.

Point Location and Clinical Tips

For ease of needling into BL-1, avoid moving the eyeball. The depth need not be great at all. The DSD instruction is relative to the point, so on BL-1 deep can be quite shallow. BL-1 occurs in a tiny area and must be needled freehand with no tube. The margin for error with a tube is much larger than the margin of error for the location of this point.

SMALL INTESTINE DIVERGENT CHANNEL

Pulses

Yin (Ye-Thick Fluids) is required for Small Intestine and Heart Divergent to be able to hold a pathogen in latency. The status of Yin in this context is revealed by the width of the moderate level of the Heart position. Add SI-4 if the pulse is thin. If the pulses are floating and rapid, Yin is not supporting Jing. You might consider Triple Heater and Pericardium Divergents instead.[5]

Key Phrases

"Thick Fluids are mobilized to support Thin Fluids and Wei Qi is internalized to the chest." "Regulates endocrine Fluids."

Small Intestine Divergent Channel brings *Wei* from the sinews to the chest and then

---

[5] Recommendations for alternative Divergent Channel treatments could not be made for the previous confluences because choices can only be made after pulse assessment. By the time the confluence of SI/HT is reached, there are fewer choices.

to the brain. Because Wei Qi is internalizing from Sinews, there is neuropathy and atrophy. Body is losing the ability to hold latency so the pathogenic factor begins to go to the organs. This can affect the entire gastrointestinal tract because three of the Sinew Confluent points including GB-22 are affected by this stage and so all the muscles are affected.

Trajectory Signs

Malar flush, lymph nodes and axillary swellings, fibrocystic breasts.

Wei Signs

Pain along the trajectory, cardiac reflux, mitral valve regurgitation, Heart fire, tongue ulceration, vertical tongue cracks, malar flush, nightmares, stiff tongue with speech affected, dry mouth and eyes with arthritis, lower abdomen pain radiating to the back because Yin does not anchor Yang. Axillary pain. Wei Qi is internalized from sinews to the gastrointestinal tract, leading to peristalsis issues, food stasis, nausea, vomiting, esophageal reflux, irritable bowel, gastritis, ulcers, cardiac regurgitation. The second trajectory brings Blood to the upper orifices, bleeding, receding gums, nosebleeds, hemoptysis, stroke, dry throat with thirst.

Mediumship Mobilization Signs

Excess mucus, excess fluid, nasal discharge.

Mediumship Depletion Signs

Depletion of Fluids in the brain, poor memory, poor day to day memory, Yin deficiency type diarrhea as body tries to flush pathogenic factor causing lost latency, seizures, angry outbursts due to Wind, tinnitus, decreased hearing, loss of vision, thinning of mucosal lining due to Wei Qi being unable to maintain coating. Irregular Menses, Addison's, Grave's disease, Hashimoto's thyroiditis. All hormonal conditions.

Points

Confluent points: **GB-22, BL-1**
Opening point: **SI-10**
Trajectory points: Part 1: **ST-12, SI-18** (to **BL-1**)
Part 2: **SI-10, HT-1**, (to **GB-22**), **CV-17** (then branch goes to **CV-4**).

Entire Channel: SI-10, GB-22, ST-12, SI-18, BL-1. Also, SI-10, HT-1, GB-22, CV-17, CV-4

Note: When using Small Intestine and Heart Divergent Channels for endogenous Fluids, needle the trajectory and then add the Mu or the He-Sea point to direct the treatment to the gland or the organ you want to affect. Examples:
- Diabetes add LR-13 or SP-9.
- Hyper- or hypothyroidism, add LU-1, LU-5, CV-12, or ST-36 depending on the origin of the condition.
- Reproductive endocrine issues, add LR-14.
- Male reproductive endocrine issues, add GB-25 or KI-10.

Adding these points will fine tune your SI/HT Divergent Channels treatment beautifully.

Small Intestine Divergent DSD Treatment Protocol

Order of Insertion
1. Confluent points
2. Opening point
3. Trajectory points

Note: If there is tightness in the shoulders, neck, paravertebral muscles, scapulae, rhomboids, etc., gua sha these areas before commencing treatment so that trapped Wei can move.

1. Needle the Confluent points (Meeting points) with DSD technique.
BL-1 both sides, GB-22 both sides

2. Needle the Opening point with DSD technique.
SI-10

3. Needle selected, appropriate Trajectory points.
SI-10, ST-12, SI-18, HT-1, (to GB-22), CV-17 with DSD technique or SDS technique or simply superficial or simply deep depending on your intention for each individual point.

Note: The trajectory points chosen here are a sample selection only. Every treatment will be different according to the finer points of the diagnosis.

Small Intestine Divergent Channel

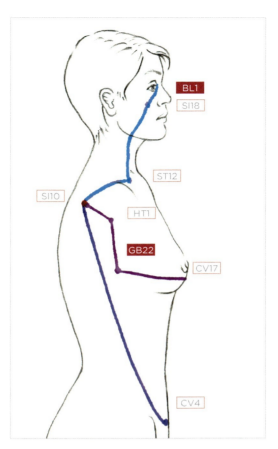
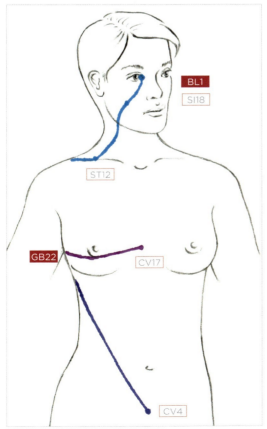
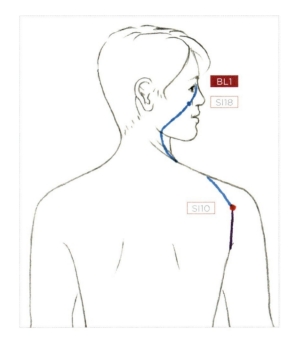

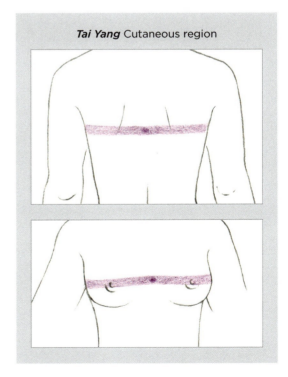
Tai Yang Cutaneous region

Small Intestine Divergent SDS Treatment Protocol

Order of Insertion

1. Gua sha cutaneous region or tight areas
2. Confluent points with cross-over
3. Opening point
4. Trajectory points
5. Jing-Well

1. Gua sha Cutaneous Regions.

If a musculoskeletal or dermatological condition, gua sha or sliding cup the Tai Yang cutaneous region "the ring around the chest" shown in the drawing or any areas of binding or tightness. If not treating a musculoskeletal or dermatological condition, begin at step 2.

2. Needle the Confluent points (Meeting points) with SDS technique.

Needle the Confluent points in a loop. Either:
  a. GB-22 (L), BL-1 (L), crossing point (e.g., GV-20), BL-1 (R), GB-22 (R), or
  b. GB-22 (R), BL-1 (R), crossing point, BL-1 (L), GB-22 (L).

3. Needle the Opening point with SDS technique.

SI-10

4. Needle selected, appropriate Trajectory points.

ST-12, SI-18, HT-1, (to GB-22), CV-17, with SDS technique or DSD technique or simply superficial or simply deep depending on your intention for each individual point.

5. Needle the Jing-Well point.

SI-1 on the same side as the last inserted Confluent point.

Frequently Asked Questions

Why does this confluence have a descending pathway?

The SI/HT confluence has both ascending and descending pathways to allow for the spectrum of depletion of Thick Fluids. By the time of the fourth confluence the body is likely no longer able to bring something up and out so the descending branch provides a trajectory to bring pathology back in (DSD). However, there may be some Thick Fluids left and so the fourth confluence also has an ascending pathway for the possibility of bringing pathology out.

HEART DIVERGENT CHANNEL

Pulses

Yin is required for Small Intestine and Heart Divergent to be able to hold a pathogen in latency. Source points of the confluence can be added. If the pulses are floating and rapid, Yin is not supporting Jing. Use Triple Heater or Pericardium Divergent instead.

Key Phrases

"Loss of Thick Fluids results in the loss of latency. Yang is unable to anchor to low back and results in the beginning of Wei atrophy." "Banks Yin to contain Heat and Wind."

Trajectory Signs

Ruddy neck with Blood showing, throbbing headaches, shoulder problems, full distended chest pain and rib pain, palpitations, stroke with loss of speech, headache with veins showing, broken capillaries on face, hemoptasis, sore throat, raw throat with Blood.

Wei Signs

Pain along the trajectory, Blood stasis leading to stroke, cardiovascular issues, palpitations, dysrhythmias, tachycardia, restlessness, insomnia, neuropathy, difficulty breathing when lying down. Heart Divergent Channel diffuses Wei to the face where it can get trapped causing constant allergies and hypersensitive face, muscular atrophy, Wei Atrophy Syndrome due to heat.

Mediumship Depletion Signs

Stroke and stroke affecting speech, seizures, disturbed sleep, dizziness on exertion, anxiety, tinnitus, speech issues, Sjogren's, Heat from the Sinews trapped in the head causing Wei atrophy, encephalitis, mania. Wei Qi trapped in limbs, Multiple Sclerosis. Heat from the Stomach and Damp from the Gallbladder dump into Small Intestine causing fermentation and malabsorption. Heat can burn intestinal lining causing autointoxication. Damp seeps into the Bladder and urination is difficult. If saturated, alternating constipation and diarrhea result. Blood deficiency signs in face, head and eyes. Severe GERD with burning hot feet, synovial fluid and cerebral spinal fluid issues. Hormonal issues.

Points

Confluent points: **GB-22, BL-1**

Opening point: **HT-1**

Trajectory points: **CV-17, CV-22, CV-23**, also from **CV-17 to CV-4**

Entire Channel: **HT-1, GB-22, CV-17, CV-22, CV-23, BL-1**. Also branch from **CV-17** to **CV-4**

Heart Divergent DSD Treatment Protocol

Order of Insertion

1. Confluent points
2. Opening point
3. Trajectory points

Note: If there is tightness in the shoulders, neck, paravertebral muscles, scapulae, rhomboids, etc., gua sha these areas before commencing treatment so that trapped Wei can move.

1. Needle the Confluent points (Meeting points) with DSD technique.

BL-1 both sides, then GB-22 both sides.

2. Needle the Opening point with DSD technique.

HT-1 either bilaterally or unilaterally on the side of the first needle inserted.

3. Needle selected, appropriate Trajectory points,

following the order of the trajectory: CV-17, CV-22, CV-23 with DSD technique or SDS technique or simply superficial or simply deep depending on your intention for each individual point.

Note: The trajectory points chosen here are a sample selection only. Every treatment will be different according to the finer points of the diagnosis.

Heart Divergent SDS Treatment Protocol

Order of Insertion

1. Gua sha cutaneous region or tight areas
2. Confluent points with cross-over
3. Opening point
4. Trajectory points
5. Jing-Well

Heart Divergent Channel

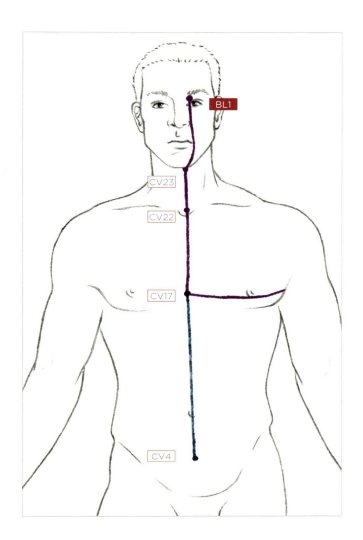

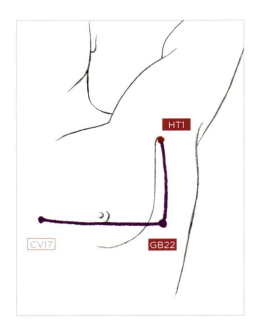

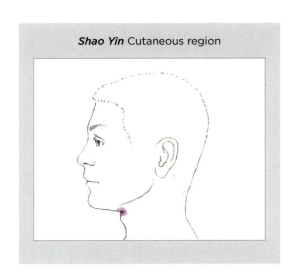

Shao Yin Cutaneous region

1. *Gua sha Cutaneous Regions.*

    If a musculoskeletal or dermatological condition, gua sha or sliding cup the Shao Yin cutaneous region: "the CV-23 area" shown in the drawing or any areas of binding or tightness. If not treating a musculoskeletal or dermatological condition, begin at step 2.

2. *Needle the Confluent points (Meeting points) with SDS technique.*

    GB-22 (L), BL-1 (L), crossing point (e.g., GV-20), BL-1 (R), GB-22 (R), or GB-22 (R), BL-1 (R), crossing point, BL-1 (L), GB-22 (L).

3. *Needle the Opening point with SDS technique.*

    HT-1 either bilaterally in the order of the sides needled in the loop, or unilaterally on the side of the first needle inserted.

4. *Needle selected, appropriate Trajectory points*

    following the order of the trajectory: CV17, CV22, CV23 with SDS technique or with different techniques on each point depending on your intention for each point.

5. *Needle the Jing-Well point.*

    HT-1 on the same side as the last inserted Confluent point.

TRIPLE HEATER DIVERGENT CHANNEL

Pulses

Floating and rapid in the chi position.

Key Phrases

"Loss of latency is complete as Fluids have been exhausted and the pathogenic factor can no longer be kept latent. Qi now has to hold the Yin in place as best it can, which also depletes the Qi." "Heat consumes structure."

What's going on at the level of Triple Heater Divergent Channel?

In the context of disease progression, the Triple Heater Divergent Channel is appropriate when the ability to maintain latency using Fluids has been lost. Two scenarios are possible at the level of Triple Heater Divergent Channel: the pathogen is moving into Marrow and causing its decline, or the pathogen is moving to the Zang Fu. Triple Heater Divergent brings Fluids to the Zang Fu to provide an emergency buffer for the pathology. Since the physiological Fluids are depleted already, Triple Heater Divergent mobilizes Dampness (pathological Fluids) to hold the pathology and slow its progression to the organs. Because Yin is absent, Heat is present in the Triple Heater scenario. When the body utilizes Dampness in the presence of Heat, Phlegm results. With Triple Heater Divergent Channel treatments we are directing some extra Qi to the body to keep that Damp around the pathogen so it doesn't spread to the organs. This is why nodules appear. At the same time, Qi is being used to transform Phlegm so that some Yin can be freed to hold onto the pathogen. SDS is not advised because we don't want to break up these nodules yet and there is no fluid to release them anyway.

Triple Heater Divergent Channel addresses the four regions which are often the first areas affected when latency is lost: the chest (especially the breasts), the neck, the throat and sensory orifices, and the bone. If a pathogen cannot be held in latency it can easily spread to these areas, creating pathology such as cancer, especially if the pathogen is a fire toxin.

Heat combined with the deficient Yin also results in Wind. Wind stirs and Yang ascends because there is not enough Yin to anchor Yang down. GV-20 which is the first point on the trajectory of Triple Heater Divergent Channel consolidates Yin in the Lower Jiao, especially the uterus, and holds Yin in place, again using Qi. Loss of appetite and shortness of breath occur at Triple Heater because there is little or no Qi remaining at CV-12, so the descending pathway of Triple Heater Divergent Channel connects to the Middle Jiao. As Heat attempts to ventilate itself, chills and fever or Wind-Heat signs can emerge intermittently. Here the pathogenic factor is out of control and Triple Heater breaks down the Marrow (including the brain, bone, Curious Organs, Marrow) because until the point of death, there is always Jing available. Triple Heater directs fluid in response to heat and utilizes Stomach Fluids to cool off the heat. Because Fluids are the easiest medium to bank, you might on occasion choose to use ST/SP DSD concurrently.

Trajectory Signs
Nodules and swellings

Wei Signs
Pain along the trajectory, neuropathy, earache, difficulty lifting arms and head, tinnitus, hot Phlegm in throat, lateral neck pain, poor appetite, loss of appetite, chronic Damp-Heat in the joints, limbs, sinews, and connective tissues. Tight throat, dry lips

Triple Heater Divergent Channel

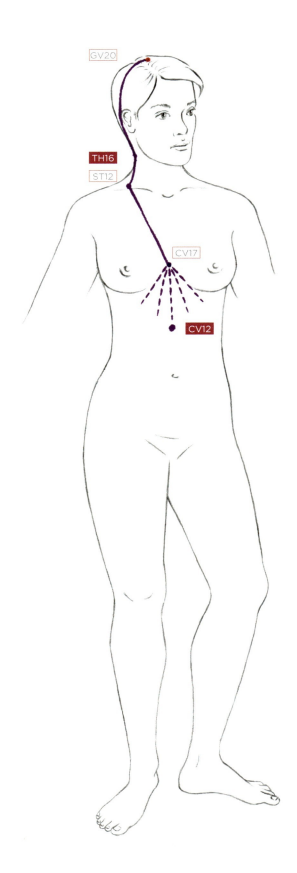
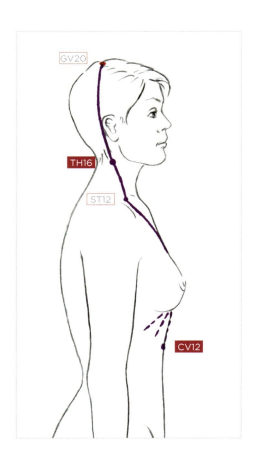
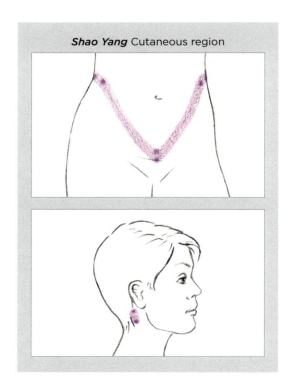

Shao Yang Cutaneous region

and mouth, difficulty swallowing, pain along trajectory. Damp-Heat leads to Wei atrophy, Wei Qi becomes trapped in the limbs, paralysis. Atrophy of the limbs, inflamed joints, rheumatoid arthritis, fibromyalgia, chronic hepatitis, pancreatitis, gastritis, inflammation of the Zang Fu, Wei Atrophy Syndrome due to Damp-Heat.

Mediumship Mobilization Signs

Excess mucus, Phlegm accumulation, excess fluid, nasal discharge.

Mediumship Depletion Signs

Disturbed Shen, restlessness, irritability, malar flush, delirium, seizures, organ inflammation, ORGAN FAILURE, visceral and constitutional changes, chronic Damp-Heat issues (Multiple Sclerosis, fibromyalgia, rheumatoid arthritis), heat exhaustion, non-healing sores, ulcers, joint inflammation and deformity, infections that are difficult to treat, head numbness due to heat, heat stirs chronic seizures and delirium, inability to engage with the world. Cancers can begin here.

Points

Confluent points: **TH-16, CV-12**
Opening point: **GV-20**
Trajectory points: **GB-12, ST-12, CV-17**
Entire Channel: **GV-20, TH-16, GB-12, ST-12, CV-17, CV-12**

This channel is usually needled DSD if used in the context of a pathological progression because latency has been lost. If needled for a musculoskeletal condition diagnosed on the basis of the trajectory, it can be needled SDS.

The neck and pelvis must be released every treatment in order for Triple Heater Divergent to work. "Windows to the Sky"[6] and "Doorways to the Earth" points can be used to do this. This is true whether needling DSD or SDS because the channel must be free to move Qi. You are freeing up Yin to create latency.

---

[6] Windows to the Sky is a European term; it does not appear in Chinese Medical literature. Doorways to the Earth is a term coined by Dr. Yuen.

Triple Heater Divergent DSD Treatment Protocol

Order of Insertion
1. Confluent points
2. Opening point
3. Trajectory points

Note: If there is tightness in the shoulders, neck, paravertebral muscles, scapulae, rhomboids, etc., gua sha these areas before commencing treatment so that trapped Wei can move.

1. Needle the Confluent points (Meeting points).
TH-16 both sides, then CV-12 with DSD technique.

2. Needle the Opening point.
GV-20 with DSD technique.

3. Needle selected, appropriate Trajectory points following the order of the trajectory.
GB-12, ST-12, CV-17 with DSD technique or SDS technique or simply superficial or simply deep depending on your intention for each individual point.

Note: The trajectory points chosen here are a sample selection only. Every treatment will be different according to the finer points of the diagnosis.

Note: Triple Heater Divergent Channel does not connect to the Lower Jiao.

Triple Heater Divergent SDS Treatment Protocol

Order of Insertion
1. Gua sha cutaneous region or tight areas
2. Confluent points
3. Opening point
4. Trajectory points
5. Jing-Well

1. Gua sha Cutaneous Regions.
If a musculoskeletal or dermatological condition, gua sha or sliding cup the three Shao Yang cutaneous regions shown in the drawing or any areas of binding or tightness. If not treating a musculoskeletal or dermatological condition, begin at step 2.

2. Needle the Confluent points (Meeting points).

Needle the Confluent points in a loop with SDS technique. Either:
- a. TH-16 (L), CV-12, TH-16 (R), or
- b. TH-16 (R), CV-12, TH-16 (L)

3. Needle the Opening point.

GV-20 with SDS technique.

4. Needle selected, appropriate Trajectory points

following the order of the trajectory: GB-12, ST-12, CV-17 with SDS technique or DSD technique or simply superficial or simply deep depending on your intention for each individual point.

5. Needle the Jing-Well point.

TH-1 on the same side as the last inserted Confluent point.

Clinical Tips

The neck and pelvis can be released with Sinew releases which are not described in this text, or with gua sha or cups on GB-30 and TH-16.

In the *Su Wen* the Triple Heater Divergent Channel has a different trajectory: GB-22, CV-17, ST-12, TH-16, GV-20, out to chest, and three Jiao's. It lists the Confluent points as GB-12 and GB-22.

PERICARDIUM DIVERGENT CHANNEL

Key Phrases

"Severe loss of Fluids and Blood. Regulates Blood by regulating Qi."

Trajectory Signs

Hot palms, malar flush, chest fullness or oppression, axillary pain, chest pain.

Wei Signs

Pain along the trajectory, chest fullness or oppression.

Mediumship Depletion Signs

Disturbed Shen, restlessness, irritability, palpitations, mania and depression (heat and Qi deficiency), confusion, insomnia, hot Phlegm, hot palms, malar flush, chest fullness, chest oppression, infections, hemorrhage, visceral and structural constitutional change, gut hypersensitivity, severe tooth decay, Carpal Tunnel Syndrome, opportunistic infections, inability to support Yin, inability to confront external pathogenic factors. EPFs go to the bloodstream, infections, heat along the clavicle, hot hands, sub-axillary swellings, dry throat, mouth, loss of Essence, heat consumes the structure, constant thirst.

Points

Confluent points: **TH-16, CV-12**
Opening point: **GB-22**
Trajectory points: **PC-1, CV-17, ST-12, CV-23, GB-12**
Entire channel: **GB-22, PC-1, CV-17, CV-12** and **ST-12, CV-23, TH-16, GB-12**

This channel is usually needled DSD if used in the context of a pathological progression because latency has been lost. If needled for a musculoskeletal condition diagnosed on the basis of the trajectory, or if used to move a pathogen out of the Pericardium, e.g., pericarditis, it can be needled SDS.

Opening the Neck and Pelvis

Opening the neck and the pelvis is important in a treatment of the fifth confluence which uses Qi to try to assist in latency. If Qi is blocked it's not available for use by the Triple Heater Divergent Channel. A very effective way to open the neck and pelvis is to use the "Windows to the Sky" and "Doorways to the Earth" points.

Choose the WTS and DTE points according to the point function. Below is a condensed list of these functions. If you choose this method, be sure to gua sha if the point is very tight. Or, you could gua sha instead of needling altogether. Also, you might consider pairing up your choices with a zonally related point in the series to enhance the opening, e.g., if you choose TH-16, pair it with the Shao Yang DTE point, GB-30, or e.g., SP-12 with a Tai Yin WTS point, LU-3.

Pericardium Divergent Channel

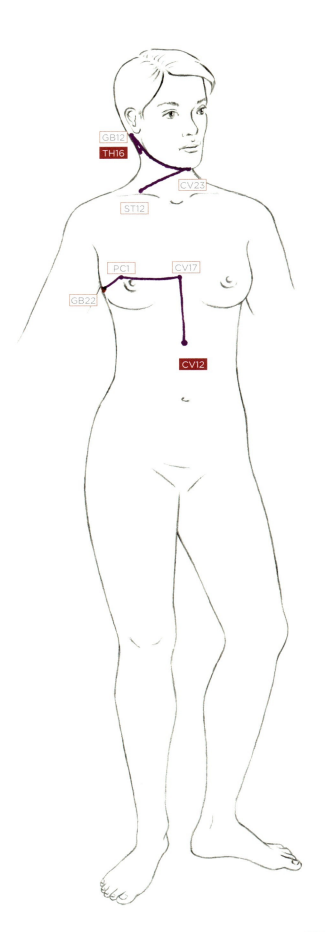
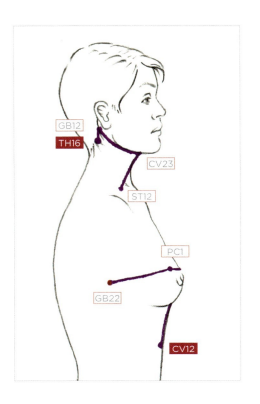
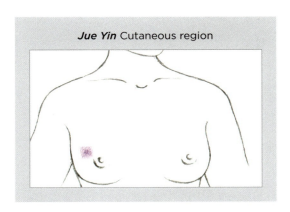

Jue Yin Cutaneous region

10 Windows to the Sky Points		12 Doorways to the Earth Points	
BL-10	descends excess Yang from head to chest	BL-40	descends excess Yin from the pelvis
SI-16	ascends Yang to the head	KI-11	for rigidity in the Lower Jiao
SI-17	ascends Yin to the head	GB-30	descends Yin to the pelvis
TH-16	descends excess Yin from the head and neck. Allows the neck to turn	LR-12	treats blockages at the genitalia
ST-9	ascends Yang to the head	ST-30	ascends Yin to the pelvis from the legs
LI-18	ascends Yang to all sensory orifices to encourage expression	SP-12	moves Blood stasis
LU-3	ascends Yang to the chest	GV-4	treats deficient Yang
PC-1	descends Yin from the head	GV-1	treats collapse of Yang
CV-22	ascends Yang to the head from the chest and descends Yin	BL-35	treats deficient Yang resulting in systemic cold
GV-16	descends Yang to the Lower Jiao	CV-1	treats empty heat
		CV-2	builds Blood
		CV-4	treats deficient Yin

Pericardium Divergent DSD Treatment Protocol

Order of Insertion

1. Confluent points in descending order
2. Opening point
3. Trajectory points

Note: If there is tightness in the shoulders, neck, paravertebral muscles, scapulae, rhomboids, etc., gua sha these areas before commencing treatment so that trapped Wei can move.

1. Needle the Confluent points (Meeting points).

TH-16 both sides, then CV-12 with DSD technique.

2. Needle the Opening point.

GB-22 either bilaterally or unilaterally on the side of the first needle inserted with DSD technique.

3. Needle selected, appropriate Trajectory points following the order of the trajectory.

E.g., PC-1, CV-17, ST-12, CV-23 with DSD technique or SDS technique or simply superficial or simply deep depending on your intention for each individual point.

Note: The trajectory points chosen here are a sample selection only. Every treatment will be different according to the finer points of the diagnosis.

Pericardium Divergent SDS Treatment Protocol

Order of Insertion

1. Gua sha cutaneous region or tight areas
2. Confluent points with cross-over
3. Opening point
4. Trajectory points
5. Jing-Well

1. Gua sha Cutaneous Regions.

If a musculoskeletal or dermatological condition, gua sha or sliding cup the *Jue Yin* cutaneous region: "the PC-1 area" shown in the drawing or any areas of binding or tightness. If not treating a musculoskeletal or dermatological condition, begin at step 2.

2. Needle the Confluent points (Meeting points).

TH-16 both sides, then CV-12 with SDS technique.

3. Needle the Opening point.

GB-22 either bilaterally in the order of the sides needled in the loop, or unilaterally on the side of the first needle inserted with SDS technique.

4. Needle selected, appropriate Trajectory points following the order of the trajectory.

E.g., with selected points (if the Confluent points were started on the left): PC-1 (L), CV-17, ST-12 (R), CV-23 with SDS technique or DSD technique or simply superficial or simply deep depending on your intention for each individual point.

5. Needle the Jing-Well point.

PC-9 on the same side as the last inserted Confluent point.

LARGE INTESTINE DIVERGENT CHANNEL

Pulses

At the sixth confluence, the Large Intestine and Lung Divergents, Yang is nearly lost. The pulses will be slow and the tongue could be purple or blue.

Key Phrases

"End stage. Yang is nearly lost. Full-blown Jing deficiency. Movement and warmth are compromised."

At the Large Intestine Divergent Channel Yang is lost. Therefore the swellings cannot be expelled by the Lungs, transformed by the Spleen or dissolved or dissipated by the Kidneys because each of these processes requires Yang.

GV-14 is a crucial point here as a convergence of Yang; it brings what Yang might be available in the Du Channel to hold the pathology away from the Primary Channel sequence where it has access to the organs.

Trajectory Signs

Abdominal pain, as Wei and Jing try to carry out the pathogenic factor, nodules and cysts or nodules in shoulder, inflamed shoulder, chest and flank fullness, breast lumps.

Wei Signs

Pain along the trajectory, rhinitis, sinusitis, sense of pressure in the ears with intermittent inability to hear, alopecia, severe reflux and nausea, heat sensation in Lungs, failure of Wei Qi, hives, cockcrow diarrhea, ascites, shingles, itch, shortness of breath, asthma, dyspnea, wheezing, late stage Crohn's disease, abdominal pain, shoulder pain, chest and flank fullness and tightness, inflamed shoulder.

Mediumship Mobilization Signs

Excess mucus, excess fluid, nasal discharge. Nodules and cysts in the shoulder as Wei and Jing try to move. Abdominal lumps, cysts, polyps, abscesses, dysentery, tiredness after bowel movements.

Mediumship Depletion Signs

Hair loss as Jing cannot traverse the neck, failure to grow hair, pressure in ears, inability

Large Intestine Divergent Channel

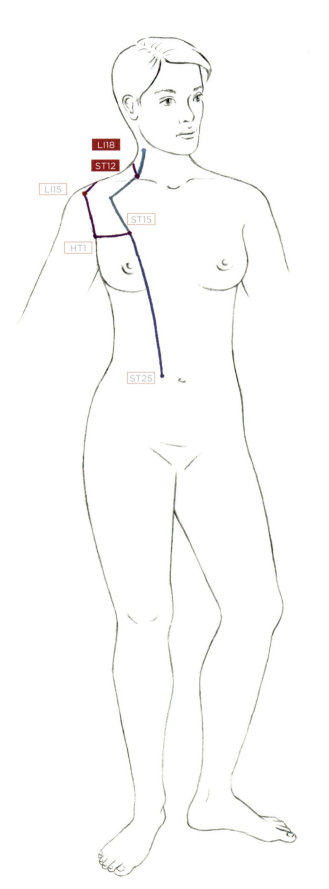
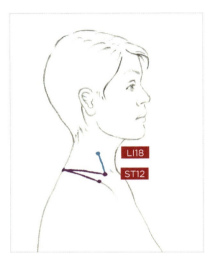
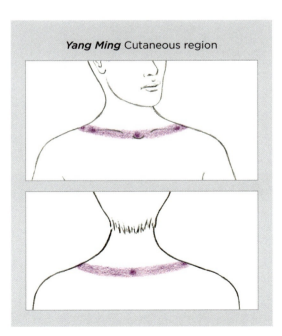

Yang Ming Cutaneous region

to hear well, chronic post nasal drip, poor growth in Upper Jiao, heat in Upper Jiao, chronic allergies, wheezing, distention fullness, congestion in chest, goiter, lumps in breast, chest, throat, abdomen, intestinal polyps and abscesses.

Points

Confluent points: **ST-12, LI-18**

Opening point: **LI-15**

Trajectory points: **GV-14.** Branch 1: **LI-15, HT-1, ST-15.** Branch 2 from **ST-15** to **ST-25.** Branch 3 from **ST15** to **LU-1, ST-12, LI-18.**

Entire channel: **LI-15, GV-14, ST-12, LI-18.** Branch 1: **LI-15, HT-1, ST-15.** Branch 2 from **ST-15 to ST-25.** Branch 3 from **ST15 to LU-1, ST-12, LI-18.**

Note: This channel is usually needled DSD if used in the context of a pathological progression because latency has been lost. If needled for a musculoskeletal condition diagnosed on the basis of the trajectory, or if using it to remove a pathogen from the Large Intestine, it can be needled SDS unless you're seeking latency for that pathogen. Add the lower He-Sea point for the Large Intestine (ST-37) in the case of the latter.

Large Intestine Divergent DSD Treatment Protocol

Order of Insertion

1. Confluent points
2. Opening point
3. Trajectory points

Note: If there is tightness in the shoulders, neck, paravertebral muscles, scapulae, rhomboids, etc., gua sha these areas before commencing treatment so that trapped Wei can move.

1. Needle the Confluent points (Meeting points).

LI-18 both sides, then ST-12 both sides with DSD technique.

2. Needle the Opening point.

LI-15 with DSD technique.

3. Needle selected, appropriate Trajectory points.

E.g., GV-14, CV-23, LI-15, HT-1, ST-15 with DSD technique or SDS technique or simply superficial or simply deep depending on your intention for each individual point.

Large Intestine Divergent SDS Treatment Protocol

Order of Insertion

1. Gua sha cutaneous region or tight areas
2. Confluent points with cross-over point
3. Opening point
4. Trajectory points
5. Jing-Well

1. Gua sha Cutaneous Regions.

If a musculoskeletal or dermatological condition, gua sha or sliding cup the Yang Ming cutaneous regions shown in the drawing or any areas of binding or tightness. If not treating a musculoskeletal or dermatological condition, begin at step 2.

2. Needle the Confluent points (Meeting points).

Needle the Confluent points in a loop with SDS technique. Either:
ST-12 (L), LI-18 (L), crossover point (e.g., GV20), LI-18 (R), ST-12 (R) or
ST-12 (R), LI-18 (R), crossover point (e.g., GV20), LI-18 (L), ST-12 (L).

3. Needle the Opening point: LI-15

4. Needle selected, appropriate Trajectory points

following the order of the trajectory with selected points: GV-14, CV-23, LI-15, HT-1, ST-15 with SDS technique or DSD technique or simply superficial or simply deep depending on your intention for each individual point.

5. Needle the Jing-Well point.

LI-1 on the same side as the last inserted Confluent point.

Note: The trajectory points chosen here are a sample selection only. Every treatment will be different according to the finer points of the diagnosis.

Note: If there is tightness in the shoulders, neck, paravertebral muscles, scapulae, rhomboids, etc., gua sha these areas before commencing treatment so that trapped Wei can move.

LUNG DIVERGENT CHANNEL

Pulses

At the sixth confluence, the Large Intestine and Lung Divergents, Yang is lost. The pulses will be slow and the tongue could be purple or blue.

Key Phrases

"Brings Wei Qi to join the Primary Channels and the Zang Fu at ST-12 where the Primary Channels meet, and at LU-1 where the Primary Channel sequence begins. This channel, the final Divergent Channel, then goes to the breast, and to GB-8 where it siphons Yang from Du Mai in an attempt to move the pathogenic factor. The pathogenic factor enters the Primary Channels and therefore the organs. Wei Qi is severely depleted. Chronic failure of Wei Qi to defend on a longterm basis because Wei Qi is trapped, stagnant or severely depleted. Yang starts to collapse altogether and latency is gone. The pathogenic factor is revealed and unchecked. End-stage disease."

As Qi collapses, the patient could have spontaneous sweat while trying to move the pathogenic factor out. The last remaining Yang Qi (Wei Qi) is sent to the Primary Channels in an effort to save the organs.

Trajectory Signs

Rapid breathing, chest fullness, cough and wheeze, chest oppression, pain down Lung Channel.

Wei Signs

Pain along the trajectory, inflamed shoulder and clavicle, swollen lymph nodes, goiters, epilepsy, seizures, convulsions, madness, chronic respiratory tract infections, pneumonia, cardiac and respiratory failure, facial edema, cellulitis, axilla pain, pain at GB-22, *Running Piglet Qi*, swellings on the breast, increased susceptibility to Wind-Cold conditions, nasal congestion, chills and fever with great weakness underlying them.

Mediumship Depletion Signs

Dry cough with blood, restlessness, anemia, leukemia, degeneration of the organs, heat in palms, hemoptysis, spontaneous sweat, Heart failure, pulmonary failure, wasting of internal organs, escaping Yang.

Lung Divergent Channel

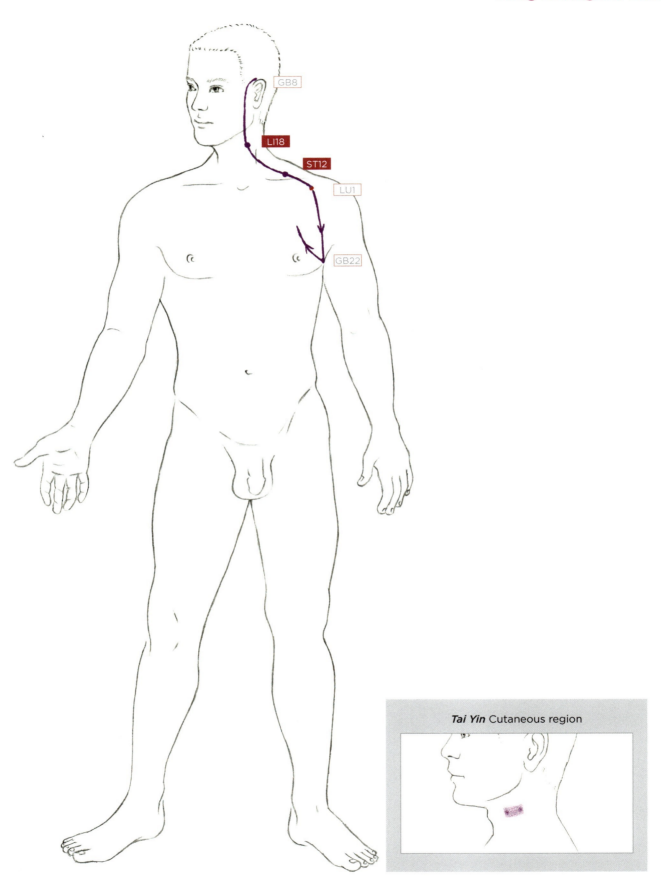

Tai Yin Cutaneous region

Points

Confluent points: ST-12, LI-18
Opening point: LU-1
Trajectory points: GB-22
Entire Channel: LU-1, GB-22, LU-1, ST-12, LI-18, GB-8 (temple)

Note: This channel is usually needled DSD if used in the context of a pathological progression because latency has been lost. If needled for a musculoskeletal condition diagnosed on the basis of the trajectory, or for the removal of a pathogenic factor from the Lungs, it can be needled SDS. Add the He-Sea point to support the Lung organ in the latter case.

Lung Divergent DSD Treatment Protocol

Order of Insertion

1. Confluent points
2. Opening point
3. Trajectory points

Note: If there is tightness in the shoulders, neck, paravertebral muscles, scapulae, rhomboids, etc., gua sha these areas before commencing treatment so that trapped Wei can move.

1. Needle the Confluent points (Meeting points).

LI-18 both sides, then ST-12 both sides with DSD technique.

2. Needle the Opening point.

LU-1 either bilaterally or unilaterally on the side of the first needle inserted with DSD technique.

3. Needle GB-22 and release holding areas around the breast with DSD technique.

Note: Needle around the breast because the trajectory goes there. Palpate where Wei Qi is pooling around the breast (or use ST-12 if breast is to be avoided). Also palpate BL-13 and BL-41 for sensitive points to release the pooling of Wei Qi so that it can circulate. Lung Divergent is used when there is much Phlegm.

Lung Divergent SDS Treatment Protocol

Order of Insertion

1. Gua sha cutaneous region or tight areas
2. Confluent points with cross-over
3. Opening point
4. Trajectory points
5. Jing-Well

1. Gua sha Cutaneous Regions.

If a musculoskeletal or dermatological condition, gua sha or sliding cup the Tai Yin cutaneous region: "the band at the throat area" shown in the drawing or any areas of binding or tightness. If not treating a musculoskeletal or dermatological condition, begin at step 2.

2. Needle the Confluent points (Meeting points) with SDS technique.

Needle the Confluent points in a loop with SDS technique. Either:
ST-12 (L), LI-18 (L), crossover point, LI-18 (R), ST-12 (R) or
ST-12 (R), LI-18 (R), crossover point, LI-18 (L), ST-12 (L).

3. Needle the Opening point.

LU-1 either bilaterally (in the order of the sides needled in the loop if looping), or unilaterally on the side of the first needle inserted with SDS technique.

4. Needle GB-22 and release holding areas around the breast with SDS technique.

5. Needle the Jing-Well point.

LU-11 on the same side as the last inserted Confluent point.

Note: In cases of the collapse of Yang Qi, moxa the Jing-Well points.

Essential Oils and Divergent Channel Treatments

Essential Oil Complementary Treatments (Simple)

A minuscule amount of essential oil is applied to the Confluent points only. A good way to achieve this is to give the patient a toothpick and instruct them to simply touch the toothpick to the rim of the bottle to pick up the tiniest amount possible and touch it to all the points without re-touching the bottle. It's often difficult to impress upon the patient how small an amount is needed. The skin should not glisten with oil at all. There are a number of reasons for using tiny amounts of oil, including:

A minuscule amount of oil provides the maximum amount of stimulation to the point. More than a tiny amount floods the nerve receptors and the body switches them off, rendering the oil relatively useless.

More than a minuscule amount on BL-1 can be dangerous as it can migrate to the eye on naturally oily skin. If you are really worried about oil at BL-1, use LI-20.

Many oils will burn the skin if the skin is moistened by the oil.

If you think the patient is likely to apply too much oil, prescribe a 10% dilution of the essential oil in caulophyllum oil if SDS or in sesame or jojoba oil if DSD.

	SDS	DSD
BL/KI DC	Peppermint or Pine	Fennel
GB/LR DC	Lemon	Rosemary
ST/SP DC	Ginger or Mugwort	Petitgrain
SI/HT DC	Ylang Ylang	Frankincense
TH/PC DC	Blue Chamomile or Myrrh	Rosewood or Ho Leaf
LI/LU DC	Eucalyptus or Cypress	Pine

Essential Oil Complementary Treatments (Complex)

This selection of oils is not necessarily more desirable than those on the simple list above. Choices between simple and complex should be made on the basis of diagnosis and knowledge of the oils so that you can determine the ratios of the oils within the blend. Generally speaking, in SDS treatments the higher of the two notes, the top (T) or middle (M) are mixed at double the volume of the lower note, often a base note (B). In DSD treatments the reverse is true; the lower note is mixed at double the volume of the higher note.

	SDS	DSD
BL/KI DC	Jasmine (B) and Pine (T)	Celery Seed (M) and Basil (T)
GB/LR DC	German Chamomile (M) and Bergamot (T)	Angelica Seed (B) and Fir (M)
ST/SP DC	Coriander Seed (M) and Clove (T)	Carrot Seed (M) and Cypress (B)
SI/HT DC	Myrrh (B) and Tangerine (T)	Caraway Seed (M) and Pine (T)
TH/PC DC	Frankincense (B) and Peppermint (T)	Spikenard (B)
LI/LU DC	Elemi (B) and Peppermint (T)	Cinnamon Bark (B) and Benzoin (B) (two bases)

Zonal Divergent Channel Treatments

A Zonal Divergent Channel treatment connects the zonally corresponding Divergent Channels:

Tai Yang:	BL and SI Divergent Channels
Shao Yang:	GB and TH Divergent Channels
Yang Ming:	ST and LI Divergent Channels
Tai Yin:	SP and LU Divergent Channels
Shao Yin:	HT and KI Divergent Channels
Jue Yin:	LR and PC Divergent Channels

A Zonal Divergent Channel Treatment

a. Involves releasing the cutaneous regions associated with the individual Divergent Channel, using gua sha or sliding cups.
b. Always includes the confluent/meeting points.
c. Is used to release a musculoskeletal or dermatological condition.

Generally speaking, chronic conditions require elemental Divergent treatments and acute conditions (especially those that involve more than one location) require Zonal Divergent treatment. Acute is difficult to define outside the context of specific clinical presentations because each case is unique. Very generally, in terms of Divergent theory, a condition of less than three weeks duration is acute. Use your clinical judgment on a case-by-case basis.

THE CUTANEOUS REGIONS
(Illustrated with the Divergent Channels)

Historically, the cutaneous regions are most often depicted as a shield over the body. They are used to release a pathogenic factor that has not impeded movement, and are treated simply by needling the Jing-Well related to the cutaneous region and the ah shi along the channel. They are not diagnosed through movement assessment as the Sinew Channels are.

The cutaneous regions used in conjunction with the Divergent Channels, however, are different, smaller and more complex. These cutaneous regions are subsets of the historically earlier, broader, all-enveloping cutaneous regions. Like the Sinew Channels, all cutaneous regions conduct Wei Qi. In the Divergent arena, they are the Wei Qi level connection of the zonally paired Divergent Channels (BL/SI, GB/TH, ST/LI, SP/LU, HT/KI, LR/PC). They are gua sha'd or treated with a sliding cup in zonal and looping treatments. The patient is preferably sitting for gua sha. This position yields the greatest amount of sha.

The Cutaneous Regions
(of the Divergent Channels)

Note: The points listed below are just for guidance in location. The cutaneous regions have no points and are not point-specific, rather, they are relatively wide areas.

Tai Yang   "The ring around the chest" that begins at GB-22 and wraps all the way around the chest via CV-17, BL-44, BL-15, GV-11, back to GB-22.

Shao Yang   Two or three areas:
- a. The mastoid process: the area encompassing GB-12 and TH-16. This zone is sometimes said to go up to TH-18 and even TH-19.
- b. The area delineated by the floating ribs: LR-13 and GB-25
- c. Sometimes an additional area is referred to: a band from GB-25 to CV-2 and CV-3.

Yang Ming   "The ring around the collar." It begins at GV-14, then to GB-21, towards SI-12, ST-12, CV-22 and then back to where it began, at GV-14.

Tai Yin   "The Band at the Throat" that encompasses ST-9, LI-18 and SI-16.

Shao Yin   An area the size of a postage stamp at CV-23.

Jue Yin   An area the size of a postage stamp at PC-1.

Zonal Divergent Protocol

1. Gua sha or sliding cup the cutaneous region pertaining to the Divergent Channel. These regions are shown in each Divergent Channel drawing as a shaded area.
2. Follow the directions for a regular SDS Divergent treatment and add the Jing-Well point of both zonally related Divergent Channels: e.g., BL-67 and SI-1.
3. Release ah shi points along the trajectory of the Sinew Channel to which the Jing-Wells belong, without retaining the needle.

If it helps with intention, the Confluent points of the Sinew Channels can be added to prevent transmission to the next zonal pair. For example, in BL/SI, one could needle (even) SI-18 to prevent transmission to the Shao Yang zonal confluence.

Frequently Asked Questions about Zonal Divergents and the Cutaneous Regions

1. *Why is gua sha done before the insertion of the needles?* Gua sha summons Wei Qi to the surface, making it ready for the instructions imparted to it by the Divergent Channel needling.

2. *How can I gua sha the front of the chest during a BL/KI or BL/SI Divergent treatment?* Gua sha of the cutaneous regions is done before the treatment, so ideally the patient is sitting at that time. It's quite astonishing how much more sha emerges when the zones are gua sha'd with the patient in sitting position. If the patient is unable to sit, either gua sha the anterior aspect of the ring first and flip them over. If the patient can only be prone for the entire treatment, just make sure that you really get into GB-22 on both sides as you gua sha the posterior half of the ring around the chest. Gua sha on only the posterior aspect is adequate in those cases because GB-22, as a Sinew Confluent point, is a major Sinew release point and governs the Tai Yang cutaneous region.

3. *What if no sha emerges when I gua sha or cup?* If no sha comes out (if no Blood becomes visible under the surface of the skin) the patient is Qi or Blood deficient and fewer needles must be used in the Divergent treatment in order to avoid exhausting the patient.

4. **What do I do if I've followed the protocol and the pain is not fully resolved in any zonal treatment?** Strongly reduce BL-63.

5. **Is it possible to gua sha the zones and do an SDS treatment within an hour?** Yes, an SDS treatment including gua sha of the cutaneous regions can be completed within an hour as long as only pertinent points on the trajectory are chosen.

The Eight Extraordinary Channels

THE EIGHT EXTRAORDINARY CHANNELS TREATMENTS

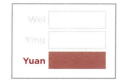

Also known as the Curious Channels, the Mysterious Channels

Historical References to the Eight Extraordinary Channels

Chapter 27 of the *Nan Jing* states clearly that the Eight Extraordinary Channels (hereafter called the Eight Extras) are beyond the reach of the twelve Primary Channels. It says, "The ancient sages [the Kidneys] constructed ditches and reservoirs for the waterways [the Primary Channels] in the event of something extraordinary [the overflow of resources or overflow of pathology]. When rain pours down from Heaven, the ditches and reservoirs [the Eight Extra Channels] become full. The ditches are beyond reach of the Primary Channels." This means that surplus resources are stored in the Eight Extras but we can't access that richness (in good health) or the pathology (in compromised health) with the 12 Primary Channels.

Until the 11th century, although practitioners had the knowledge to be able to tap into the Eight Extras (the ancient practices of Yang Sheng were focused on transmuting Jing and longevity), it was strongly believed that it was unethical for a practitioner to tap into them because they contain the sacred blueprint of our existence including the sequence of its realization or unfolding. To interfere by treating the Eight Extras was considered hubris. To be playing Creator was considered unethical medical practice. There is still a resonance of these issues of ethics in modern medicine in the debates we have now about stem cell use and DNA manipulation.

Prior to the 11th century, the Eight Extras were discussed theoretically only; they were revered as the channels of transformation. But in the Song Dynasty, during the neo-Confucianist period—after the Tang Dynasty saw a decline in Daoism and Buddhism—the philosopher Zhu Xi said that since Ming-Destiny[1] is in one's own hands, we must be able to tap into destiny and its carrier, Jing. At this point, the Eight Extras ceased being viewed only as channels of transformation and began to be seen as channels of intervention. The idea that we may be able to retard aging and direct postnatal Qi to the prenatal level to replenish Essence, began to proliferate. So the actual practice of

---

[1] Ming actually translates as fate and refers to the genetics we have been given. Yun is the term commonly used in Chinese Medicine meaning destiny and refers to cosmic influences. Here I am using the word destiny in its more informal sense.

the Eight Extras originates from that time. Later, in the Ming Dynasty, Li Shi Zhen (1518-1593) summarized treatment methodology and the Eight Extras not only became accessible, they became channels of practical intervention.

Zhu Xi developed and promoted the idea that pre-determined destiny—which can elicit passive acceptance of one's limiting facets—was equally balanced by the notion of free will. That notion allows for the taking of responsibility for one's actions and being able to change one's nature through one's will. We can change our destiny by needling into the Eight Extras and altering the genetic code, altering our nature. This is the essential gravity of these remarkable channels. To enter into that code is an action to be taken with great reverence, by invitation, and with extreme care.

WARNING: *The Eight Extra Channels are only for the treatment of Yuan-level (Constitutional level) imbalances and illnesses. Surprisingly, some acupuncturists elect to use Eight Extra Channels in the treatment of exterior conditions such as the common cold. It is in plain violation of the principles of acupuncture to do so. There is no need or reason to tap into the most precious level of Qi, the Yuan-Source (constitutional) Qi—the deepest level of an individual's existence—when a simple Wei Qi level treatment will suffice. Similarly, the use of the Eight Extra Channels in vanity treatments, including certain currently popular (but not all) facelift treatments, gravely disrespects Yuan Qi. Utilizing this Qi by bringing it and its Fluids to the surface ultimately shortens life and speeds aging through the exhaustion of Yuan Qi. These practices should be strictly avoided for the health of patients and for the health of the practice of acupuncture itself.*

Mechanisms of the Eight Extraordinary Channels

The Eight Extras are conduits of constitutional Qi (Yuan Qi). Yuan Qi contains our ancestral inheritance, our nature. The Eight Extras therefore govern the creation of form. The first Eight Extra, the Chong, is the blueprint; it's like a set of construction drawings. The Ren Channel is like a warehouse that stores or provides the materials (Yin) for the building. The Du is like the construction crew that provides the energy (Yang) to build the being, according to the blueprint stored in the Chong. The building performs its function in space, aging and changing through time. The Wei Channels govern the assimilation of these changes. The Qiao Channels reflect the present.

The building inspector can give a report on the building's current status (Yin Qiao) and also how the building now fits into the streetscape, its current context (Yang Qiao).

The Wei Channels record the way in which the building came to be the way it is. The building inspector might document the changes the building has undergone in its long history (Yin Wei Mai) and make predictions about how it will age in the future, and what the building will need (Yang Wei Mai). The Dai Mai would function as storage, sanitation, and a clearing house for trash.

The Eight Extras treat issues relating to gender, sexual identity, ethnicity, humanity, growth, maturity, development, sexual function, conception and pregnancy. They derive their Qi from the Essence of the Kidneys.

The Eight Extras are also reservoirs of surplus Qi. Excess Blood and Qi can be banked back into these channels.

Since the Eight Extra Channels are responsible for the replication of RNA and DNA, they are responsible for the management or latency of factors that affect the DNA and RNA reproduction. These factors include all carcinogens, xenobiotics, all plastics, heavy metals, vaccines, saccharine, aspartame, petroleum derivatives, and anything else that can affect the DNA. The Eight Extras either hold the pathogenic factor in the Jing-Essence, or they produce changes in the DNA to enable the body to tolerate the pathogen. These changes can take generations to complete.

Evolutionary pressure is responded to at the level of the Eight Extras. The Eight Extra Channels govern evolution. Interestingly, the major evolutionary differences between apes, early humans and modern humans are not in the Zang Fu organs as much as in the Curious Organs, particularly the skeleton, and the brain and uterus it houses. It's the skull, brain, stance and gait that show the characteristics of evolutionary change, while Liver and Kidney function, for example, change very little.

In a given lifetime we experience a micro evolution. Changes occur in the structure, the brain, the reproductive organs, and the Blood vessels when we experience, for example, osteoporosis, arthritis, Alzheimer's Disease, or changes in fertility and circulation. All these changes occur in the presence of pathology, under the influence of the Eight Extra Channels.

The Eight Extras also govern the cycles of birth, maturity and death and the rate at which maturity occurs. This includes pathological growth at the level of Yuan-Source

Qi which in common terms would be considered cancer.

As the Eight Extraordinary Channels are vessels of evolution, they allow for the perpetuation of the species through procreation and adaptation. When a new life is conceived, the fetus receives the imprint of the pathology residing in the parents' Marrow. This happens because the Jing offered to create a new life contains the Shen (the Spirit) of the parents and also their Marrow which in turn holds the experiences of their lives thus far. This is how illnesses can be seen to run in the family. These can include asthma, allergies, dermatological, digestive, organ, and even psychological issues. Inherited and congenital issues are treated with the Eight Extras.

Chapter 71 of the *Ling Shu* explains that the Eight Extra Channels bring Zong-Ancestral Qi up from the chest, enabling it to express through the throat, larynx, and the Heart as it manifests in the eyes. They allow our eyes and our voice to beam the inner light that glows when we are living our destiny. In the greatest sense, the freeing of Eight Extras enables us to accept ourselves and to view our circumstances at all times as opportunities for our spirit to shine.

Indications for the Use of the Eight Extraordinary Channels

The Eight Extraordinary Channels are used for intervention in:

1. Physical, psychological or emotional issues that originated in childhood in the first cycle of seven or eight years.
2. Issues arising at birth, issues resulting from birth trauma.
3. Issues relating to the cycles of birth, growth, maturity, decline, aging.
4. Conditions affecting the DNA, retroviral diseases, cancer, HIV, AIDS, genetic diseases, the dying process.
5. Issues relating to the Curious Organs: the Gallbladder, uterus, prostate, bone, bone marrow, spine, blood vessels, brain.
6. Life-threatening illnesses.
7. Threatened miscarriage or threatened maternal death during pregnancy.
8. Congenital defects: e.g., Down's Syndrome, Heart defects, infantile seizures, convulsions, epilepsy, results of a smoking/drug-addicted/alcohol-consuming mother, encephalitis, meningitis. The dissemination of Yin and Yang.
9. Impotence, infertility, issues with sexual Fluids, the preservation of the species.
10. Illness contracted in childhood.
11. A complaint that runs in the family, e.g., heart disease, arthritis, Parkinson's disease.

12. Acute flare ups of anything that originated in childhood, e.g., allergies, asthma.
13. Giving the elderly an opportunity to extend life.
14. Issues with the cycles of seven and eight: premature aging, premature growth, issues during menopause, andropause.
15. Abnormal growth such as cancer.
16. Conflict related to gender identity, ethnic identity.
17. Achieving latency of a pathogenic factor at the Yuan level.
18. Disparity between above and below, and between left and right
19. Imbalance of Yin and Yang: floating Yang with Yin deficiency, sinking Yin with Yang deficiency, the regulation of fire and water.
20. Issues pertaining to the realization of one's life purpose and self-acceptance.

The Names of the Eight Extraordinary Channels

Chong Mai	Penetrating Channel
Ren Mai	Conception Channel, Bonding Channel
Du Mai	Governing Channel
Yin Qiao Mai	Yin Heel Stance Channel
Yang Qiao Mai	Yang Heel Stance Channel
Yin Wei Mai	Yin Linking Channel
Yang Wei Mai	Yang Linking Channel
Dai Mai	Belt Channel

The Three Ancestries

The Eight Extra Channels are grouped into three *ancestries* or chronologically ordered groups, which can be seen as differing states of Yuan Qi. The First Ancestry is the foundation of Yin and Yang, originating as prenatal Qi. It comprises Chong, Ren and Du and unfolds from the moment of conception until the end of the first seven or eight years. The Second and Third Ancestries relate to postnatal Qi.[2] The Second Ancestry comprises the Wei Channels which describe the unfolding of Yin and Yang. The Third Ancestry comprises the Qiao Channels and Dai Mai. The Qiao Channels allow us to be self-embodied, physically present and experiencing the present moment; Dai Mai allows us to release unwanted experience and matter. Life is said to unfold in clearly demarcated cycles lasting seven years in females and eight years in males according to the *Su Wen*, or in cycles of ten years according to the *Ling Shu*. Each of these cycles features a major transitional period in one's life.

---

[2] Given the description of the First Ancestry in the Classics, the labels Second and Third evolved later.

Note: Given the current prevalence of the use of hormones in agriculture, the amount of contact we have with plastics, and other recently introduced violations to the Jing (overdosing of vaccines, the constant closeness of strong electromagnetic fields with personal phones and computers, etc.), the physical manifestation of these cycles has recently become shortened. This is why we are seeing a prevalence of the early onset puberty, and of abnormal growth (cancers in children).

The First Ancestry: Chong Mai, Ren Mai, and Du Mai
The Second Ancestry: Yin Wei Mai and Yang Wei Mai
The Third Ancestry: Yin Qiao Mai, Yang Qiao Mai and Dai Mai

The Chong Channel is created in utero. Ren and Du spring from the Chong. The Ren Channel is complete by the end of the second year. The Du Channel nears completion at the end of the first cycle of seven and eight. The first ancestry is entirely complete by puberty when we are able to reproduce. Throughout life, Chong remains the bridge between pre- and postnatal Qi. The second ancestry (the Wei's), records the unfolding of one's life through space and time. The third (the Qiao's), records the way in which we feel about ourselves and the outside world in the present moment. The channels of all three ancestries deal with pathologies that accumulate during our lives.

Considerations when Beginning any Eight Extraordinary Treatment

Needling into the Eight Extras is a very serious endeavor. If a patient is not ready for such treatments, they will feel violated to his or her very core. It's important, after having chosen to go the Eight Extra route, to tread lightly at first, to test the waters, to make sure the patient is on board with the treatment. It's a good idea to begin with either a Chong or a Dai Mai treatment. Decide whether, in general terms, you're helping the patient clear a pathway for pathology (Dai) or helping them build resources (Chong).

Eight Extraordinary Channel Treatment Tool Kit

Opening Points

The Opening points are not part of the Classical tradition, but originate in the 11th Century and initially are the work of Xu Feng who wrote *The Manual of Acupuncture, Zhen Jin Ju Ying*.[3] They are not compulsory. When standardized medicine came into being in the mid-twentieth century, all that remained of the Eight Extras were the Ming Dynasty Opening points. The function of the Opening points is simply to probe the level of Yuan

---

[3] In the third century, Wang Shu-He wrote commentaries on the Eight Extra Channels (still untranslated) which postulates different Opening points.

Qi; *they do not treat the channel.* Some of the Opening points are Shu-Stream points used in cases where excess prevails and needs to be drained. Some of the Opening points are Luo points (all Luo points connect to Yuan-Source Qi). The Opening points must be needled with vibrating, shaking or listening technique in order to establish energetically that an Eight Extra treatment is taking place. If a Luo point is merely needled, for example, the body will understand that the Luo point on the primary Channel is being needled; if the Luo point is bled, the body will understand that the Luo Channel is being treated. Neither of these techniques indicate Eight Extra to the body.

Channel	Point	Name
Chong Mai	SP-4	*Grandfather Grandchild*
Ren Mai	LU-7	*Lightning Strike*
Du Mai	SI-3	*Back Ravine*
Yin Wei Mai	PC-6	*Inner Pass*
Yang Wei Mai	TH-5	*Outer Pass*
Yin Qiao Mai	KI-6	*The Illuminating Sea*
Yang Qiao Mai	BL-62	*The Extending Channel*
Dai Mai	GB-41	*Foot Overlooking Tears*

Opening Point Principles

1. In the second and third ancestries, the Opening point is needled unilaterally on the right side in females and the left side in males.
2. Ren is always opened on the *left* regardless of gender. Du is always opened on the *right*, regardless of gender. This is because prenatally, left is Yin and right is Yang.
3. In Chong treatments intended to nourish postnatal Qi, the Opening point is on the right in females and left in males. If intended to replenish prenatal Qi, the Chong is opened on the left in females and the right in males.
4. Alternatively, the Opening point and the channel could be needled on the same side that the Eight Extra pulse for that channel is found.

Trajectory Points

Trajectory points are points other than the Opening points that delineate the trajectory and actually treat the Eight Extra Channel.

Coupled Pairs

Paired points are usually Opening points of another Eight Extra Channel sometimes chosen to enhance the treatment. They are needled last. They are only included if their function is required in the treatment, if that function is not covered in the points already needled. They are often not required.

The coupled pair theory originated in the 17th century and is the work of Yang Ji Zhou who wrote *Great Accomplishments of Acupuncture*. Coupled pairs were also developed by Zhen Jiu Da Cheng who frequently did not use them. The Ming Dynasty coupled pairs are: SP-4 with PC-6, LU-7 with KI-6, BL-62 with SI-3, GB-41 with TH-5. The classical application of the Eight Extraordinary Channels does not include the coupled pair unless there is a specific reason for doing so according to the point function of the coupled pair point.

If coupling the Eight Extras is desired, it should be noted that any Eight Extra Channel can be coupled with any other. The Ming Dynasty designated pairs comprise just one model.

Eight Extra Needling Techniques

Needling technique is of utmost importance in Eight Extra Channel treatments. For example, if you were to needle KI-6 with lifting and thrusting technique, the body understands your intention is to address KI-6 as a primary Channel point. If you were to use circular technique on KI-6 the body would understand your intention is to address KI-6 as an ah shi on a Sinew Channel. Vibrating and shaking are the most commonly used techniques for Extraordinary Channel needling. The aim is to create deep but subtle ripples in a huge thick sea of Jing.

1. *Vibrating*: Hold the needle with one hand and vibrate the top of the handle with the PC-8 of your opposite hand. This forces movement in the channel. This technique can be done at the moderate or at the deep level and depends on your intention. Or, simply hold the needle by the handle between thumb and forefinger and vibrate the needle. When done correctly, it creates a very subtle sensation of humming throughout the body. It's essential that the practitioner be calm and grounded, feeling their weight through the floor.
2. *Shaking*: This is equal to rocking or jostling and has a wider arc than vibrating. It's also easier than vibrating but not as potent. Use shaking if vibrating is too difficult.
3. *Listening*: This means being receptive to the Qi after needling the point. Needle to

the deep level (prenatal level) by lifting and thrusting, then bring the needle up to the moderate (postnatal) level. This technique is applied to Opening points which are also Luo points.

4. *Reduction*: To reduce a point, vibrate it *quickly*.
5. *Tonification*: To tonify a point, vibrate it *slowly*.
6. Needle the Yin Channel Opening points in the biggest dip or crevice.
7. Needle the Yang Channel Opening point where the skin and fascia bundle the most.
8. As with all acupuncture points, the Opening point will sometimes not be found in its textbook location.

Duration of Treatment

Needles should be retained for 40 minutes measured from the time of the insertion of the first needle.

Treatment Course

Eight Extra treatments should be performed once a week for a while at first. When it becomes clear that the patient is changing, the treatments begin to be spaced further apart to two and then three weeks. The duration of the entire course is three months or one hundred days which is the length of time it takes to change or mobilize the Jing. In emergency situations, Eight Extras are treated three days on and three days off until the desired change is achieved.

Unilateral Needling in the Eight Extraordinary Channels

Historically, the Eight Extras were needled unilaterally. Li Shi Zhen said it is disrespectful to needle the Eight Extras bilaterally and would needle the side on which he found the pulse for that Eight Extra Channel. Sun Si Miao said the Eight Extras would only be treated bilaterally if the Eight Extra pulse was found bilaterally.

In my own practice, I find uniformly that needling unilaterally produces a stronger result in the body than bilateral needling. The reason is that it is natural for the body to seek balance and symmetry. When you stimulate an acupuncture point, the body stimulates the contralateral point in an attempt to produce the same effect to balance both sides. The body is teaching itself to produce a healing effect within. This is extremely powerful. Most often, patients will report feeling the same sensations on the un-needled side. Sometimes they will report that the sensation on the other side is stronger. The fact that the body is producing this effect on its own means that the healing or the movement of Qi can be and is being learned, and the body is much more likely to be able to reproduce that effect after the treatment.

Combining Eight Extraordinary Channels

If it is necessary to combine two Eight Extra Channels in one treatment the needling order is as follows:

1. The Opening point of the channel of focus (on the side according to gender or pulse, whichever is preferred).
2. Selected trajectory points of that channel on that side of the body.
3. Selected trajectory points of the second Eight Extra on the opposite side of the body
4. The Opening point of the second Eight Extra on the second side, the side of its own trajectory points.

Points Added to Eight Extraordinary Treatments

Most often, there is no need to add points to Eight Extra treatments. The channels and their trajectories are comprehensive and highly potent. Points that can be added are Yuan level points: He-Sea, Mu, Shu, Influential, Triple Heater, Kidney, Ren and Du points, Divergent Confluent points, and Luo points (because they connect to the Yuan-Source level). It is quite inadvisable to add a point that is not in or connected to the Yuan level. These points would present a distraction, blur the intention of the treatment, and likely ruin the treatment.

Moxa in Eight Extraordinary Treatments

If using moxa in Eight Extra treatments, three cones are used on the moxibustioned point(s). The exceptions are the Ren Channel where seven cones are used and the Du Channel where one cone is used. A cone is the equivalent of one rice grain-sized piece of moxa.

Strong Connections between the Eight Extra Channels and the Curious Organs

Du Mai, the Qiao Mai's and Wei Mai's connect strongly to the brain and Marrow.

Chong, Ren, Du, Dai Mai connect strongly to the uterus.

Dai and Yang Wei Mai connect strongly to the Gallbladder.

Ren, Du, and the Qiao Mai's connect strongly to the bone.

Chong and Yin Wei Mai connect strongly to the Blood vessels.

Diagnosis of the Eight Extra Channels

Diagnosis of the Eight Extra Channels is made by assessing:

1. Physiological signs and symptoms
2. Psychological signs and symptoms
3. Pulses taken in Eight Extra style

Pulse Diagnosis of the Eight Extraordinary Channels

The technique of pulse-taking for the Eight Extra Channels should be taught one to one. Here I'll do my best to explain how it feels, but as with everything in this manual, it's best to learn hands-on.

Assess one wrist at a time, starting with either side.

1. Press all pulse positions down simultaneously until the flow of Blood is halted in the radial artery. This is called *15 Mung beans* of pressure.
2. Release the pressure very slightly, enough to allow the minimum possible amount of Blood through. The force is now said to be *14 beans* of pressure.
3. Write down the location(s) of any pulse felt pushing upwards into your finger at that *14 beans* position.
4. Increase the pressure again to *15 beans*.
5. Note whether the pulse you felt at *14 beans* is still there, in the same position(s) now at *15 beans*.
6. If the pulse is still there at *15 beans*, you have found a pulse of Eight Extra indication, "an Eight Extra pulse".

(If the pulse you found disappears at 15 beans, you've found a Divergent Channel pulse.)

7. Match the pulse to the descriptions in the table below and treat that channel.
8. If the pulse is felt in all three positions, release pressure on all the pulses simultaneously very, very slowly. If the pulse follows you:

    a. all the way to the superficial level, it's a Du pulse

    b. to the moderate level and stops following you, it's a Chong pulse.

    c. only within the deepest level and stops following you before you get to the cusp of the deep and moderate levels, or if it doesn't follow at all, it's a Ren pulse.

If the pulse is felt here	Treat this channel
Cun only	Yang Qiao Mai
Chi only	Yin Qiao Mai

Guan only	Dai Mai
Cun and Guan	Yang Wei Mai
Guan and Chi	Yin Wei Mai
Cun but extending into the thenar eminence	Yang Wei Mai
Chi but extending proximally	Yin Wei Mai
Cun, Guan and Chi and floats to Wei level	Du Mai
Cun, Guan and Chi and floats to Ying level	Chong Mai
Cun, Guan and Chi and does not float	Ren Mai

If a pulse is found simultaneously in the cun and chi positions, it may indicate an interplay of the Qiao Channels.

Essential Oil Complementary Treatments (simplified)

A minuscule amount of essential oil is applied to the Opening point and, if necessary, to selected points on the trajectory. A good way to achieve this is to give the patient a toothpick and instruct them to simply touch the toothpick to the rim of the bottle to pick up the tiniest amount possible and touch it to all the points being treated without re-touching the bottle. It's often difficult to impress upon the patient how small an amount is needed. The skin should not glisten with oil at all. Here are three reasons for using tiny amounts of oil:

a. More than that floods the nerve receptors and the body switches them off, rendering the oil useless.
b. More than a minuscule amount on BL-1 can be dangerous as it migrates to the eye via the skin's natural oils.
c. The tiniest amount provides the maximum amount of stimulation to the point.

Channel	Point/s	Essential Oil/s
Chong Mai	SP-4	If only treating Opening point: Patchouli, or Patchouli and Angelica blend. If treating SP-4 with trajectory points, use the following oils on the trajectory points after applying Patchouli on SP-4.
	1st trajectory	Savory
	2nd trajectory	Violet PC-6 must close the second trajectory: Clary Sage
	3rd trajectory	Cedarwood
	4th trajectory	Savory
	5th trajectory	Patchouli

Ren Mai	LU-7	Oakmoss, or Neroli and Ginger blend
Du Mai	SI-3	Cedarwood and Rosemary blend or Cedarwood and Cinnamon Leaf blend. If treating SI-3 as a coupled pair with BL-62, use blend of Fennel, Cinnamon Leaf and Mugwort on SI-3.
Yin Wei Mai	PC-6	Clary Sage or a blend of Vetiver, Frankincense and Vanilla, or a blend of Rose and Melissa
Yang Wei Mai	TH-5	Rosalina and Rosemary blend, or Rosemary and Citronella blend
Yin Qiao Mai	KI-6	Jasmine or Narcisscus, or Narcissus, Jasmine and Juniper blend
Yang Qiao Mai	BL-62	Cinnamon Leaf, or Cinnamon Leaf and Basil blend
Dai Mai	GB-41	Mugwort for Damp-Cold, or a blend of Sage, Roman Chamomile and Basil for Damp-Heat, or a blend of Mugwort, Niaouli and Sandalwood

Essential Oil Treatment Protocol for the Eight Extra Channels

Apply a minuscule amount of oil to the Opening point every day for 100 days. The application of oil to trajectory points is optional if acupuncture is being performed as a principal modality. If trajectory points are being oiled, the amount of oil applied is again barely detectable.

Eight Extraordinary Channel Treatment Protocol

1. Needle the Opening point with vibrating/shaking or listening technique. *(This step may be omitted; opening points are not Classical practice, but an 11th Century addition.)*
   The remaining points are needled with vibrating or shaking technique.
2. Needle the first point on the trajectory, if you've chosen to needle that point.
3. Needle the landmark points you've chosen.
4. Needle the remaining points you've chosen from the trajectory.
   Note: If you feel it's necessary to treat two Eight Extras, after Step 4, needle the selected trajectory points of the second channel on the opposite side of the body and then needle the Opening point of the second channel on that second side.
5. Needle any additional points you've chosen, if any (from the Yuan-Source level).
6. Suggest to the patient they be quiet and reflective.
7. Leave the needles in for 40 minutes from the time of the first insertion.
8. Remove needles in the order opposite to that of insertion, i.e., the last needle is the first to be removed.
9. Leave the patient lying down for a few minutes before asking them to dress.

Openings, First Points, Landmark Points Reference List

Landmark points are those near major articulations, orifices, or prominences. A well-formulated Eight Extra treatment will include landmark points because they serve to clearly delineate the channel and resonate strongly with the treatment principle for that channel.

Channel	*Opening point*	*First Point on Trajectory*	*Landmark points*
Chong Mai	SP-4	CV-2	CV-2, KI-11, ST-30, KI-16, KI-21
Chong 2nd	SP-4	KI-22	KI-27, ST-1
Chong 3rd	SP-4	ST-30	GV-1, GV-4
Chong 4th	SP-4	KI-10	KI-10, BL-40
Chong 5th	SP-4	ST-30	ST-30, ST-36, ST-42
Ren Mai	LU-7	CV-2	CV-2, CV-8[4], CV-15, CV-22, CV-23, ST-4, ST-1
Du Mai	SI-3	GV-1	GV-1, GV-14, GV-20
Yin Wei Mai	PC-6	KI-9	SP-15, CV-22, CV-23
Yang Wei Mai	TH-5	BL-63	BL-63, GB-35, GB-29, LI-14, SI-10, GB-21, GB-20, GB-13
Yin Qiao Mai	KI-6	KI-6	KI-6, KI-11, KI-16, KI-21, ST-12, BL-1, GB-20
Yang Qiao Mai	BL-62	BL-62	BL-62, GB-29, LI-15, BL-1, GB-20
Dai Mai	GB-41	LR-13	LR-13, GB-27, GB-28

---

[4] CV-8 is not needled.

Frequently Asked Questions about Eight Extra Channel Treatments

1. *Does needling the Opening point constitute an Eight Extra treatment?* No, Opening points with or without the coupled pair do not constitute treatment of an Extraordinary Channel. Opening (probing) an Eight Extra Channel by needling the Opening point without completing the treatment can be dangerous as many of the Opening points are Luo points which provide direct passage to the constitution. That means that a pathogen that has not been dealt with properly can be given entrée to the constitution via Opening points. Avoid that issue by needling points on the trajectory.

2. *But don't the Source points on the Primary Channels connect to the Eight Extra Channels?* Chapter 27 of the *Nan Jing* says that the Eight Extra Channels are beyond the reach of the 12 Primary Channels. The Yuan-Source points connect to the Triple Heater mechanism and stimulate it to distribute Jing-Essence from the left Kidney via the right Kidney, along Du Mai to the Zang Fu, into the Yuan-Source points. Therefore one is reaching into Triple Heater and its pathway by using the Yuan-Source points, not the Eight Extra Channels.

3. *How do I locate the Kidney Shu's?* The Kidney Shu's on the chest are 0.5 cun lateral to the anterior midline. They are right on the edge of the depressions made by the intercostal spaces. The needle is inserted transversely.

4. *Why does an Eight Extra treatment cause my patient to become cold or to have flashes of cold?* The Eight Extra Channels access the Jing which is a cold medium. When the Jing is changed or moved through an Eight Extra treatment, cold can move through the body. This is not pathological, but a response to the treatment, unless the Jing is harboring pathological cold, in which case the Cold may be scattering.

5. *Isn't PC-6 the paired point for any trajectory of the Chong?* PC-6 is used as a paired point with the *second* trajectory because it invigorates Blood and opens the chest which is the intention for the second trajectory.

6. *If needling the Opening point is optional, how does the body know an Eight Extra treatment is being performed?* The Opening points were introduced nearly two thousand years after the initial discussions of the Eight Extra Channels and, with the exception of the Qiao Channels, are not even on the trajectories. The action of vibrating or shaking the needles makes the treatment of the Eight Extras unequivocal to the body.

CHONG MAI TREATMENTS

The Penetrating Channel, The Thrusting Vessel, The Sea of Blood, The Sea of the 12 Primary Channels, The Sea of Postnatal Qi, The Sea of the Five Zang and Six Fu, The Central Axis, The Union of Yin and Yang.

These names reflect that Chong is the foundation of all Yin and Yang.

Mechanisms of Chong Mai

Chong Mai contains the Jing we need to carry out our destiny. The role of the Chong Channel is to bring Yuan Qi in the form of Yin and Yang, to the Ren and Du Channels to support postnatal Qi and Blood. Chong Mai's development is complete at the end of the first cycle of seven or eight years and deeply affects the entire life.

Needling into the Chong is profoundly revealing. It's like inviting the patient to look right into the deep ocean of who they really are. When working with the Chong, we are working with one's *nature*–that which is born into your Heart. The Chong's role is to express one's nature through one's Heart. To do that, we must first understand the Source of our nature, our temperament, which in turn determines our behavior as well as our medical conditions. Discomfort with one's racial, ethnic and cultural identity and discomfort with one's gender or sexual identity are treated with the Chong Channel.

The Heart houses the Shen (Spirit) and carries out the life's curriculum, which is stored in the Kidneys. Because of this essential relationship between the Heart and the Kidneys, open communication between the two centers is absolutely crucial for a healthy life. The Heart is the sovereign ruler of the individual and allows us to be in control of our destiny. The Heart shines the Spirit outward while carrying out this lifetime's curriculum, generating complete satisfaction with our destiny.

Chong Mai, from which an individual's postnatal Yin and Yang are derived, is also known as the *Blueprint of Life*. Hence Chong Mai is the origin of the Ren and Du Channels. The Chong contains the formula for one's nature, the way in which Yin and Yang interplay to create a life. It contains the genetic material for the unfolding of an individual life. This material has a direct impact on fertility and is transmitted to the next generation.

Chong Mai treats damage done to the constitution, inherited or not, direct or indirect, whether from xenobiotics, vaccines, pesticides, aging, sexual abuse or trauma, shock, birth trauma, chromosomal abnormalities or birth defects. In cases where destiny requires the presence of a chromosomal abnormality, the role of Chong Mai is to regulate Yin and Yang to mediate the imbalance.

Chong Mai represents the sum of our emotional and physiological experiences in utero and sets the tone for the remainder of that lifetime. If Chong Mai has been well-nourished it is able to provide confidence at the deepest level in future relationships. If basic emotional and physiological needs are not met, if the Chong Mai is neglected, through limited or conditional love, limited loving touch, cradling, rocking, soothing, nurturing, and/or if there is limited nourishment given the baby (limited contact with the breast, for example), rectus abdominis becomes tight (known as the hidden beam) and the child is programmed to withdraw or to set up barriers to prevent the formation of close relationships. Treatment of the Chong gives the patient an opportunity to sense these barriers, opening up the realm of personal and interpersonal confidence.

Chong Mai is the bridge between the pre- and postnatal environments. It is responsible for bringing prenatal Qi to support postnatal Qi. Chong Mai supports the Spleen via Kidney Yang. Therefore the Chong treats pathology related to assimilation, such as conditions arising from long-term Spleen Qi deficiency. These conditions may manifest as diarrhea, malabsorption syndromes, food allergies, leaky gut, borborygmus and wasting diseases.

Chong treats the five accumulations. Each of the accumulations is associated with one of the five Zang organs. The accumulation of the Heart is the hidden beam; of the Lung, dyspnea; of the Liver, fatty deposits; of the Spleen, focal distention of the abdomen; of the Kidney, *Running Piglet Qi*.

The natural support Chong gives the Spleen establishes confidence and boundaries in relationships. It makes a connection with the Pure Yang of the Stomach, ascending Fluids to the sensory orifices.

Chong Mai communicates Heart and Kidneys through one of its inherent mechanisms: the Great Luo of Shao Yin. (See detail on page 241.)

Chong is largely complete by age 2 (age 3 in Chinese chronology, which includes the gestation period). It is entirely complete by the end of the first cycle of seven or eight years.

Prenatal and Postnatal Chong

The first—or prenatal—manifestation of Chong occurs during the formation of the embryo. It runs through the deep midline of the body; its function is to separate Yin and Yang. Once born, we have the postnatal Chong to which we can gain access through points on the surface of the body. Our discussion in this chapter is about the postnatal Chong.

Chong Signs and Symptoms

If the Chong Channel is not functioning well, a selection of these signs and symptoms may arise:

Heart pain, *Running Piglet Qi*, difficulty concentrating or relaxing, sleep issues, panic attacks, anxiety, knotted chest, digestive issues, food stasis, nausea and vomiting, diarrhea, colitis, esophageal reflux, hemorrhoids, borborygmus, navel pain, pain below sternum with vomit, cockcrow diarrhea, difficulty storing Blood, long periods, a feeling of being weighed down, Shen imbalance, hot flashes, high blood pressure due to renal insufficiency.

Tongue sign: Chong Mai often has a very specific tongue presentation, called the "hidden beam" or "chopstick Qi" tongue. On either side of the midline and close to it, the tongue will have two beams, or rails that are narrow and raised and extend from the Upper Jiao to the Lower Jiao. These bands reflect accumulations of trauma that have affected the Chong and which the body is trying to hold at bay in the Chong. They indicate that hidden beam—the abdominal muscles between the Stomach and Kidney Channels—is tight. Consequently, Heart and Kidneys are not communicating. The color of a typical Chong Mai tongue is purple and shiny or pale purple.

Psychological Presentation

Chong Mai can be used to help people discover their own true nature if that has been obscured, suppressed by training, or forgotten through distraction. Chong Mai helps patients determine which of their habitual responses are the product of social or familial conditioning and which are born of true nature. Chong treatments help people understand who they really are and helps patients access their deepest desires so they can determine how to achieve fulfillment in life. Discomfort with one's racial, ethnic and cultural identity as well as discomfort with one's gender or sexual identity are treated with the Chong Channel.

Just as the Chong has trajectories that ascend Yuan Qi, it also has trajectories that descend and ground it back to earth to balance and conserve Yin and Yang Qi. In this way, Chong Mai can be used to treat patients who have driven themselves to the point of exhaustion of resources. It enables the patient to retreat and replenish those resources by detaching from the outside world for an appropriate period of time. If a patient is not ready for this period of comparative retreat, treatment of the Chong will cause him or her to interpret the treatment's effect as lethargy when, in fact, the treatment offers an invitation for necessary rest and retreat.

Needling the Opening Point

Gong Sun, the name of SP-4, means *Grandfather Grandchild*. This point gives access to that which is inherited, that which runs in the family. It requires deep and long palpation before it's needled. Very often this point is bound and tight, so dig into it with your palpating finger to begin to break up the adhesions before needling deep into it. This point is either needled deeply, or needled deeply and then immediately brought to the moderate (Luo) level. The patient may feel rebellious Qi; this is a common response and usually settles after the insertion of ST-30. The Opening point is needled on all five trajectories.

Coupled Pair

There is no need to add a coupled pair except when needling the second trajectory of Chong. PC-6 is used only as a coupling point in the second trajectory of the Chong. It will compromise the treatment intention of the other trajectories.

The Five Chong Trajectories

Chong Mai has five trajectories, each with very different functions. It is important to assess the signs and symptoms in terms of the five trajectories, choose one or perhaps two of those trajectories and focus the treatment there. Three trajectories ascend and two descend. Needle ascending trajectories in ascending order and descending trajectories in descending order.

Chong First Trajectory

The Sea of the 12 Primary Channels, the Sea of Postnatal Qi, the Sea of the Five Zang and Six Fu Organs

Indications of Chong (First Trajectory)

This trajectory deals with deficiency and excess issues of postnatal Qi. It treats birth trauma, issues related to deficient Spleen Qi from the time of birth, cockcrow diarrhea, watery stools, weak digestive function, improperly digested food, allergies originating in early childhood, chronic fatigue with depression, Celiac disease. It addresses the results of physiological and emotional needs unmet since birth.

Classical Principal Sign: Cockcrow diarrhea (early morning diarrhea).

General Pulse Picture: Kidney Yang will not be felt to nourish the Spleen. See also, Eight Extra pulses, page 228.

Points of Chong (First Trajectory)

Begins in the lower abdomen, emerges at the axis of the pubic bone **CV-2, KI-11**, then **ST-30** where the Qi of Chong emerges, **SP-12,** moves back toward the midline before going up the Kidney Channel **KI-11, KI-12, KI-13, KI-14, KI-15,** to the landmark point **KI-16,** then on to **KI-17, KI-18, KI-19, KI-20, KI-21** (all 0.5 cun from the midline), diffuses into **chest**. (As the Jing disseminates upwards and reaches the chest, it scatters.)

Landmarks: **CV-2, KI-11, ST-30, KI-16, KI-21.**

Entire trajectory: Lower abdomen, **CV-2, KI-11, ST-30, SP-12, KI-11, KI-12, KI-13, KI-14, KI-15, KI-16, KI-17, KI-18, KI-19, KI-20, KI-21**.

Point Translations and Indications of Chong (First Trajectory)

CV-2	*Curved Bone*	Nourishes Blood.
KI-11	*Bend at the Pubic Bone*	Genital pain.
ST-30	*The Qi of Chong*	Brings Essence to support postnatal Qi.
SP-12	*Chong Doorway*	Ascends the Qi of the Spleen.
KI-12	*Great Manifestation*	Treats leukorrhea, prostatitis, incontinence.
KI-13	*Point of Qi*	Genital itch, stagnation of Wind-Cold.
KI-14	*The Four Fullnesses*	Treats stagnated Qi in the Lower Jiao: fibroids, undigested food, mucus, blood or Phlegm in the stools, pain on defecation, regulates waterways, painful menses with clots.

Chong Mai

First Trajectory

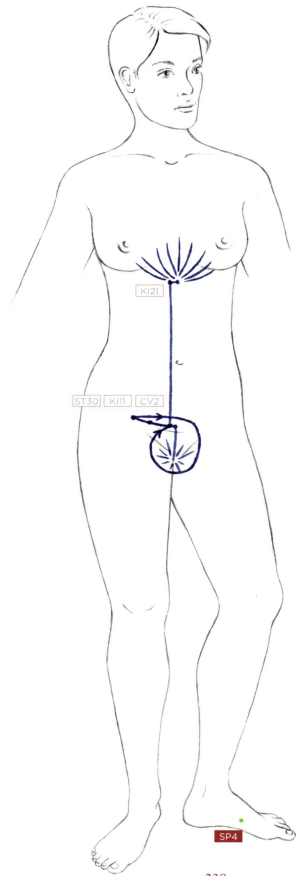

KI-15	*Central Director*	Regulates Damp-Heat blockages: constipation, urinary blockage, prostatitis.
KI-16	*Membrane Transport*	Leaky gut, edema, too much water or too little hydration, harmonizes Spleen and Stomach, endometriosis.
KI-17	*Shang Bend*	Strengthens Spleen, Damp Bi.
KI-18	*Stone Pass*	Strengthens Spleen. Moves accumulations and concentrations (food, Blood, Qi, fluid, Phlegm). Fullness after eating.
KI-19	*Yin Metropolis*	Strengthens Spleen for Blood related issues, Blood deficiency, Blood stagnation, hemorrhage.
KI-20	*Abdomen Connecting Valley*	Strengthens digestion, fatigue after eating, food stagnation, poor digestion and appetite.
KI-21	*Mysterious Gate*	Assists in exploring the mystery of one's self. Eating disorders, regulates Liver when Liver invades Spleen. Treats eating to ease emotional stress. Enables internal contemplation, self-discovery.

The first trajectory has no paired point.

Treatment Principles for Chong (First Trajectory)
1. To bring Kidney Yang to assist Spleen Yang.
2. To strengthen Spleen Qi via Kidney Qi.
3. To bring surplus postnatal Qi to the Kidneys to replenish prenatal Qi.

Point Selection Method for Chong (First Trajectory)
Choose points from both Lower and Middle Jiao's.
1. Choose points in the Lower Jiao (up to KI-16) to break up stagnation. These points are often dispersed.
2. Choose point in the Middle Jiao (KI-17 to KI-21) for deficiencies, to fortify the Spleen. (To *fortify* means to resolve Dampness in order to allow the Spleen to become stronger as opposed to *tonifying* the Spleen which means to strengthen the Spleen directly.)

Example of Point Selection for Chong (First Trajectory)
SP-4, KI-11, ST-30, KI-16, KI-21

Needling Technique for Chong (First Trajectory)

As you palpate the Chong, you'll find areas that are tight. Needle these to release all the bound areas (ah shi's) in rectus abdominis before needling.

Your treatment strategy in the first trajectory will involve either tonifying Spleen Qi via Kidney Qi, or tonifying prenatal Qi by banking postnatal Qi to the Source. Needle from the Kidney Channel towards or away from the Stomach Channel depending on which of these two intentions you chose.

If bringing postnatal Qi to the Kidneys, insert the needle one inch from the anterior midline and angle towards the midline so that when you reach the Yuan level, the tip of the needle is 0.5 cun from the midline.

If bringing Kidney Yang to support Spleen Yang, needle Kidney points pointed towards the Stomach Channel.

Treatment Protocol for Chong (First Trajectory)

All points are needled with vibrating technique.

1. Needle the Opening point, SP-4, right for females, left for males.
2. Needle the landmark points chosen, e.g., ST-30, KI-16, KI-21.
3. Needle the remaining chosen trajectory points distal to proximal.
4. Revisit each point in the order needled and check that the patient feels at least a very subtle vibration in each point.
5. Ask the patient to visualize or to imagine the feeling of the connection of all the points. Often they will report that they already feel this connection vibrating.
6. Take the pulses in the Eight Extra position. The pulses will have moved deeper into the wrist. If they have not, re-vibrate the needles, ensuring that connection with the Yuan level has been made. This is done by intention rather than literal depth.
7. (*Optional*). Give the patient an affirmation to repeat aloud or silently while they have needles in, e.g., *My natural energy is restored, and I am calm and free.*
8. Leave needles in for 40 minutes after the insertion of the first trajectory point.
9. Take the pulses in Eight Extra style, note the change and report it to the patient.
10. Remove the needles in the following order:
    a. Opening point
    b. other needles in the order opposite that of insertion
11. Allow the patient five minutes on the table, preferably alone, to reflect.

Chong Second Trajectory

The Great Luo of Shao Yin, the Sea of Blood

Mechanisms of Chong (Second Trajectory)

The second trajectory of Chong Mai is the link between Jing-Essence and all other humors. In this sense, it is known as the Sea of Blood. The Stomach is the origin of Blood and Fluids. The second trajectory moves the "Pure Yang" of the Stomach (pure, Thin Fluids originating in the Stomach) up to the sensory orifices for the maintenance of sensory perception.

The second trajectory also communicates Kidneys and Heart. In this context, it is known as the *Great Luo of Shao Yin*, the connecting passage between the Kidneys and the Heart. The second trajectory ends in the face and therefore brings Blood to the face.

Note: The *Great Luo of the Spleen* connects to this trajectory at CV-15. A third Great Luo, the *Great Luo of the Stomach*, which is really the heartbeat (and known as the *Empty Mile*) also connects to the second trajectory of the Chong. All the Great Luos connect in the chest, where Essence, Blood and Fluids link together. These connections are accessible using the second trajectory of the Chong, at the Kidney Shu points on the chest. The three Great Luos (which are Source-to-Blood connectors, as opposed to the standard Luos which are Blood-to-Source connectors) play a key part in the manufacture, management and movement of Blood. Therefore Chong's second trajectory treats Blood stagnation. It is particularly indicated for Cold in the Blood. (Cold in the Blood is often contracted in the post-partum period, but also through walking on cold floors and not keeping the feet warm in general.)

As the second trajectory connects to the chest, it connects to Ancestral Qi, (Zong-Gathering Qi), and therefore affects the diaphragm.

Indications of Chong (Second Trajectory)

Physiological: Heart pain with fullness and knotting behind or below the sternum leading to vomiting, or the feeling of wanting to vomit. Chest oppression. Blood stasis in the Heart and Liver. Splenomegaly. The *hidden beam*, Heart pain, *Running Piglet Qi*, panic attacks (failure of Heart and Kidneys to communicate), pale face, pale tongue sometimes with a purplish hue.

Chong Mai

Second Trajectory

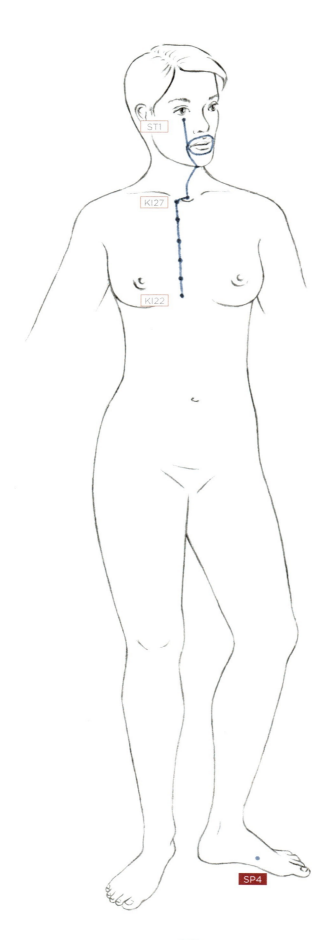

Psychological: Lack of sense of self. The inability to feel nourished within the self. Psychosomatic panic attacks.

Classical Principal Signs: The hidden beam, Heart pain, *Running Piglet Qi* (panic attacks), Blood stagnation.

General Pulse Picture: Choppy, especially in the Middle Jiao. See also, Eight Extra pulses, page 228.

Points of Chong (Second Trajectory)

All Kidney Shu points (KI-22 to KI-27) are located half a cun from the midline.

KI-22, KI-23, KI-24, KI-25, KI-26, KI-27, CV-22, CV-23, encircles the mouth, **ST-1.**

The second trajectory connects back to the Ren Channel at CV-22, CV-23, and ST-1.

Point Translations and Indications of Chong (Second Trajectory)

Note: In the context of the Eight Extraordinary Channels, where prenatal Qi is being protected or conserved, the Kidney Shu points are in reverse order to the Bladder Shu points. Of the Bladder Shu points, those of the water element are the most inferior and the metal most superior, but of the Kidney Shu points as Eight Extra Channel points, the metal is the most inferior and the water most superior. If the principal aim of the treatment is to support Spleen Qi (postnatal Qi), however, the order of the Kidney Shu points is the same as the Bladder Shu points, i.e., KI-26 becomes metal and KI-22 becomes water.

KI-22 (metal)	*Stepping Along the Gallery*	For seeing our own intrinsic meaning and beauty. Diffuses Lungs and treats cough.
KI-23 (fire)	*Spirit Seal/Heart Seal*	Invites forward the spirit that resides in the chest. For those who feel a sense of emptiness when reflecting on their life's purpose. Inability to catch breath, depression, anxiety, the feeling of pressure weighing on the Heart.
KI-24 (wood)	*Spirit Burial Ground*	Assists in letting things go. Moves patient into wanting to put life in order, or "affairs in order" if dying. Assists in letting go of life without feeling that life is decaying or that life was not complete. Treats stress-related breast lumps (fibrocystic breasts) due to failure to let go of stagnation in the chest.

KI-25 (earth)	*Spirit Storehouse*	For revealing the true nature of the spirit which has been buried. Loss of appetite or pleasure in eating. Treats a sense of emptiness and the inability of the patient to identify something precious about themselves. Treats irritability, bitterness, refusal to reflect on the self, and treats the feeling of being a victim.
KI-26 (water)	*Lively Center*	Loss of animation of Spirit. Lethargy, boredom. Invigorates Kidney Yang to assist Spleen Yang and connects that up to the Lungs to "enliven the center".
KI-27 (Master Kidney Shu)	*Warehouse of Transportation*	Strengthens Spleen to support respiratory and Heart function. Treats Heart valve prolapses including mitral valve prolapse.
CV-22	*Celestial Chimney*	Resolves Phlegm in the throat and chest.
CV-23	*Ridge at the Spring*	Opens throat. Descends rebellious Qi.
ST-1	*Supporting Tears*	Accepts the Pure Yang of the Stomach for the sensory orifices. Enhances sensory perception.

Coupled Pair: If wishing to add a paired point, PC-6 is needled last. It is inserted on the opposite side of the Opening point.

Treatment Principles of Chong (Second Trajectory)

1. To nourish and invigorate Blood while regulating Ancestral-Zong-Gathering/Chest Qi.
2. To communicate the Heart and Kidneys.
3. To bring Blood to the face.
4. To enable the patient to find meaning in their experiences. The second trajectory brings Jing to the level of the spirit.

Example of Point Selection for Chong (Second Trajectory)

SP-4, then the appropriate Kidney Shu point/s, then PC-6.

The second trajectory of Chong is the only trajectory that requires the use of PC-6 as a paired point.

Treatment Protocol for Chong (Second Trajectory)

All points are needled with vibrating technique.

1. Needle the Opening point, SP-4, right for females, left for males.
2. (*Optional*). Choose at least one point to needle from the first trajectory, e.g., ST-30.
3. Needle the landmark points you have chosen from the second trajectory, e.g., KI-27, ST-1.
4. Needle the remaining selected second trajectory points.
5. Needle PC-6 on the side opposite SP-4.
6. Revisit each point in the order needled, vibrate the needle, and check that the patient feels at least a very subtle vibration in each point as you are doing the manipulation.
7. Ask the patient to visualize or to imagine the feeling of the connection of all the points. Often they will report that they already feel this connection vibrating.
8. Take the pulses in the Eight Extra position. The pulses will have moved deeper into the wrist. If they have not, re-vibrate the needles, ensuring that connection with the Yuan level has been made. This is done by intention rather than literal depth.
9. (*Optional*). Give the patient an affirmation to repeat while they are in treatment, e.g., *I feel content, complete and comfortable with who I am.*
10. Leave needles in for 40 minutes after the insertion of the first trajectory point.
11. Take the pulses in Eight Extra style, note the change and report it to the patient.
12. Remove the needles in the following order:
    a. Opening point.
    b. other needles in the order opposite that of insertion.
13. Allow the patient five minutes on the table, preferably alone, to reflect.

Chong Mai

Third Trajectory

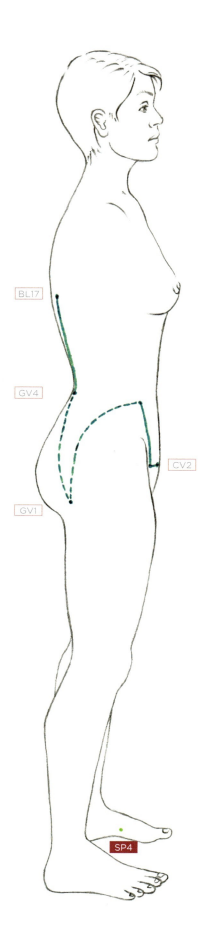

Chong Third Trajectory

Mechanisms of Chong (Third Trajectory)

The third trajectory of the Chong Channel is responsible for the ascension of Yang from Chong, (which is the origin of all Yin and Yang), to the beginning of Du. The connection to Du Mai is made via Dai Mai, to which Chong connects. The trajectory moves Yang Qi to invigorate Blood which, when stagnant or deficient, causes pain.

The third trajectory has an impact on the Bladder Shu points beginning at BL-17 which is the influential point of Blood and also the Shu point of the diaphragm. Therefore the third trajectory treats Blood stagnation and the accompanying pain that arises when Liver is tight due to Cold or Blood deficiency. The Liver is then unable to control the smooth flow of Qi in smooth muscle, particularly the uterus.

Indications of Chong (Third Trajectory)

Physiological: Seemingly intractable bi syndrome, pain in joints, blockage of the sensory orifices, stiffness of the lumbar region, disc herniations, fractures, Blood stasis, prolapses, leakages from the orifices of the lower abdomen, leaky gut, Crohn's disease, Irritable Bowel Syndrome, Damp-Heat in the Lower Jiao (especially Bladder and Large Intestine), gynecological issues involving the inability to uphold (miscarriages, spontaneous abortions, leukorrhea, chronic vaginal discharge), yeast infections, fibroids, endometriosis, premenstrual syndrome, urogenital issues, prostatitis, incontinence, stabbing pain in the Lower Jiao, Addison's disease.

Psychological: The third trajectory allows one to keep things mentally in place because it is Yang which provides the energy needed to hold things in their place, and memory is stored in the Blood. (Chong Mai is the Sea of Blood, and the third trajectory connects to Du Mai, the Sea of Yang.) The third trajectory treats Alzheimer's Disease, dementia, and the inability to retrieve from the memory.

Points of Chong (Third Trajectory)

CV-2, ST-30, GB-26, GV-1 (or GV-4), BL-17.

Treatment Principles for Chong (Third Trajectory)

1. To invigorate Yang.
2. To invigorate Yang to move Bi-Obstruction due to Blood stasis.

Example of Point Selection for Chong (Third Trajectory)

SP-4, GB-26(-), GV-4 (+), BL-17(+). (+ means tonify, - means reduce)
- BL-11 the upper transporting point for Blood and influential point of the bone can be added. It treats Bi syndrome due to Blood stagnation.
- When treating issues of the Lower Jiao, it is essential to open the chest with GB-22 or LU-1.

Coupled Pair Choices

If needed, add SI-3 to enhance the movement of Yang. Or add GB-41 to relax the ancestral sinews (due to its connection to Dai Mai).

Treatment Protocol for Chong (Third Trajectory)

All points are needled with vibrating technique.

1. The patient is side-lying with the foot to be needled positioned to allow easy access to SP-4.
2. Needle the Opening point, SP-4, right for females, left for males.
3. Needle the landmark points chosen, e.g., CV-2, ST-30, GV-1 or GV-4.
4. Needle the remaining chosen trajectory points.
5. Revisit each point in the order needled and check that the patient feels at least a very subtle vibration in each point.
6. Ask the patient to visualize or to imagine the feeling of the connection of all the points. Often they will report that they already feel this connection vibrating. In a trajectory that is meandering such as this one, you might elect to show them a drawing of the trajectory.
7. Take the pulses in the Eight Extra position. The pulses will have moved deeper into the wrist. If they have not, re-vibrate the needles, ensuring that connection with the Yuan level has been made. This is done by intention rather than literal depth.
8. *(Optional).* Give the patient an affirmation to repeat while they are in treatment, e.g., *I feel invigorated; I feel my Blood moving.*
9. Leave needles in for 40 minutes after the insertion of the first trajectory point.
10. Take the pulses in Eight Extra style, note the change and report it to the patient.
11. Remove the needles in the following order:
    a. Opening point
    b. other needles in the order opposite that of insertion
12. Allow the patient five minutes on the table, preferably alone, to reflect.

Chong Fourth Trajectory

Mechanisms of Chong (Fourth Trajectory)

The fourth trajectory is the first to travel downward. It creates the Qiao Channels and is therefore responsible for supporting the structure of the body. It brings Jing to the dorsum of the foot to support the structure and the bone. This trajectory encourages the Kidneys to support the posture and bones and to ascend Qi to raise that which is weakened or prolapsed from the loss of resources. The fourth trajectory brings Yang Qi to the Spleen.

Indications of Chong (Fourth Trajectory)

Physiological: Loss of Yang affecting the posture, asthma, Yang deficiency due to Blood stasis, gastrointestinal problems, stunted growth, being small for one's age, dwarfism.

Psychological: Poor perception of oneself in the present moment. Poor equilibrium in the psyche. A desire in a child to walk too early, before they have capability. Failure of the child to walk by age two. (Walking must not be taught; walking will begin when the musculoskeletal system and the Yang energetics develop sufficiently.)

Points of Chong (Fourth Trajectory)

KI-11, KI-10, BL-40, (through KI-6 and KI-3) **Kidney Prime** (posterior to KI-1, see drawing).

Note: Moxa is used on all these points.

Coupled Pair

(not required): KI-6

Treatment Principle of Chong (Fourth Trajectory)

1. To ascend Spleen Qi via Kidney Yang.
2. To support the posture by raising Spleen Qi via Kidney Yang.

Treatment Protocol for Chong (Fourth Trajectory)

All points are needled with vibrating technique.

    1. Needle the Opening point, SP-4, right for females, left for males.
    2. Needle the trajectory points: KI-10, BL-40, Kidney Prime.
    3. Revisit each point in the order needled and check that the patient feels at least a

Chong Mai
Fourth Trajectory

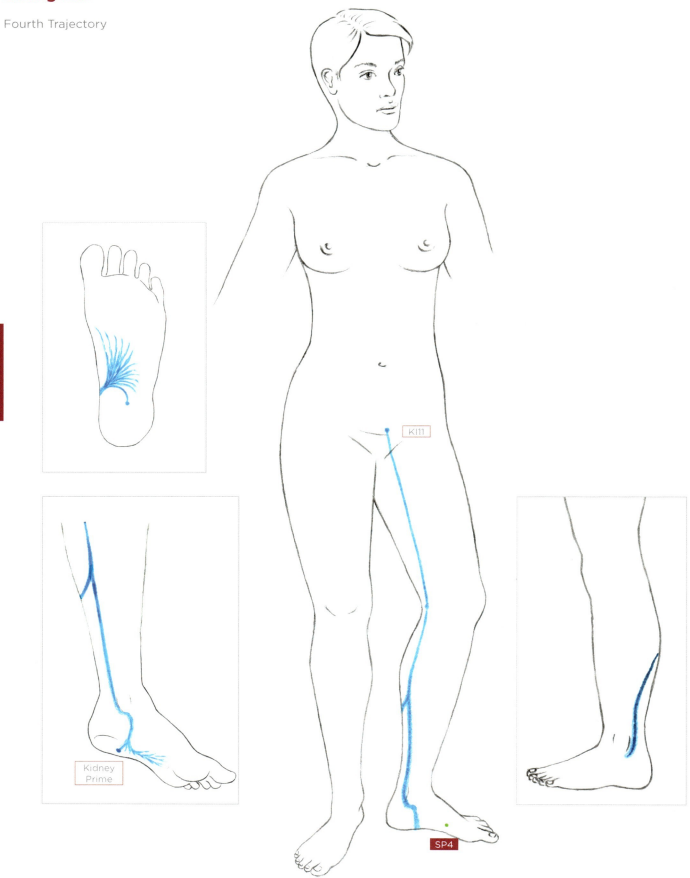

very subtle vibration in each point.
4. Moxa all trajectory points safely until the heat is felt to be penetrating. (I use pole moxa against the needle.)
5. Ask the patient to visualize or to imagine the feeling of the connection of all the points. Often they will report that they already feel this connection vibrating.
6. Take the pulses in the Eight Extra position. The pulses will have moved deeper into the wrist. If they have not, re-vibrate the needles, ensuring that connection with the Yuan level has been made. This is done by intention rather than literal depth.
7. *(Optional)*. Give the patient an affirmation to repeat while they are in treatment, e.g., *I brim with enthusiasm which ignites me.*
8. Leave needles in for 40 minutes after the insertion of the first trajectory point.
9. Take the pulses in Eight Extra style, note the change and report it to the patient.
10. Remove needles in the following order:
    a. Opening point
    b. other needles in the order opposite that of insertion
11. Allow the patient five minutes on the table, preferably alone, to reflect.

Frequently Asked Question

How deeply should I needle Kidney Prime? Use a one inch needle, press the tube very firmly, press (ease, don't tap) the needle in, insert the needle as deeply as you can. Often, with this point, the deeper you go, the milder the sensation.

Chong Fifth Trajectory

Mechanisms of Chong (Fifth Trajectory)

The fifth trajectory of the Chong tonifies postnatal Qi by strengthening the Spleen and by nourishing Liver Blood so that postnatal Qi is able to support Kidney Yin without causing a deficit in Blood. If the Liver were to become deficient in Blood, it would tax the Spleen. The fifth trajectory includes the upper and lower transporting points of the *Sea of Food and Drink*, ST-30 and ST-36 respectively. The fifth trajectory ensures adequate nutrients are extracted from food so the *Four Seas* (the *Sea of Food and Drink*, the *Sea of Qi and Blood*, the *Sea of Marrow* and the *Sea of Zang Fu and Postnatal Qi*) are fully supported. The trajectory goes to the beginning of both the Spleen and Liver Channels to balance Qi in the event Liver invades Spleen when Spleen is deficient.

Chong Mai

Fifth Trajectory

8 EXTRA

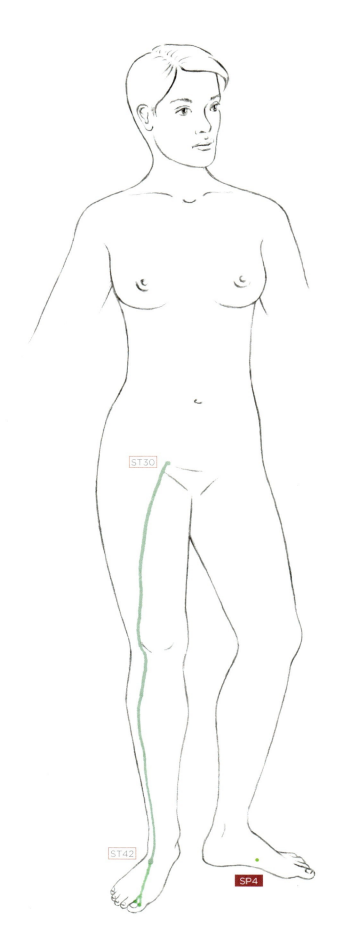

Indications of Chong (Fifth Trajectory)

Difficulty assimilating nutrients due to Spleen Qi deficiency, food stasis, nausea, vomiting, diarrhea, intestinal Wind, ulcerative colitis, Celiac disease, esophageal reflux, hemorrhoids, borborygmus, navel pain, fermentation (Damp-Heat), the Five Jaundices which arise due to food (hepatitis, food poisoning), alcohol, excess sex, limbic jaundice. The fifth trajectory transports nutrients to the flesh.

Points of Chong (Fifth Trajectory)

ST-30, ST-36, ST-37, ST-39, ST-42, LR-1, SP-1.

ST-37 and ST-39 are Blood transporting points.

ST-30 and ST-36 are transporting points for the *Sea of Food and Drinks*.

ST-42 ascends the Pure Yang of the Stomach; transports nutrients to the flesh.

Note: Use both LR-1 and SP-1 if Liver is invading Spleen. Choose SP-1 for Shen disturbances or bleeding (reckless Blood); choose LR-1 for Blood stagnation, to regulate Blood, Fluids and Qi.

Coupled Pair

Use Yuan-Source points if choosing to add a channel.

Treatment Principles of Chong (Fifth Trajectory)

1. To tonify Spleen Qi and nourish Stomach Yin.
2. To assist in bringing the Pure Yang of the Stomach (Fluids) to nourish the sensory orifices.

Treatment Protocol for Chong (Fifth Trajectory)

All points are needled with vibrating technique.

1. Needle the Opening point, SP-4, right for females, left for males.
2. Needle the landmark points chosen, e.g., ST-30, ST-36, ST-42.
3. Needle the remaining chosen trajectory points in the direction of the trajectory.
4. Revisit each point in the order of insertion and check that the patient feels at least a very subtle vibration in each point.
5. Ask the patient to visualize or to imagine the feeling of the connection of all the points. Often they will report that they already feel this connection vibrating.

6. Take the pulses in the Eight Extra position. The pulses will have moved deeper into the wrist. If they have not, re-vibrate the needles, ensuring that connection with the Yuan level has been made. This is done by intention rather than literal depth.
7. *(Optional).* Give the patient an affirmation to repeat while they are in treatment, e.g., *I am calm, and deeply nourished.*
8. Leave needles in for 40 minutes after the insertion of the first trajectory point.
9. Take the pulses in Eight Extra style, note the change and report it to the patient.
10. Remove needles in the following order:
    a. Opening point
    b. other needles in the order opposite that of insertion
11. Allow the patient five minutes on the table, preferably alone, to reflect.

REN MAI TREATMENTS

Conception Vessel (CV), The Channel of Bonding, The Sea of Yin

Ren Mai is a member of the first ancestry. As the Sea of Yin, Ren Mai provides the materials for the Sea of Yang (Du Mai) to create the structure of the body. As the Channel of Bonding, Ren Mai enables us to feel whole and complete in ourselves.

Mechanisms of the Ren Mai

The severing of the umbilical cord instantly activates Ren Mai. Now that nourishment is no longer provided through the umbilicus, Ren Mai causes the baby to seek nourishment from the only Source it has yet known, its mother. Ren Mai governs and is affected by the symbiotic bond between mother and child. The rhythms of survival: breathing, heartbeat and sleeping patterns are all set by the Ren. The entire channel is delineated and active in the process of nourishment. Breastfeeding is a bonding ritual, a ritual of Ren. When the mother holds the baby, they are Ren-to-Ren and the baby's mouth encircles the nipple. The baby looks into mother's eyes and synchronizes with the energy of her heartbeat and her breathing. There's an instinctual yearning toward union. If bonding is delayed, curtailed or does not happen at all, the child does not experience the natural effect of being brought into a state of union. As a result, the child's capacity to bond appropriately during its entire lifetime can be greatly affected. If Ren Mai is well-formed through natural, full engagement with the mother especially during the period between the moment of birth and the time Du Mai opens, the individual will not ultimately see the world as a place of disappointments and hurt. Appropriate bonding with the Ren is important throughout childhood, but during the first developmental period it is essential.

During the Ren Mai development period the child has not realized the idea that they are separate beings from their mother. The child feels what the mother feels as though those feelings are originating within the child. The feelings a baby experiences during the very first experience of nourishment at the breast, and to a slightly lesser extent the feelings the baby experiences through breastfeeding thereafter, are those the child will associate with nourishment (in every sense) on an unconscious level for the remainder of his or her life. Therefore a baby being breastfed by an anxious mother will associate anxiety with love and form love relationships that have anxiety as a key feature because the Ren has been calibrated that way. This is why some people think they are not really in love unless the relationship is challenging or is creating some kind of stress. In treating Ren Mai conditions, it is important to inquire about separation at birth and breastfeeding. Ren Mai treatments re-program imbalances in past bonding (or lack of bonding) allowing for healthy bonding in the present and future.

Note: In practice we see many clinical presentations in adults that are ultimately rooted in Ren Mai issues. That being said, once Ren Mai is established, Du Mai must also be allowed to flourish. When it's time for Du Mai to be activated—as the child acquires the ability to stand, note where mother is and walk a safe distance away—it's essential that while continuing to nourish Ren appropriately, the mother, for the first time, begins the process of letting-go, of allowing the next stage of childhood to unfold. This is sometimes difficult for the mother.

The integrity of the Ren Channel is profoundly affected by the birth environment. The abdomen, chest, mouth and eyes are all part of the Ren trajectory; these regions are activated shortly after birth, in terms of creating the bond. For the Ren to be healthy, its activation at birth should be close to seamless, without stress, minimizing the sense of breaking from a whole. Birth should take place in conditions that mimic the in utero environment. The room should be very warm, calm and dimly lit. Some elect to give birth in body-temperature water. The umbilical cord should only be cut after it has stopped pulsating. This is easy to feel when holding the cord. When the pulsing has stopped, the gradual and sometimes lengthy process of the handover of respiration has concluded and the Lungs are finally ready to assume full responsibility for breathing. Although occasionally necessary, to sever the cord before it has stopped pumping gravely insults the Ren as the baby is abruptly placed into emergency survival mode, the

Lungs having been unnaturally shocked into full responsibility. The modern practice of giving birth in cold rooms, under bright lights, in frantic environments with an expectation of emergency, creates untold damage. To mend our society, we must take steps to re-humanize standard birthing practice as much as possible.

Non-Pathological State of Ren Mai

When Ren Mai is in good balance the person feels whole and complete in themselves. Partnerships, friendships and relationships are created free of a sense of neediness and free of the desire to be needed.

Pathological State of Ren Mai

In the absence of the feeling of being complete and whole in oneself, the body accumulates and stagnates Yin, in response to that feeling of need. As Yin is shifted to meet this need, it forms Yin stasis which leads to a state of Yin deficiency as Yin is no longer in free currency. On a physical level, inadequate nourishment results in a Yin deficiency which the body responds to by accumulating pathological Yin. Ren Mai treatments enable the patient to see the world in a more grounded way, as healthy Yin provides ballast.

Destiny (the child's or the mother's) may require the experience of over-dependence and therefore a Yin deficient state is created, leading to the compensatory accumulation of Yin in such a way that the baby is incapacitated: Down's Syndrome, mental retardation, retracted neck, spinal tumors.

Indications of Ren Mai

Classical Principal Sign: Yin deficiency due to Yin stasis.

Post delivery issues: retention of lochia, lumbago, post-partum depression, food stasis, vomiting, constipation, diarrhea, hemorrhoids, wasting and thirsting, the five neck nodules.

General pulse picture: Thin, or thin and rapid, and slippery as the body accumulates pathological Yin in the absence of Yin. See also Eight Extra pulse methodology on page 228.

Physical Indications of Ren Mai

Below, the physical and psychological indications of the Ren are separated for easy reference. As with any channel, in clinical practice there is no separation between the two groups of signs and symptoms.

- Yin deficiency with Yin stasis. Yin accumulates as compensation for a deficiency of Yin. This can be seen in countless ways, for example, buffalo hump, fatty deposits along the spine as in Down's Syndrome, club fingers and toes, fibroids, endometriosis, tumors, ovarian cysts, diaper rash, scrotal swellings. Also, masses or tumors in areas that are key to nourishment and procreation: breasts, uterus, ovaries, thyroid, prostate, testicles.
- Testicular pain, genital dysfunction.
- The feeling that something is weighing on the self, Dampness, chest oppression.
- Valve or sphincter issues: around eyes, mouth, digestive tract, esophagus, intestines, anus, and urethra. Mitral valve prolapse, stenosis, hardening of the heart valves, long-term constipation, difficulty with orbicularis oris and oculi, digestive issues and asthma all involve sphincters and/or valves. Yin contains Yang and enables Yang to anchor, so the Ren Mai controls the movement of the sphincter muscles and valves. If a child is weaned before the child is ready, the orbicular muscle around the mouth will tighten.
- If breast milk is replaced too early by food or formula, the digestive sphincter muscles will tighten, leading to colic, gastric reflux, and food allergies or gluten sensitivities as the child rejects the replacement food. Later in life, the grief experienced in what is felt to be rejection through early weaning manifests as strain in the orbiculus oculi muscles as the eyes become strained in an unconscious suppression of emotion. If the child is forced to toilet train, the strain can impact on other orbicular muscles and result in impaired vision, and a lifetime of constipation.
- Difficulty swallowing.
- Constant Dampness and Cold.
- Dryness, dehydration.
- Back pain with profuse sweating and straightening of the arch of the low back.

Psychological Indications of Ren Mai

- Difficulty bonding to the breast and to the mother.
- Resistance to early weaning, as seen in attempts to control the environment by tightening sphincter muscles. A child who feels they cannot control what's going on around them might develop constipation; the child feels it can at least impose control

on the functions of its own body.
- Difficulty with commitment; difficulty in making or keeping relationships at any age. Feeling scared or feeling cardiovascular responses when encountering bonding or relationship opportunities.
- Fear of commitment due to an unwillingness to take care of somebody else.
- Habitually forming inappropriate relationships.
- Feeling incomplete, never feeling completely whole, the inability to feel contained. Feeling something is missing. Never feeling content or full. Feeling barren.
- Feeling incomplete in the absence of a partner; believing that the presence of somebody else is necessary for the feeling of wholeness. Searching for a soul mate in order to feel complete. Holding the belief that there is a soul mate.
- Dependence and over-dependence issues. The need to feel protected or touched at all times. This occurs on a broad spectrum from needing a blanket in all weather in order to sleep to being reluctant to leave mother's side in middle childhood.
- A tendency to be controlling or controlled in relationships.
- Feeling disconnected or unconnected.
- A tendency to feel victimized.
- Inability to be comfortable responding to people.
- Always wanting something in the mouth, addiction to talking.
- Ren can be over-stimulated and over-nourished, causing over-bonding, expressed as neediness, lack of independence, a preference for being pampered, the inability to make decisions for one's self, the tendency to enter into relationships enabling total dependence. Over-nourishment leads to excess Yin (Phlegm, Dampness, Yin stasis) and a tendency toward illness to secure the person on whom one is depending.
- Ren can be under-stimulated and deficient, leading to the inability to connect with anyone.
- Insufficient Yin (often occurs in premature babies).
- Eating without a feeling of satiation, bulimia.
- Addictions.
- Accumulating excess Yin after deeply felt loss (such as loss of a child or the premature death of parent) because that which defines Ren (a feeling of deep belonging) is missing.
- Difficulty with understanding one's identity. Difficulty in identifying with one's gender, ethnicity, group consciousness.

Ren Mai

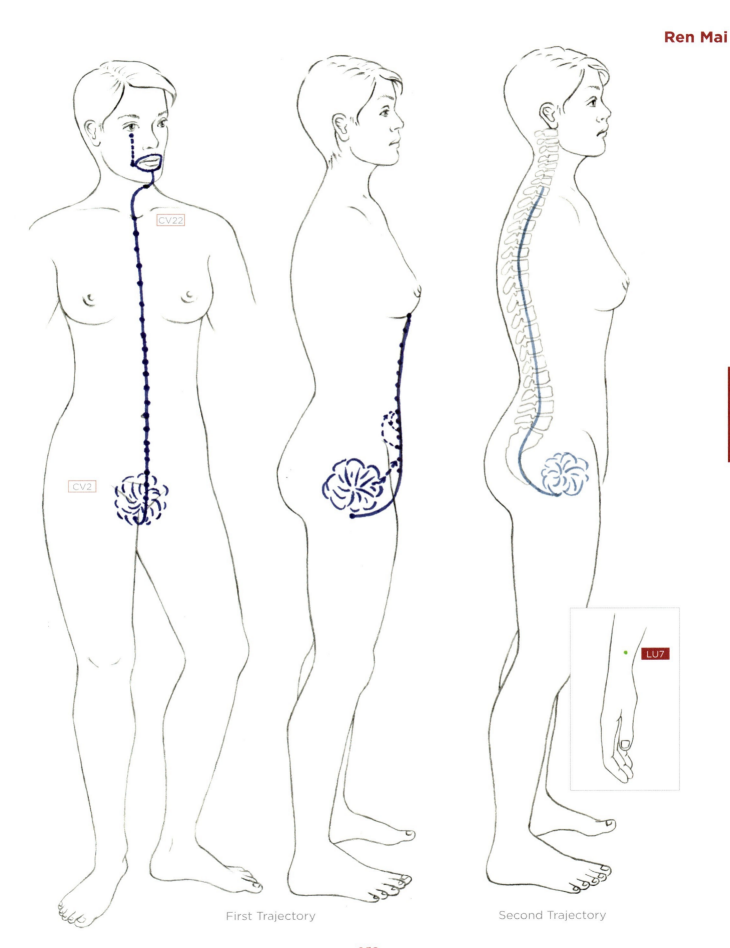

First Trajectory

Second Trajectory

Points of Ren Mai

Ren Mai First Trajectory

Begins in the Lower Jiao behind *Zhong Ji* (CV-3)[5] then **CV-1, CV-2, CV-3, CV-4, CV-5, CV-6, CV-7, CV-8, CV-9, CV-10, CV-11, CV-12, CV-13, CV-14, CV-15, CV-16, CV-17, CV-18, CV-19, CV-20, CV-21, CV-22, CV-23, CV-24, ST-4, ST-1.**

Ren Mai Second Trajectory

Originates in the pelvis and travels up the spine to GV-14:

GV-1, GV-2, GV-3, GV-4, GV-5, GV-6, GV-7, GV-8, GV-9, GV-10, GV-11, GV-12, GV-13, GV-14.

Opening Point of Ren Mai

In the uterus, in the sea of amniotic fluid, the "breath" is provided through the umbilicus and is seamless. LU-7, *Broken Sequence*, refers to the moment of the beginning of the first breath, the very first interaction with the outside world. The baby has broken from the whole and begins the process of finding self-containment. Because LU-7 is a Luo point, it connects the prenatal and postnatal arenas (the Luo to Source connection).

Point Translations and Indications - Selected Points of Ren Mai

CV-1	*Yin Convergence*	Nourishes Yin and drains Dampness. Clears Empty Heat manifesting in the genitals as genital itch or sweat. Regulates the Chong, Ren and Du Channels. Moves Yin stasis. Clears Wind, treats genital swelling. Resuscitates after drowning. Meeting of Chong and Du.
CV-2	*Curved Bone*	Cold in Liver, impotence, hernia, discharges. Meeting of the Liver Channel.
CV-3	*Central Pole*	Damp-Heat in Lower Jiao. Nourishes Yin and breaks up Yin accumulation. Generally used for excess conditions. Meeting of the three Leg Yin Channels.
CV-4	*Origin Pass*	Tonifies Yang for longevity. Treats amenorrhea due to Cold. Warms the interior to move emotions. Treats food stagnation. Treats Yin stasis having impacted on the Shen. Used in deficiencies. Tonifies Kidneys. Meeting of the three leg Yin Channels.
CV-5	*Stone Gate*	Treats Damp-Heat in the Lower Jiao.

[5] The *Ling Shu* says Ren Mai begins in the uterus. Wang Shu-He says Ren Mai begins at ST-30.

CV-6	*Sea of Qi*	Treats Yin stasis, heaviness of the limbs, Coldness, frigidity. Supports the Spleen.
CV-7	*Yin Exchange*	The principal point for infertility. Chong Mai and Ren Mai meet here. Regulates the exchange of Blood and Essence. Disperse for Yin accumulations: fibroids, cysts, tumors.
CV-8	*Spirit Tower Gate*	The first scar. This point is not needled, moxa only. Damp-Cold in the Lower Jiao. Resuscitation point. Stimulates consciousness, stops diarrhea, regulates the intestines. Principal point for issues related to identity.
CV-9	*Fluid Separation*	Assists in the separation of pure and turbid Fluids as indicated by Damp conditions such as ascites. Treats Dampness and Phlegm when moxa'd. Promotes urination. Does not nourish Yin. Moxa for the closure of the fontanelle. Contraindicated during pregnancy.
CV-10	*Lower Receptacle*	Promotes peristalsis and elimination. Treats distention, undigested food; descends Qi for nausea, vomiting, reflux. Meeting of the Spleen Channel.
CV-11	*Strengthening Distance*	Aids digestion, rotting and ripening; descends Stomach Qi, tonifies Spleen Qi. Impaired digestive movement. Food stasis. Failure to derive nutrients from food.
CV-12	*Central Vessel*	Opening of the Stomach organ, beginning of Lung Channel. Regulates entire digestive system. Treats digestive issues and Yin stasis. Helps promote urination. Influential point of the Fu-Bowels. Stimulates the origin of Fluids and Blood. Meeting of the Stomach, Small Intestine and Triple Heater Channels.
CV-13	*Upper Vessel*	For rebellious Qi of the Stomach and Lung resulting in vomiting and coughing. To calm digestive tract after stressful eating practices: eating on-the-go, rushing meals. Meeting of the Stomach and Small Intestine Channels.
CV-14	*Gigantic Tower Gate*	Clears Stomach Fire and Heart Fire disturbing the Shen. Mu point of the Heart.
CV-15	*Turtledove Tail*	Source point of all Yin. Nourishes Yin, calms the

		Shen. Treats abdominal pain due to Blood stagnation. Blood stagnation, mania and withdrawal. Transforms Phlegm. Moistens dryness. Treats *dian-kuang* (mania and withdrawal). Luo point of the Ren Channel.
CV-16	*Central Court*	Relaxes the chest.
CV-17	*Center of the Altar*	Transforms Phlegm. Promotes lactation. Regulates the Qi in the chest. Supports Gu Qi and De Qi in their production of Ancestral-Zong-Gathering/Chest Qi. Chronic respiratory conditions. Mu point of the Pericardium. Influential point for the Sea of Qi.
CV-18	*Jade Hall*	Descends rebellious Qi of the Lung and Stomach. Respiratory distress with disturbed Shen.
CV-19	*Purple Palace*	Descends rebellious Lung Qi. Respiratory distress with disturbed Shen.
CV-20	*Chest Canopy*	Relaxes the chest; treats chest, clavicular and flank pain.
CV-21	*The Jade Axis*	Clears plum pit Qi and Stomach Fire. Treats the feeling of guilt. No moxa.
CV-22	*Celestial Chimney*	Resolves Phlegm in the throat and chest and Wind-Phlegm in the voice. Breaks up goiters. Windows to the Sky point.
CV-23	*Ridge at the Spring*	Opens throat, activates tongue for acute and sudden loss of voice. Head Wind, Bell's Palsy. Descends rebellious Qi. Meeting of Yin Wei Mai.
CV-24	*Sauce Receptacle*	Nourishes Yin and body Fluids. Hydrates the mouth. Subdues Wind in the face.
ST-4	*Earth Granary*	Treats a feeling of being hollow or empty.
ST-1	*Supporting Tears*	Teary, red, itchy, swollen eyes, visual distortion, floaters. Deviation of the mouth. Tinnitus. Accepts the Pure Yang of the Stomach for the sensory orifices.

Treatment Principles of Ren Mai, First and Second Trajectories

1. To resolve Yin stasis appearing with Yin deficiency.
2. To nourish Yin to anchor Yang.
3. To expel Yin stasis.
4. To anchor the Shen, Yang and Qi.
5. To warm the interior, to dry Damp and expel Cold.

Differentiating between the First and Second Trajectories of Ren Mai

Reducing the second trajectory (Du Mai) has the effect of tonifying the first trajectory (Ren Mai). Reducing the first trajectory tonifies the second trajectory. Hence Ren issues can be addressed by working with Du Mai and Du Mai can be addressed through the Ren. (In my practice, I work directly with the trajectory I feel is most affected because it feels simpler.)

The diagnosis of the trajectory indicated is done by taking the pulses in the Eight Extra style (see page 228.) If the Ren pulse is found on the left side (regardless of gender), the first trajectory is indicated. If a Ren pulse is found on the right side, the second trajectory is indicated because the pulse tells us Ren Mai is trying to support Du Mai. Yin is transforming into Yang. Select points on the second trajectory (Du Mai) that nourish Yin.

Point Selection Method for Ren Mai

The Lower Jiao Ren points treat uneasiness about one's form, ethnicity or gender. These issues create problems in the Lower Jiao: reproductive and intestinal issues. The Middle Jiao Ren points treat long-term food sensitivities and loss of appetite control. The Upper Jiao Ren points treat respiratory and Shen issues and enable trust and faith in the divine, as a baby trusts that its needs will be met without asking.

The abdominal and chest points of Ren are considered in three groups of seven to reflect the cycles of seven and eight years. It should be noted that Ren treatments, like all Eight Extras, are equally applicable to men and women.

Ren begins: Lower Jiao, then CV-1

The first set of seven, the Lower Jiao:	CV-2, 3, 4, 5, 6, 7, 8	Deficiencies
The second set of seven the Middle Jiao:	CV-9, 10, 11, 12, 13, 14, 15	Deficiencies
The third set of seven the Upper Jiao:	CV-16, 17, 18, 19, 20, 21, 22	Yin Stasis
The trajectory continues:	CV-23, 24	The culmination of Yin
	ST-4, ST-1	The distribution of Yin to the sensory orifices

Needling Techniques for Ren Mai

Since all Eight Extra points are vibrated (or shaken), abdominal points are generally needled with a slow vibration (tonified) and chest points are needled with a fast vibration (dispersed). This is because, generally speaking, the abdominal points of the Ren Channel are used to tonify deficiency and the chest points are used to disperse excess, since the chest can tend to accumulate Yin in order to compensate for the Yin deficiency.

Points on Ren Mai that treat Cold should be treated with seven moxa cones.

Needling the Opening Point of Ren Mai

Gently press the thenar eminence to stretch the Lung Channel out. The Opening point will be more easily palpable. Release the stretch. Needle towards the thumb. The patient may become quite sleepy.

Example of Point Selection for Ren Mai

To resolve Yin stasis with accompanying Yin deficiency: LU-7, CV-1, CV-7, CV-12, CV-15, CV-17, CV-22, CV-24, ST-1

To nourish Yin to anchor Yang: LU-7, CV-1, CV-7, CV-12, CV-15, CV-24

To expel Yin stasis: LU-7, CV-3, CV-4, CV-9, CV-17, CV-22

To anchor the Shen, Yang and Qi: LU-7, CV-23, CV-18, CV-15, CV-4

To warm the interior, dry Damp and expel Cold: LU-7, CV-6, CV-8, CV-9, CV-21

Treatment Protocol for Ren Mai

All points are vibrated.

1. Needle the Opening point, LU-7, left for females, right for males. (Sides are reversed in Ren and Du). Or, open Ren on the left and Du on the right regardless of gender.
2. Needle the landmark points chosen, if any, in ascending order. Landmark points are CV-2, CV-7, CV-9, CV-15, CV-17, CV-22, CV-23, CV-24.
3. Needle the remaining chosen points in ascending order for the first trajectory and descending order for the second trajectory.
4. Revisit each point in the order needled and check that the patient feels at least a very subtle vibration in each point.
5. Ask the patient to visualize or to imagine the feeling of the connection of all the points. Often they will report that they already feel this connection vibrating.

6. Take the pulses in the Eight Extra position. The pulses will have moved deeper into the wrist. If they have not, re-vibrate the needles, ensuring that connection with the Yuan level has been made. This is done by intention rather than literal depth.
7. *(Optional)*. Give the patient an affirmation to repeat while they are in treatment, e.g., *I am whole and complete within*.
8. Leave needles in for 40 minutes after the insertion of the Opening point.
9. Take the pulses in Eight Extra style, note the change and report it to the patient.
10. Remove the needles in the following order:
    a. Opening point
    b. other needles in the order opposite that of insertion
11. Allow the patient five minutes on the table, preferably alone, to reflect.

DU MAI TREATMENTS

The Governing Channel/Vessel (GV), the Sea of Yang, the Channel of Individuality

Mechanisms of Du Mai

The Du Channel is the origin of all Yang and as such it warms, upholds and moves. Du Mai governs the separation from the maternal matrix, the functioning of the sensory-motor tracts and the development of reflexes, the achievement of the upright posture, and the development of curiosity, individuality, independence and disposition. Du Mai allows for the construction of the body via the movement and warmth of Yang Qi. It creates the curves of the spine, enabling the child to engage with the world. The child's thoughts and emotions are conveyed along this route, stimulating exploration and experimentation. Du Mai animates the Shen and governs orientation to the world. It reveals meaning and purpose in life through its generation of the Triple Heater mechanism at birth.

Du Mai is activated after birth with the first movement of the head and is mature at the age of two when a child is ready to wean and has fully established the upright posture. It controls the oral cavity and phonetics. When Du Mai is in balance, the child can be harmonious even when told "no".

Du Mai provides the Yang to enable the body to transform, transport, ascend, consolidate, bank, prevent leakages, scatter Cold and expel pathological Yin.

Du Mai's chief function is to support postnatal Qi. The rotting and ripening of food occurs under the auspices of Kidney Yang which is ascended to the digestive tract by the Spleen. The origin of this Yang is Du Mai.

Du Mai provides the Yang for the formation of Wei Qi, supporting Wei Qi via the Du branch that goes to BL-1.

Du Mai is a member of the first ancestry of Eight Extra Channels and as such is involved in the origin of life. Du allows for fertility through the warming effect of Yang Qi.

Du Mai governs the Yang humors: Qi and Shen.

Non-Pathological State of Du Mai

When Du Mai is in balance the person feels free and fully independent. They are able to walk away from that which does not serve them.

Pathological State of Du Mai

When Du Mai is not in balance, there is conflict with moving forward. This is often accompanied by either a lack of independence or rebellion with hyperactivity. Curiosity and the desire to learn are impeded.

Indications of Du Mai

Classical principal signs and symptoms: Chronic swollen eyes. Epilepsy, loss of voice, throat Bi, head Wind, numbness of the limbs.

General pulse picture: Floating and long. See also Eight Extra pulse technique on page 228.

Physical Indications of Du Mai

- Exuberant Wind signs: Neurological signs - infantile seizures, Parkinson's disease, epilepsy, stroke, Bell's palsy, hemiplegia.
- Disturbed Shen, restlessness, high fevers, Malaria.
- Deficient Yang signs: Stiffness, Cold, frigidity, numbness.
- Low libido, decreased sexual function, impotence, sterility or infertility. Low motility of the egg or sperm.

- Amnesia, "feeble-mindedness".
- Balance and gait issues, lack of coordination.
- Deficient Yang resulting in deficient Wei Qi maintaining the Sinews and the sensory orifices, manifesting in the failure to resolve issues in those regions, e.g., polyps, dermatological issues, chronic Phlegm congestion.
- Back pain as though having been "hit by a sledgehammer". Excruciating pain in the back.
- Rebellious Qi in the lower abdomen causing Heart pain and difficulty in urination and defecation.
- Hemorrhoids, incontinence.
- Dry throat.
- Throat Bi affecting language, difficulty articulating ideas. Stuttering.
- Loss of voice.
- Prolapses.

Psychological Indications of Du Mai

Du Mai in a State of Excess:
- Strong aversion to commitment and responsibility.
- Over-independence.
- Early independence with an accompanying difficulty with commitment and a dissatisfaction with current status.
- Over-achievement without happiness.
- Hyperactivity. Behaving as though over-stimulated.
- Always searching for something better.
- Holding the view that the world is separate from self. Wei Qi pushes world away resulting in Wind and Heat pathology.
- Seeing the world as perverse and not allowing it in, resulting in rebellious Qi, throat issues, allergies, respiratory conditions and Stomach Fire.
- Attention Deficit Hyperactivity Disorder (ADHD), especially in children, caused by overexposure to stimuli (noisy toys, too many objects in the room, bright paint colors, toys with lights, electronic screens of all kinds, and electronic toys).
- Allergies or seizures can develop as a result of hyper-stimulation.

Du Mai in a State of Deficiency:
- Failure to initiate action.
- A tendency to follow and never to lead.

- Timidity, shyness.
- Fear of being alone.
- A tendency to be clingy, over-dependent (over-bonded) due to excess Cold or Damp in Ren Mai.
- Language problems including stuttering or lack of speech.
- Failure to establish boundaries or a tendency to break them.
- Lack of animation, motivation and enthusiasm reflected in posture, motion and gesture.
- A child who is under-stimulated will develop a lack of motivation.
- Failure to establish independence.

Opening Point of Du Mai

SI-3   *Behind the Ravine*   (The Ravine is the Kidneys.) The Fire element, represented here as a Small Intestine point, amplifies life's curriculum, which is stored in the Kidneys. SI-3 is also a Shu-Stream point and it moves pathology to the exterior for release. Shu-Stream points can usher out or bring back in. As the Opening point of Du Mai, SI-3 facilitates Yang moving out into the world to enable curiosity and as the Yang (moving) pair of the Heart, Small Intestine brings that information back into the Heart to be owned. SI-3 treats the head, face and neck.

Main Points of Du Mai

Begins below the *pole* (*xia ji*)[6] then **GV-1, GV-2, GV-3, GV-4, GV-5, GV-6, GV-7, GV-8, GV-9, GV-10, GV-11, GV-12, GV-13, GV-14 GV-15, GV-16, GV-17, GV-18, GV-19, GV-20, GV-21, GV-22, GV-23, GV-24, GV-25, GV-26, GV-27, GV-28.**

Point Translations and Indications of the Main Points of Du Mai

GV-1	*Long Endurance*	Damp-Heat, dysentery, turbid, burning urine, prolapse of anus, hemorrhoids, stiffness of the spine, heavy head. Calms Shen, anchors Yang. Luo point of Du Mai.
GV-2	*Waist Shu*	Wind-Damp in the Lower Jiao causing frequent urination, distending pain on urination, irregular menstruation, internal Wind, epilepsy. Moves the waist.

---

[6] Wang Shu-He identifies the pole as GV-1, Li Shi Zhen says it's CV-1, and the *Nan Jing* identifies the pole as Po Men (the anus).

GV-3	Waist Yang Gate	Treats internal Cold with Yang deficiency. Warms uterus to address Blood stasis and infertility.
GV-4	Life Gate	Tonifies Essence. Tonifies Kidney Yang if moxa'd. Use only if patient is over age 21, or at least past puberty.
GV-5	Suspended Axis	Brings Yang to the Spleen to treat prolapse. Loose stools.
GV-6	Spinal Center	No Moxa. Treats hemorrhoids, Dampness, ascites, diarrhea. Massage point to help children with diarrhea.
GV-7	Essential Pivot	Visual dizziness when standing. Treats jaundice. Gallbladder and Stomach issues.
GV-8	Sinew Contraction	Treats atrophy of the sinews. Helps person change pattern of their habitual response to stress. Opens patient to possibilities. Exuberant Heat resulting in seizures, delirium, mania.
GV-9	Extreme Yang	Master point for coughing and wheezing, opens chest. Root of trapezius and master point for the diaphragm. Treats chronic Damp-Heat. Regulates Liver and Gallbladder.
GV-10	Soul Tower	No needling (needling disturbs Spirit). Cough, wheeze, depression, pessimism.
GV-11	Spirit Path	No needling (needling disturbs Spirit). Moxa only. Clears Heat in Heart, calms Shen. Anxiety, palpitations.
GV-12	Body Pillar	Tonifies Lung Qi for chronic Lung Qi deficiency. Internal Wind, fever. Straightens spine. Master point for pathology in the brain which is affecting the spine.
GV-13	Kiln Path	Point at which excess Heat is moved to the scapula rather than allowing it to go into BL-11, the influential point of the bones, which is adjacent. Treats Lung Heat and Steaming Bone Syndrome. Cup the point. Meeting of the Bladder Channel.
GV-14	Great Hammer	Moxa to tonify Wei Qi and to bring Yang to the upper limbs. Bleed to clear internal Heat. Meeting of all six Yang Channels.
GV-15	Mute Door	Stimulates speech. Yang Wei Mai meeting.
GV-16	Wind Mansion	Expels Wind from the Marrow/brain for stroke, seizures and epilepsy. No retention. Engage Wind and withdraw needle. Clears Heat in throat. Opens and relaxes the four

		limbs. Ghost point. Yang Wei Mai meeting.
GV-17	*Brain Door*	Expels Wind affecting brain. Massage for Wind. Treats poor memory and Wind in the head. Swelling of head and orifices. Meeting of the Bladder Channel.
GV-18	*Enduring Space*	Expels Wind. Moves bowels.
GV-19	*Behind the Vertex*	Calms Shen and subdues Yang.
GV-20	*Hundred Meetings*	Meeting of all six Yang Channels and Liver Channel. Opens consciousness to clear the mind. Moxa to ascend Yang only if there are no Heat signs. Lifts the Shen. Upper point of the Sea of Marrow. Treats loss of sensation. Moves Yang Qi.
GV-21	*Before the Vertex*	Subdues Wind and swelling on the face, especially the nose.
GV-22	*Meeting of Arrogance*	Subdues Wind. Needle away from the dominant side.
GV-23	*Upper Star*	Opens nose and eyes. Stops bleeding in head and face. Treats polyps, Phlegm trapped in sinuses, and allergies. Ghost point.
GV-24	*Spirit Court*	No needle. Calms Shen. Meeting of the Bladder and Stomach Channels.
GV-25	*White Bone Hole*	No moxa. Opens nose to release Heat and congestion.
GV-26	*Center of Man*	Resuscitates consciousness, clears Heat. Ghost point. Meeting of the Large Intestine and Stomach Channels.
GV-27	*Mouth Extremity*	No moxa. Clears empty Heat. Gum and lip swellings. Loss of voice and throat bi.
GV-28	*Gum Intersection*	Clears Heat on the face. Bleed for red face, headaches, Stomach Fire manifesting in gums and sensory orifices. Meeting of the Stomach Channel and Ren Mai. Loss of voice and throat bi.

Du Mai

First Trajectory

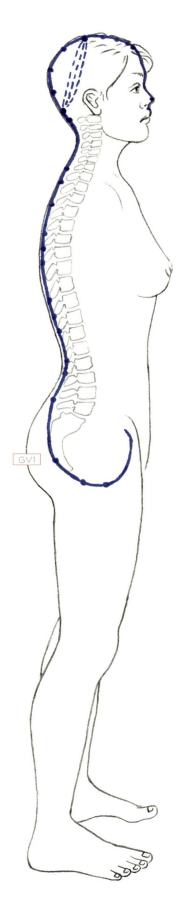
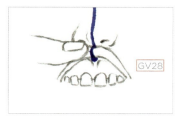
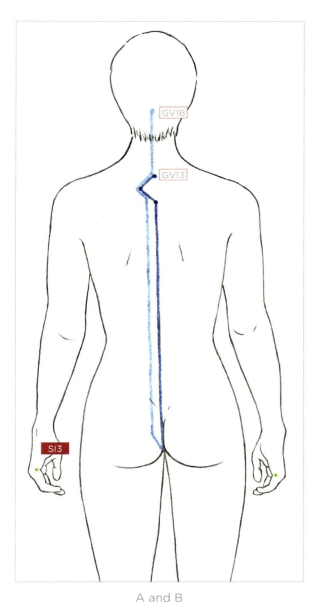

A and B

Du Mai First Trajectory

Du Mai First Trajectory Characteristics

The first trajectory creates the ability to be independent: it forms the upright posture and propels the structure and the psyche forward. It governs the desire to explore and allows risk-taking to occur in that process.

Du Mai First Trajectory Points

Begins in the pelvis, then to CV-1, GV-1, then travels up the spine diverting to BL-12 from GV-12 before returning to GV-13, over posterior midline of the head and down anterior midline into the philtrum, ending inside the mouth on the gum at GV-28, where it connects to Ren Mai. This trajectory creates the upright posture.

Points: **CV-1, GV-1, GV-2, GV-3, GV-4, GV-5, GV-6, GV-7, GV-8, GV-9, GV-10, GV-11, GV-12, GV-13, GV-14 GV-15, GV-16, GV-17, GV-18, GV-19, GV-20, GV-21, GV-22, GV-23, GV-24, GV-25, GV-26, GV-27, GV-28.**

Du takes two additional paths between GV-1 and GV-16 (shown as A, B). A: GV-1 to GV-12, then BL-12 and ending at GV-13. B: GV-1, then along Hua To line to GV-12, BL-12, GV-13, to GV-16.

Du Mai First Trajectory Pathology

Shyness, disinterest in learning.

Males: Rebellious Qi emanating from the lower abdomen causes Heart pain and difficulty in urination and defecation.

Females: Infertility, hemorrhoids, incontinence, dry throat.

Du Mai First Trajectory Treatment Principle

To articulate Yang.

Du Mai First Trajectory Sample Point Selection

SI-3, GV-4, GV-14, BL-23, BL-52.

Du Mai Second Trajectory

Du Mai Second Trajectory Characteristics

The second trajectory invites morality to temper the reach into the outside world. Without this aspect of Du Mai, we would constantly be "stepping on toes", feeling guilt at having overstepped and rage at being held back by structures imposed from the outside. This tempering of "rampant Yang" is achieved not only by Yin (weighing down or

Du Mai

Second Trajectory

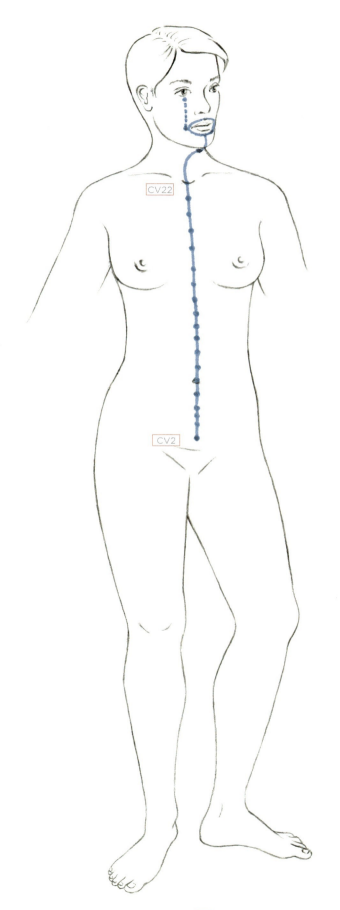

corralling the Yang) but by an aspect of Yang itself. There must be an *action* of tempering within Yang itself, an active capacity of tempering the strength to move or reach forward. This aspect of Du Mai, expressed in the second trajectory, is the instinct and ability to move toward home, toward what is true for us.

Du Mai Second Trajectory Points

Begins in the lower abdomen, goes to the navel, chest, throat, encircles the mouth and terminates at the eyes. This trajectory is identical to Ren Mai.
Points: **CV-1, CV-2, CV-3, CV-4, CV-5, CV-6, CV-7, CV-8, CV-9, CV-10, CV-11, CV-12, CV-13, CV-14, CV-15, CV-16, CV-17, CV-18, CV-19, CV-20, CV-21, CV-22, CV-23, CV-24, ST-4, ST-1.**

Du Mai Second Trajectory Pathology

Overachieving, over-independence, inability to commit and be satisfied.

Du Mai Second Trajectory Treatment Principle

To anchor Yang.

Du Mai Second Trajectory Sample Point Selection

SI-3, CV-4, CV-5, LU-7

Du Mai Third Trajectory

Du Mai Third Trajectory Characteristics

Governs the sensory-motor tracts. Allows for stimulus to create action. Brings Wei Qi to the Sinew Channels. Communicates with Yang Qiao Mai.

Du Mai Third Trajectory Points

Begins at BL-1, ascends to the forehead, then to GV-20, enters the brain, and emerges at GV-16 where it divides in two and travels along the Hua To Jia Ji points, then enters the Kidneys at BL-23.

Du Mai Third Trajectory Pathology

Classical Symptoms: Red swollen eyes, head Wind, numbness of the limbs, epilepsy. Also Parkinson's disease, seizures. Sensory-motor tract issues. Wei Qi issues.

Du Mai

Third Trajectory

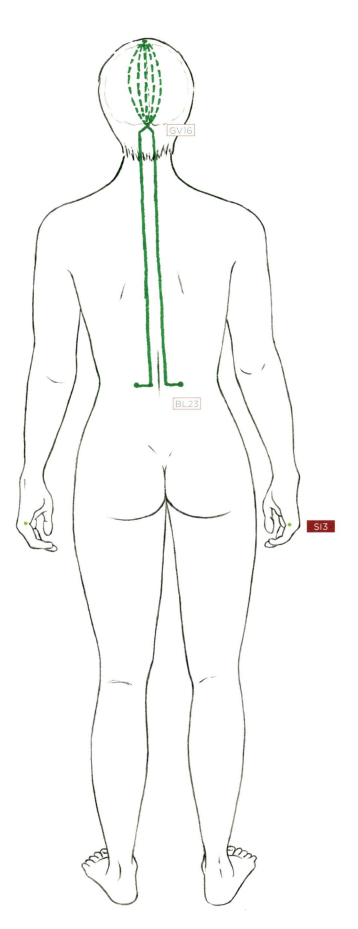
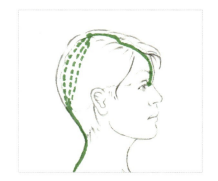
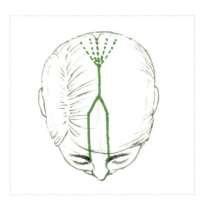

Du Mai Third Trajectory Treatment Principle

To subdue Wind in the portals.

Du Mai Third Trajectory Sample Point Selection

SI-3, BL-1, GV-20, GV-16, GV-12, sensitive Hua To Jia Ji points, BL-23.
Moxa GV-12 if the spine is rebellious (stiff).

Du Mai Fourth Trajectory

Du Mai Fourth Trajectory Characteristics

The Sea of Yang. Warms, transforms, transports, ascends and upholds Qi. Assists Spleen in ascending Qi, banks Qi to stop loss. Protects by supporting Wei-Defensive Qi. Enables the sustaining of enthusiasm.

Du Mai Fourth Trajectory Points

Begins in the lower abdomen, goes to the genitalia, CV-1, then GV-1, then to gluteus (sometimes referred to as BL-35), to the spine and ends in the Kidneys (BL-23).

Du Mai Fourth Trajectory Pathology

Hemorrhoids, sagging gluteus, prolapses, hernia. Weakness, tightness or spasms of the lower limbs, Qi stagnation. Lack of animation, enthusiasm, motivation.

Du Mai Fourth Trajectory Treatment Principle

To uphold the Yang.

Du Mai Fourth Trajectory Sample Point Selection

SI-3, GV-1, BL-35, BL-23
Add LI-11 if the upper limbs exhibit weakness, tightness or spasms.
Add GB-34 if the lower limbs exhibit weakness, tightness or spasms.

Selecting Trajectories in Du Mai Treatments

If a Du Mai pulse is found on the *right*, the first, third or fourth trajectory of the Du is indicated. Differentiate between the trajectories according to signs and symptoms and palpation. If a Du Mai pulse is found on the *left*, it's a second trajectory pulse. The Yang of Du Mai is supporting the Yin of Ren Mai. Use points on the Ren that tonify Yang.

Du Mai

Fourth Trajectory

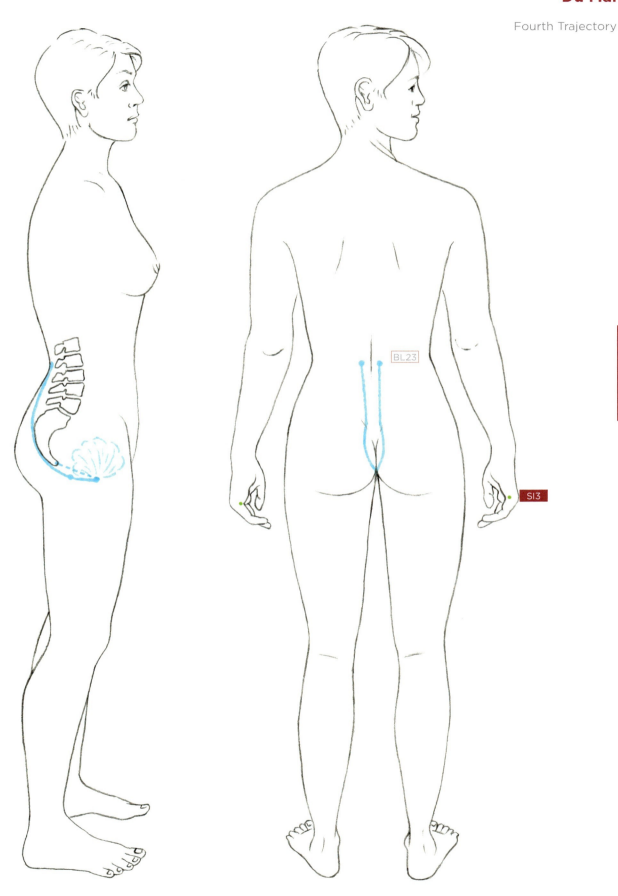

Treatment

Needling the Opening Point of Du Mai, SI-3.

Create a loose fist, so that the little finger is curled toward the palm. Needle into the bundle of fascia. The patient may feel as though floating.

Landmark Points of Du Mai

GV-1, GV-4, GV-9, GV-14, GV-20, GV-26 (These may or may not be included in a treatment.)

Point Selection for Du Mai

Point selection is often thought of in terms of the three curves of the spine.

The points of the lower curvature, GV-1 to GV-4 treat Du-related intestinal, reproductive and urogenital issues.

The points of the middle curvature, GV-5 to GV-9 treat Du-related digestive issues.

The points of the upper curvature, GV-10 to GV-16 treat Du-related respiratory, cardiovascular and throat issues.

Du points on the head, GV-17 to GV-28 treat Du-related Shen, neurological and sensory orifice conditions.

Lower Du points tend to treat Dampness.

Upper Du points tend to treat Wind issues.

Tonify points chosen to address loss or weakness.

Reduce points chosen to address excess.

WARNING

GV-6	cannot be moxa'd. Scoliosis would result.
GV-10 and GV-11	cannot be needled. Departure of Shen would result.
GV-4	is strictly contraindicated before puberty and best only used in adulthood. The Bladder Shu points are contraindicated until the end of the first cycle of seven at the earliest, but are best not used on children under the age of 10. Needling the Bladder Shu's or GV-4 before adulthood, or at least before puberty interrupts the dissemination of Yuan Qi and disorients it. The exception to this rule would be extreme conditions at the level of the Constitution involving pathological Yin, such as Down's Syndrome.
GV-24	is not needled. The Shen would be disturbed.

Children with Wind

Insert and remove immediately, leaving the point open if treating Wind. Be sure to use a needle with a coiled handle and a loop on the top of it. Alternatively, non-insertable needles can be used, with light pressure.

Treatment Protocol for Du Mai

Assess the signs and symptoms and identify which trajectory of Du Mai is to be treated.

1. Needle the Opening point, SI-3, left for females, right for males. (Sides are reversed in Ren and Du.) Alternatively, open Du Mai on the right for both genders and Ren Mai on the left for both genders.
2. Needle the landmark points chosen, if any, in the order they occur on the trajectory you are needling.
3. Needle the remaining chosen trajectory points.
4. Revisit each point in the order needled and check that the patient feels at least a very subtle vibration in each point.
5. Ask the patient to visualize or to imagine the feeling of the connection of all the points. Often they will report that they already feel this connection vibrating. In a trajectory that is as complex as some of these branches, you might elect to show them a picture.
6. Take the pulses in the Eight Extra position. The pulses will have moved deeper into the wrist. If they have not, re-vibrate the needles, ensuring that connection with the Yuan level has been made. This is done by intention rather than literal depth.
7. *(Optional).* Give the patient an affirmation to repeat while they are in treatment, e.g., *I am calm, grounded, strong, focused and motivated.*
8. Leave needles in for 40 minutes after the insertion of the Opening point.
9. Take the pulses in Eight Extra style, note the change and report it to the patient.
10. Remove the needles in the following order:
    a. Opening point
    b. other needles in the order opposite that of insertion
11. Allow the patient five minutes on the table, preferably alone, to reflect.

The Wei Channels

Weaving the Cloth of Life

The Wei Channels are analogous to a silk cloth depicting the images and actions of one's life. The Chinese word for Wei contains the characters *silk* and *network*, just as the warp and weft on the loom is a network. The Wei Channels are like a historical record to which we could refer, to inquire about the events and actions of a life lived.[7]

The *substance* of the cloth and the *images* on the cloth are analogous to the collection of *events* in our lives and the perceivable *changes* that those events have made in our bodies and minds. This is Yin Wei Mai, the record of changes imparted to the bodymind.

Yang Wei Mai is analogous to a record of the *actions* taken to *create* the cloth. When you look at a tapestry you can imagine the actions that took place to make it. The threads could only have been woven a certain way in order for the cloth to appear the way it does. The movement of the threads is recorded as the cloth is formed, that is, we can see the result of the past actions of the weaver.

Yang Wei Mai records past actions; Yin Wei Mai records changes to substance (and events during the course of the lifetime that altered the way structure was formed.)

By contrast, the Qiao Channels represent a snapshot of the tapestry (and it's context) in the present moment.

GB-29 and SI-10 represent the shuttle and the foot pedals of the loom, which are active and potent in the present moment. These two points connect the Qiao and Wei Channels. Whatever we feel and decide to do in a given moment is a reflection of the Qiao's and manifests in the Wei's.

The part of the cloth woven so far can govern the tone of what we decide to weave in the remainder of the tapestry, although at any moment we can make a choice which would alter the tapestry as a whole.

---

[7] This Wei means linking and is not related to the word Wei which translates as defensive. They are different characters in Chinese; in English the distinction is identified by context.

YIN WEI MAI TREATMENTS

The Yin Linking Channel, The Vessels of Aging and the Cycles of Seven and Eight
(Yin and Yang Wei Mai)

Yin Wei Mai links Yin to create substance. Yang Wei Mai links Yang to create movement.

Mechanisms of Yin Wei Mai

The Wei Channels, as a pair, record the impact of the major transitions we undergo in time and space. Yin Wei Mai records the changes in our structure (in the physical body), and Yang Wei Mai records the activities the body was engaged in that resulted in those physical changes. Together they form a tangible and intangible autobiography–a physical, mental and emotional record of all that we have experienced.

When a person is consistently living in the present moment, the Wei Channels are in balance. The Wei Channels become imbalanced when they stagnate as the patient longs for that which is past (a pathology of Yin Wei Mai), or fears or fantasizes about what is to come (a pathology of Yang Wei Mai). Obsessions about the past and future and resistance create images which, in order to exist, require financing by Blood and Qi. Over time Qi and Blood become exhausted through their support of these images which inhibit our movement through the stages of life. The body responds to the depletion of resources by trying to conserve these commodities through stagnating them. If Blood is stagnated, the Shen is automatically negatively affected as it cannot be in free flow. If Qi is stagnated, pain results.

Yin Wei Mai is responsible for the integrity of the structure. It keeps Yin from disintegrating and at the same time is the mediumship of aging. Yin is conserved as it is returned to its origin at CV-22 and CV-23. This is one of the ways in which postnatal Yin replenishes prenatal Yin.

Yin Wei Mai is the channel that takes us out of the first ancestry, into the outside world. Encounters with the outside world can lead to disappointment, regret, Heart pain, even anxious anticipation about looking back at the end of life, examining our accomplishments and deeming them insufficient. These emotions inhibit the flow of Qi in the Wei Channels.

The two Wei Channels comprise the second ancestry, the second set of the Eight Extraordinary Channels.

Non-Pathological State of Yin Wei Mai

When Yin Wei Mai is in good balance the person has their attention on the present moment; the past has been let go and the future is not feared or subject to focus.

Pathological State of Yin Wei Mai

When Yin Wei Mai is not in balance, there is obsession with the past or future, with a deficiency and stagnation of Qi.

Indications of Yin Wei Mai

Classical principal signs: Heart pain, palpitations, restlessness, affected Shen. Heart pain means disappointment in not having achieved goals set. *Fei Yang* is another classical sign and refers to lumbar pain accompanied by fear and depression. This is detectable as a "flying" or palpable pulse at BL-58. Visual dizziness, sudden fainting with stiffness, and chest and rib pain can also arise.

General pulse picture: Thready, choppy, rapid. See also, Eight Extra pulse technique on page 228.

Physical Indications of Yin Wei Mai

Accumulations occur as the obsession with creating images of the past and future drain the Ren of Yin and the Du of Yang. The resulting stagnation of Yin and Yang creates pain which is both emotional and somatic.

- The Five Accumulations related to the Zang organs:
    1. Heart: *fu liang/hidden beam*.
    2. Lung: *fu xi/panting*.
    3. Liver: *peng Qi/fatty deposits*.
    4. Spleen: *pi Qi/glomus Qi (Blood)*.
    5. Kidney: *ben tun/Running Piglet Qi*.
- *Ji and Ju* (accumulations and concentrations): hernia, UTI, prostatitis. (Men-focused).
- *Zheng and Jia* (concretions and gatherings which afflict the Lower Jiao): fibroids, cysts, tumors (Women-focused).

Note: Ji and Zheng (accumulations and concretions) are fixed masses.
 Ju and Jia (concentrations and gatherings) are not fixed masses.

- Low back pain which is achy and heavy and sometimes stiff and tight.
- Alzheimer's Disease, poor memory.
- Palpitations, fibrillations, arrhythmia, tachycardia, mitral valve prolapse, restlessness, chest, rib and Heart pain (as Liver Blood is unable to nourish Heart Blood).

- Inability to accept the past resulting in shame and guilt.
- Emotional stagnation resulting in deficient Blood due to Qi stasis.
- Visceral dryness caused by Blood deficiency. (Dryness of the Zang.)
- Headaches due to Blood deficiency, especially those occurring during menstruation.

Psychological Indications of Yin Wei Mai

Longing for the past creates pain. The perceived space between the present and the past cannot be filled and is under psychic tension which becomes somatic.

- Obsession with the past. Yearning for the resolution of past trauma, past hurts, past disappointments.
- Feeling as though one is not in control of one's own life.
- A sense of lack of purpose.
- Lack of will, lack of motivation, lack of enthusiasm, cynicism, pessimism.
- Visceral dryness/visceral agitation, due to the denial of the expression of the innate personality. This denial blocks the dissemination of Jing via Triple Heater and results in a shift in personality.
- Pensiveness, obsession resulting in stagnation.
- Guilt.
- Asking the self "what if…" Spending time wondering what life would be like if one were born in a different place or time.
- Resistance to aging. Resistance to the visible and structural changes that occur with aging.
- Anxiety about life not turning out as expected.
- Anxiety about not being able to overcome the past.
- Throat Bi due to inability to talk about past trauma.
- Anxiety about contracting a disease that runs in the family. (The Zhi-Will can overcome inherited conditions.)
- Suppression of memories.
- Shen disturbance with Blood deficiency.
- Yin Wei Mai treats the Nine Heart Pains: Emotional pain related to Finances, Prosperity, Health, Career, Vocation, Relationships, Children or Creativity, Adventure, and the cultivation of a sense of Home.

Yin Wei Mai

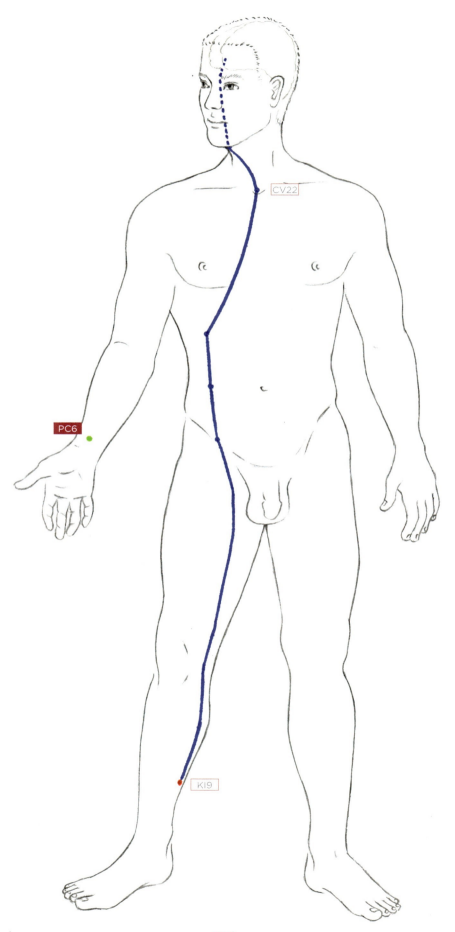

Points of Yin Wei Mai

The sequence of points is a narrative of self-examination. Yin Wei Mai's points invite examination of our life experience and the impact the self (reflected in the Kidneys) has had on society (reflected in the Spleen) and the interface between the exterior and the outside world (reflected in the Liver as the Liver controls Wei Qi). At the end of the channel, Yin Wei Mai returns to the Ren Channel, its origin.

KI-9, SP-13, SP-15, SP-16, LR-14, CV-22, CV-23, then enters the brain.

Opening Point of Yin Wei Mai

PC-6 *Inner Pass* Opens the chest to relieve Heart pain. Dredges Heat.

Xi-Cleft Points as Eight Extra Emergency Points

Xi-Cleft points are areas where Qi pools, causing pain. In the context of the Primary Channels, Xi-Cleft points are strongly reduced to relieve pain in the channel. In the context of the Eight Extras, the Xi-Cleft points have two broad functions, one for emergencies (for which they are strongly reduced and can be used alone) and one for their deep philosophical and physiological meaning (for which they are vibrated in the manner of the other points along the channel). For example, KI-9, the Xi-Cleft point of Yin Wei Mai might be strongly reduced to treat acute angina (Heart pain), but it would be vibrated if used to treat an inability to let go of the past that seems to have suddenly brought a person's life to a halt. (Later the channel could gather enough stagnation to produce that angina.) Because *these points can be used alone and for ease of reference, I have placed a special description of the Xi-Cleft points before the main description of the points of the Wei and Qiao Channels.*

Xi-Cleft Point of Yin Wei Mai

KI-9 *Guest House* Clears the Heart, clears Heart pain, clears Heat. Settles Fright.

Point Translations and Indications - Selected Points of Yin Wei Mai

KI-9 *Guest House* Presents an invitation to step outside of the self and examine the self as though one were a guest, that is, with less judgment. Allows one to choose and take on a different, freer identity, to break the cycle of obsession with past and future. Frees the patient to feel that the experiences of life are transient (guest-like). As the Xi-Cleft point of Yin Wei Mai, KI-9 is used for anxiety related to performance in society, e.g., work stress. Enables a person to step back and see the destiny they have chosen. An analgesic point, it treats trauma and grounds patients, allowing them to know who they are again. Transforms obsession. Detoxification point used in periods of cultivation, and in pregnancy.

SP-13 *The Abode of the Bowels, The Warehouse of the Residence.*

Allows patients to understand their development in society and at the same time, define their place of sanctuary, their place of rest. When we feel at home, experiences can come and go freely, and the bowels can move freely. SP-13 functions as a metaphor for the encouragement of the flow of events; they move down and are let go. Often long-term constipation can be traced to an event. SP-13 frees the bowels from this attachment. Invites freedom from sentimental attachments, physical and mental. Relieves pain and relaxes muscles. Treats abdominal accumulations, obesity, concretions and conglomerations. Rectifies, courses and regulates Qi. Enables one to define their home base. Meeting of the three leg Yin Channels and the Stomach Channel.

SP-15 *The Great Bend, The Great Curve*

Treats the "Great Wind", the feeling of chaos as things change and adjustment to the change seems unattainable. Treats fullness and distention, absorption and elimination. Allows us to own our life's experiences, and absorb and eliminate them. Treats incomplete assimilation. Treats the tendency to avoid assimilation of life's lessons (hence the "curve") and the tendency to avoidance. Moves stagnation created by obsession and Dampness. Disperses fluid accumulation.

SP-16 *Abdominal Weakness, Abdominal Lament.*

Treats sorrow, remorse about the self. Lamenting or harboring grudges can cause the loss of the ability to love again; SP-16 opens the self to be able to love for no reason. Treats the tendency to withdraw love due to an incident. Treats the tendency to measure love and not acknowledge love as greater than a reward for sacrifice. Treats dysentery, diarrhea, undigested food, blood and mucus in the stools, constipation, being stuck in time and unable to move on. Treats paraplegia, paralysis, post-traumatic stress disorder, the catatonic state that follows shock or assault, revenge or anti-social behavior following assault. Descends Qi. Breaks up Damp accumulations. Clears Heat, anxiety, irritability.

LR-14 *Gateway of Completion*

Directs us back to ourselves, rectifies and normalizes Qi. Treats obsession with time. Time is cyclical and these cycles can be deemed complete and let go. Enables the emergence of the feeling of life being complete. Allows memories to retreat. Treats perception of past, present and future. Treats irregular menses, dysmenorrhea. Regulates Qi. Governs synchronicity and treats jet-lag. Irregular, intermittent, or rapid heartbeat. Transforms Phlegm and regulates Qi. Treats Shao Yang conditions.

CV-22 *Celestial Chimney, Releasing the Chimney.*

Enables the patient to let go. Allows self-expression to rise from the chest to enable the achievement of one's visions and the realization of one's motivations. Nourishes Fluids.

CV-23 *Angular Spring* Opens the way to returning to the self, to reassume one's true identity as it connects back its partner, Bubbling Spring at KI-1. Opens and restores one's voice and allows for the articulation of one's truth as the Heart opens to the tongue. Heart pain results when we don't speak our truth, and failure to speak one's truth is an insult to the constitution; CV-23 restores this expression and nourishes Yin in the process.

Treatment

Treatment of Yin Wei Mai enables the patient to view their life as a series of events that come and go, and gives the patient the opportunity to choose to return to living in the present moment.

The main aim of a Yin Wei Mai treatment is to help the patient find a sense of satisfied happiness in themselves.

Treatment Principles of Yin Wei Mai

1. To calm the Shen.
2. To nourish Blood.
3. To regulate Qi.
4. To nourish any Yin humor (Yin, Blood, Fluids) in the absence of stagnation of the Yin humors. (If stagnation of a Yin humor exists, use Ren or Chong.)
5. To nourish any Yin humor in the presence of Qi stasis or emotional stasis.

Needling the Opening Point of Yin Wei Mai, PC-6

Flex the patient's wrist gently. Often, the point will be quite apparent. Needle where the greatest dip between the tendons is. If the tendons are too close together to needle between, needle under the tendon from the ulnar side. The patient will feel as though they are able to breathe more deeply.

Treatment Protocol for Yin Wei Mai

1. (*Optional*) Needle the Opening point, PC-6, right for females, left for males.
2. Needle the first point on the trajectory, KI-9.
3. Needle the landmark points chosen, if any, in ascending order, e.g., SP-15, CV-22, CV-23.
4. Needle the remaining chosen trajectory points.
5. Revisit each point in the order needled and check that the patient feels at least a very subtle vibration in each point.
6. Ask the patient to visualize or to imagine the feeling of the connection of all the points. Often they will report that they already feel this connection vibrating.
7. Take the pulses in the Eight Extra position. The pulses will have moved deeper into the wrist. If they have not, re-vibrate the needles, ensuring that connection with the Yuan level has been made. This is done by intention rather than literal depth.
8. (*Optional*) Give the patient an affirmation to repeat while they are in treatment, e.g., *I am calm and grounded. I live in the present moment.*
9. Leave needles in for 40 minutes after the insertion of the Opening point.

10. Take the pulses in Eight Extra style, note the change and report it to the patient.
11. Remove the needles in the following order:
    a. Opening point
    b. other needles in the order opposite that of insertion
12. Allow the patient five minutes on the table, preferably alone, to reflect.

Frequently Asked Questions

1. *Is Yin Wei Mai equally applicable to men and women?* Yes, Yin Wei Mai is equally applicable to men and women. All humans experience Heart pain. No channel in Chinese Medicine is gender specific.
2. *SP-12 is not mentioned here. Why?* SP-12 is almost identical in function to SP-16. SP-12 would be added for a patients who are having difficulty nourishing themselves and others. It would also be added for women having difficulty with lactation.

YANG WEI MAI TREATMENTS

The Yang Linking Channel

Mechanisms of Yang Wei Mai

The role of Yang Wei Mai is to reconcile the movement of Yang on the exterior with the movement or supply of Yang on the interior. The chief implication of this is that Kidney Yang—the origin of Yang—must be able to move efficiently to the exterior (as Wei Qi) to deal with EPFs. Failure of the body to coordinate this movement results in Shao Yang conditions as the pathogen is allowed past the exterior. Aversion to cold with chills or high fevers result.

The Wei Mai are collections of the experience of aging. Yang Wei Mai is the recorder of the autobiography in terms of action. At the cerebellum, at GV-16 and GV-15, Yang Wei Mai records onto the brain the activity the body has undertaken in the outside world. All the major events of life make an impact on the evolution of the channel. These events include: schooling, puberty, adolescence, college, career, career changes, marriage, divorce, children, menopause, andropause, deaths of important people, major disappointments and achievements, and retirement. Experiencing difficulty with these events and transitions creates imbalances in the Wei Channels.

Yang Wei Mai determines the way in which we connect with our external environment. In later life, Yang Wei Mai determines what we do with our structure, based on Yang Wei Mai's knowledge of the body's capabilities.

Yang Wei Mai recycles Yang. When Yang is in excess, Yang Wei Mai links up that excess and returns it to Du Mai at GV-16 and GV-15 (just as Yin Wei Mai returns excess Yin to Ren Mai at CV-22 and CV-23.)

Yang Wei Mai has the capacity to gather Yang together and concentrate it in a region on its trajectory where there is an acute need for Yang. For example, if a person were experiencing a severe draft, rather than allow the body to develop Bell's Palsy, Yang Wei Mai would concentrate Yang Qi at GB-20. Yang Wei Mai consolidates Yang Qi at the surface in general.

Yang Wei Mai enters the cerebellum at GB-20 and records physical skills, e.g., swimming, bike riding, and even socialization and how to interact with people. Yang Wei Mai therefore controls coordination. Yang Wei Mai features Gallbladder points because Gallbladder controls the Marrow and the bone.

Yang Wei Mai associates an activity with time. It produces the sense of deja vu where it feels as if we have previously engaged a certain activity.

Yang Wei Mai creates an opportunity for a cadence in time. It creates a small oasis between the past and the future and gives the patient a chance to picture a new future, clear of the encumbrances of the past. Hence, Yang Wei Mai treatments give the patient the opportunity to renew themselves, to change, to be a different person from the present onwards.

Non-Pathological State of Yang Wei Mai
When Yang Wei Mai is in good balance the patient experiences optimism.

Pathological State of Yang Wei Mai
When Yang Wei Mai is out of balance the patient is obsessed about the future and exhibits Shao Yang conditions.

Indications of Yang Wei Mai

Classical Principal Sign: Alternating chills and fevers. Aversion to cold, or high fever. Shao Yang conditions indicating a failure of Wei Qi to communicate between the interior and the exterior.

General Pulse Picture: Floating, slippery and rapid, often weak at the deep level. See also, Eight Extra pulse taking on page 228.

Physical Indications of Yang Wei Mai

Yang Wei Mai pathology arises when the channel is unable to support and direct Yang, causing the signs and symptoms listed below. Whether Wei Qi appears to be excess or deficient, the treatment of Yang Wei Mai can be indicated.

- Sudden fainting, stiffening, disorientation, dizziness, visual dizziness, lack of clarity of thought (brain fog), blockage of the upper orifices, and loss of consciousness as Wei Qi is unable to reach the head.
- Lumbar swelling and pain or sudden lumbar swelling and swayback as fear locks Yang into the lower back causing pain.
- Intermittent or alternating chills and fever, a bitter taste in the mouth, nausea, vomiting, jaundice, malabsorption syndromes, loose stools, temporal headaches, migraines, otitis media, chronic ear infections, all due to insufficient Yang to transform Dampness.
- Chronic respiratory conditions due to insufficient Wei Qi.
- Chronic Sinew and skin conditions due to insufficient Wei Qi.
- Wei Atrophy Syndrome due to the insufficient circulation of Yang which results in Yang becoming lodged in the musculature causing the muscles to become burnt or scorched.
- Wind signs and symptoms.
- Head Wind conditions such as Bell's Palsy, Tourette's syndrome, epilepsy, meningitis, encephalitis, TMD, Multiple Sclerosis.
- Problems with decision making and other Gallbladder issues as Heat is created to burn off the Damp. Damp-Heat can then rise to the upper Gallbladder Channel affecting the brain.
- Migraines (one-sided due to indecision), Liver fire, hypertension, skin conditions, ear, nose, throat issues, muscular and neurological conditions, chronic respiratory conditions due to excess Wei Qi.
- Herpes, low grade fevers, intermittent fevers.
- Excess Yang signs and symptoms. If the patient is constantly living outside of the

present moment, the musculature is constantly firing. Du will become exhausted as it tries to continually feed this expenditure of Yang.
- Lack of certainty.
- Post-traumatic stress disorder resulting in perceived injury even in the absence of actual injury, as the memory of the incident remains somatized. The pain is there because the memory is unconscious and unprocessed. For example, the patient was in a car accident and was not injured, but gripped the wheel very hard and now has chronic hand pain. The memory of the trauma has been stored in the bone. Yang Wei Mai is stuck and is keeping the past manifesting in the present.
- Consumption of the Marrow.

Psychological Indications of Yang Wei Mai
- Being scattered, over-extended, as Yang Qi is not consolidated.
- A tendency to over-commitment: too many appointments, too many people to relate to, having long "to do" lists.
- Failure to prioritize.
- Difficulty managing a major life change.
- Difficulties with socialization.
- Engaging in a regular behavior as a result of trauma or needing to act in a certain way when reminded of a trauma, e.g., every time I think of that, I have to go for a drive.
- Obsession with the future. Fear of the future and acting upon that fear.
- Fear and Fright. Paralyzing fear.
- Depression as Yang is stagnant in the lower back.
- The feeling of being empty and hollow.
- The feeling of never being comfortable doing what one does, feeling unable to master anything.
- The feeling of never being able to reach one's fullest potential.
- Failure to achieve a sense of direction, a sense of quest, or momentum.
- The disappointment of having settled for second best, not having achieved one's dreams.
- Inability to accept death. Yang Wei Mai can bring about an emotional transformation during the end-stage of a disease. Useful in hospice settings. Pair with Yin Wei Mai for transitioning through death.

Yang Wei Mai

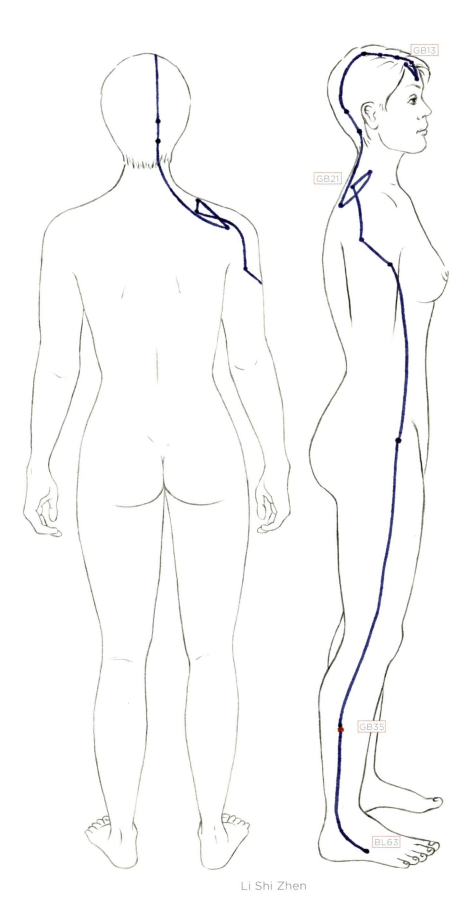

Li Shi Zhen

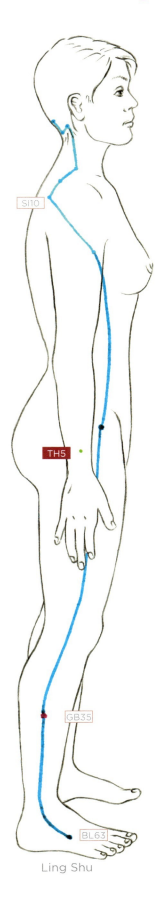

Ling Shu

Points of Yang Wei Mai

BL-63, GB-35, GB-29, LI-14, TH-13, TH-14, TH-15, GB-21, SI-10, GB-20, GB-19, GB-18, GB-17, GB-16, GB-15, GB-14, GB-13. (Li Shi Zhen.)

Li Shi Zhen contended the channel ends there because what follows is the act of choice. He postulated that change is possible because we are in control of our choices, and the way in which we do things does not have to be brought to the brain through Du Mai where it would become constitutional and therefore transmissible to the next generation.

Alternative Trajectories of Yang Wei Mai

BL-63, GB-35, GB-29, LI-14, SI-10, TH-15, GB-21, GB-20, GV-16, GV-15. (Shown on right side of p. 293.)

BL-63, GB-35, GB-29, LI-14, SI-10, TH-15, GB-21, GB-20, GB-13, GB-14, GB-15, GB-16, GB-17, GB-18, GB-19, GV-16, GV-15.

BL-63, GB-35, GB-29, LI-14, SI-10, TH-15, GB-21, GB-13, GB-14, GB-15, GB-16, GB-17, GB-18, GB-19, GB-20, GV-16, GV-15. (From the *Great Accomplishments of Acupuncture and Moxibustion*.)

Opening Point of Yang Wei Mai

TH-5 *Outer Gate* This point is used when fire toxins are present. Clears emotional stagnation, particularly fear (in Yang Wei Mai context.) Frees emotion to enable change to occur.

Xi-Cleft Point of Yang Wei Mai

GB-35 *Yang Exchange* Strong tonification for cardiac arrest. The flatliner point; it's used in trauma and as a last ditch effort in cardiac resuscitation. Use strong stimulation. Collapse of Yang, fainting. Can be combined with GB-13 if there is no pulse or breath. Used for panic about life's transitions.

Point Translations and Indications - Selected Points of Yang Wei Mai

BL-63[8] *Metal Gate, Golden Gate*

The metal element is what allows us to go outward into the world, and the action of extension into the outside

---

[8] The *Nei Jing* postulates BL-57 as the Opening point of Yang Wei Mai. Li Shi Zhen postulates BL-63 because it calms the spirit. Both points soothe the sinews.

world is a Tai Yang function. These factors are married in this point. Engenders calm about our mission, opens up appreciation of our virtues through our experience of our actions in the world. Treats seizures. Treats Fright-Wind (panic attacks). Supports Wei Qi for consistent deficiency of Wei Qi. Lethargy, suicidal tendencies. Constant pain. Soothes the sinews and calms the spirit at the same time. Opens the sensory orifices for the reprogramming of responses to past stress. Meeting of Yang.

GB-35 *Yang Exchange*   The Xi-Cleft point of Yang Wei Mai. Clears the mind of confusion. Makes one's course clear. Enables the making of decisions. Treats chills and fevers. Calms Shen. Uncontrolled or very expressive crying at loss of loved one. Leakage of Qi and humors: spontaneous sweat, wheezing and asthma, hemorrhaging, chronic diarrhea. A sense of emptiness and being hollow. Disperse GB-35 for pain. Analgesic point. Leg pain, migraines due to stress, hip pain. Single sided problems, lateral problems, chest pain, intercostal discomfort.

GB-29 *Squat Bone*   The Meeting point of Yang Wei Mai and Yang Qiao Mai. Point where beliefs about past and future enter Yang Qiao Mai and inform the gait and posture. Treats Damp in the Lower Jiao, heaviness, constipation and diarrhea. Treats short-term memory loss, absentmindedness.

LI-14 *Upper Arm*   Fosters the ability to be active and to deal with challenges in the outside world. Brings willingness to handle a new image of oneself and the responsibilities associated. Hot Bi, Heat causing spasms. Meeting of Yang on the arm. Meeting of the Stomach Channel. Clears Heat. Clears Heat for explosive temperament, agitation. Point needle proximally.

SI-10 *Upper Arm Shu*   Releases arm for extension into the outside world. Treats deformities and arthritis in the hands, inability to stretch out hands. Moves upper arm. Moves Qi and Blood. Idiopathic shoulder, arm and hand issues. Trigger fingers and thumb. Meeting of Yang Qiao Mai.

TH-15	*Celestial Liao*	Treats Wind and external pathogenic factors. Wind-Damp and Wind-Phlegm. Analgesic for chronic Bi syndrome. Physical and emotional pain. Moves Qi and Blood to treat pain.
GB-21	*The Well at the Shoulders*	Treats ascending Qi. Cup for seizures and violence. Releases Jing-Well points to open the portals, resuscitates consciousness. Moves Phlegm away from sensory orifices. Clears Phlegm on the breasts, swellings around nipple, clogged ducts. Induces labor, difficult delivery. Used after miscarriage or abortion, to clear the uterus.
GB-20	*Pool of Wind*	Courses Wind. Treats shaking, tremors, epilepsy, opens the sinuses and sensory orifices. Itchy eyes, ringing in the ears, blurred vision due to Wind (visual dizziness), runny nose, nosebleeds, difficulty with speech, headaches, low back pain. Opens awareness of aspirations and the capacity to act with clarity. Gallbladder, Triple Heater and Yang Qiao Mai meeting. Needle toward opposite side.
GB-19	*Brain Emptiness*	Indecisiveness, difficulty retrieving memory, amnesia. Drains Heat in the Gallbladder, jaundice, gallstones. Wind affecting neck and upper spine. Relaxes neck muscles to enable concentration and thinking.
GB-18	*Soul Order/Organization*	Supports the will to live. Supports positive projection into the world. Damp-Heat in Lungs. Constipation. Diffuses Lungs to expel Phlegm. Breaks up Phlegm. Opens nose, nasal polyps, deviated septum, nosebleeds, sinusitis, allergic rhinitis. Allergies arising due to stress. Treats the three ghosts: wandering, hungry and sexual. Brings motivation for life, to live life fully.
GB-17	*Upright Ying Qi*	Relaxation point, elicits the feeling of being at home, of being nourished. Brings Fluids to the brain. Shaky head. Parkinson's. Seizures with projectile vomiting. Vomiting to bring about relief. Plum blossom this point if Wind is present.

GB-16 *Window of the Eyes*

Refusal to look at the past, due to trauma. Eye conditions, blurred vision, cataracts, glaucoma, eye pressure. Treat Damp-Heat in the eyes, red, itchy, swollen eyes. Generates clear vision for understanding life's path.

GB-15 *Head Tear Receptacle*

Watery eyes from weeping, crying, being upset about the past. Tearing from allergies. Nasal congestion. Depression, loss of consciousness. Allows Qi to enter brain to clear Heat in brain. Crying with every reminder of past hurts. Bladder and Gallbladder meeting.

GB-14 *The White of Yang*

Treats Lung conditions involving Yang. Skin conditions involving Heat, prickly heat, hives with stress. Stress related cough. Emphysema. Expels Wind, tinnitus, spasms, encephalitis, meningitis. Stimulates one's creativity. Runny nose, itchy eyes, headaches. Stomach and Gallbladder meeting. Clears Heat. Treats manic episodes for people who break from reality. Needle obliquely toward eyebrow.

GB-13 *Root of the Spirit*

Calms Shen. Brings life experiences into the brain. Enables a change of mind. Extinguishes Wind. Seizures, epilepsy, mania, neurological disturbances, erratic behavior preceded by stress, Fright-Wind (insanity).

GV-15 *Mute Gate*

Treats the inability to articulate.

GV-16 *Wind Warehouse*

Expels Wind from the Marrow/Brain for stroke, seizures and epilepsy. No retention. Engage Wind and withdraw needle. Clears Heat in throat. Opens and relaxes the four limbs. Ghost point. Connection back to Du Mai. Yang returns to Du Mai at this point.

Treatment

Yang Wei Mai treatments create an opportunity for renewal, for the changing of expectations about the future.

Treatment Principles for Yang Wei Mai

1. To summon Yang
2. To articulate Yang
3. To resolve Dampness
4. To resolve Damp-Heat

Example of Point Selection for Yang Wei Mai

TH-5, BL-63, GB-35, LI-14, GB-21, GB-13 (To resolve Damp-Heat.)

Note: When a memory stored by Yang Wei Mai becomes somatized we must address where Yang Wei and Yang Qiao meet, at GB-29 and SI-10. When releasing unconscious somatized trauma, these points are cupped. This treatment is best done side-lying. Needle all the points chosen on the channel with vibrating technique and either add a cup over GB-29 and SI-10, or omit needles from those two points and cup them only. This treatment withdraws the impact of trauma from the structure, which has been causing structural, gait, postural, or self-esteem issues. The addition of more Qiao points might be considered if chronic pain is present.

Needling the Opening Point, TH-5

Extend the wrist and needle where the tendon bundles up near the textbook location. The patient may break into a light sweat.

Treatment Protocol for Yang Wei Mai

1. (*Optional*). Needle the Opening point, TH-5, right for females, left for males.
2. Needle the first point on the trajectory, BL-63.
3. Needle the landmark points chosen, if any, in ascending order, e.g., GB-29, LI-14, GB-21, SI-10, GB-20, GB-13.
4. Needle the remaining chosen trajectory points.
5. Revisit each point in the order needled and check that the patient feels at least a very subtle vibration in each point.
6. Ask the patient to visualize or to imagine the feeling of the connection of all the points. Often they will report that they already feel this connection vibrating. In a trajectory that is meandering such as this one, you might elect to show them a picture.
7. Take the pulses in the Eight Extra position. The pulses will have moved deeper

into the wrist. If they have not, re-vibrate the needles, ensuring that connection with the Yuan level has been made. This is done by intention rather than literal depth.

8. *(Optional)*. Give the patient an affirmation to repeat while they are in treatment. E.g., *My energy is wonderfully distributed through my body and I am calm.*
9. Leave needles in for 40 minutes after the insertion of the Opening point.
10. Take the pulses in Eight Extra style, note the change and report it to the patient.
11. Remove the needles in the following order:
    a. Opening point
    b. other needles in the order opposite that of insertion
11. Allow the patient five minutes on the table, preferably alone, to reflect.

YIN QIAO MAI TREATMENTS

The Yin Heel Channel, the Yin Stance Channel, the Yin Motility Channel, the Yin Bridge Channel, the Sea of the Yin Luos.

Mechanisms of Yin Qiao Mai

Yin Qiao Mai mobilizes consciousness for the purpose of self reflection: the cultivation of a natural appreciation of oneself and ease in being oneself in the present moment. It determines the concepts of identity and the orientation of the self in society. If the patient has been taught not to appreciate and love the self, Yin Qiao Mai stagnates, accumulating both Dampness and emotions. A pathological state then develops and the individual experiences emotions along a spectrum from "humorous" self-deprecation to self-loathing.

The Qiao Mai address weaknesses in postnatal Qi in order to prevent Dampness settling into the ditches, the Qiao's themselves. Hence the use of moxa is essential in Yin Qiao Mai treatments.

The Qiao Mai maintain integrity of the muscles in order to maintain integrity of the structure.

When Yin Qiao Mai is in excess, Yang Qiao Mai is automatically deficient and vice versa.

Differentiating between Ren Mai and Yin Qiao Mai

Yin Qiao Mai treats Yin stasis and Yin stagnation: Blood stagnation, Phlegm stagnation, Damp stagnation. Yin Qiao Mai will not treat Yin deficiency (though it will treat empty Heat signs.)

Tonifying Yin Qiao Mai allows it to overcome a pathological influence coming from Yang Qiao Mai.

Note: Stasis denotes a palpable mass, stagnation implies no mass.

Ren Mai treats Yin stagnation due to Yin deficiency. Ren does treat Yin deficiency. Ren Mai is the channel of choice for Yin deficiency in an Eight Extra context.

Differentiating between the Wei Channels and the Qiao Channels

In general, the Wei Channels deal with deficiencies and the Qiao Channels deal with excesses.

The Wei Channels deal with the past (Yin Wei) and the future (Yang Wei).

The Qiao Mai deal with the present moment, with how the patient feels about themselves in the present (Yin Qiao) and how they feel they fit into the outside world at present (Yang Qiao).

Non-Pathological State of Yin Qiao Mai

When Yin Qiao Mai is in good balance the person is pleased to be who they are.

Indications of Yin Qiao Mai

Classical principal sign: Heaviness of eyes, difficulty opening the eyes. A strong desire to be asleep. Inability to find interest in anything.

General pulse picture: Very often, and in advanced cases, none of the pulses can be located. The practitioner can often dig down and find nothing. Often the wrist itself will feel very Damp. Sometimes, you feel that you can't find the pulses even after pressing in deeply, but when you come back up to the Wei level, the pulses appear, floating and thready, because the patient is always trying to run away from themselves; they are unable to go within themselves. In other cases, the pulses will be very, very deep in all positions with no superficial pulse at all. See also, Eight Extra pulse taking technique on page 228.

Yin Qiao Mai

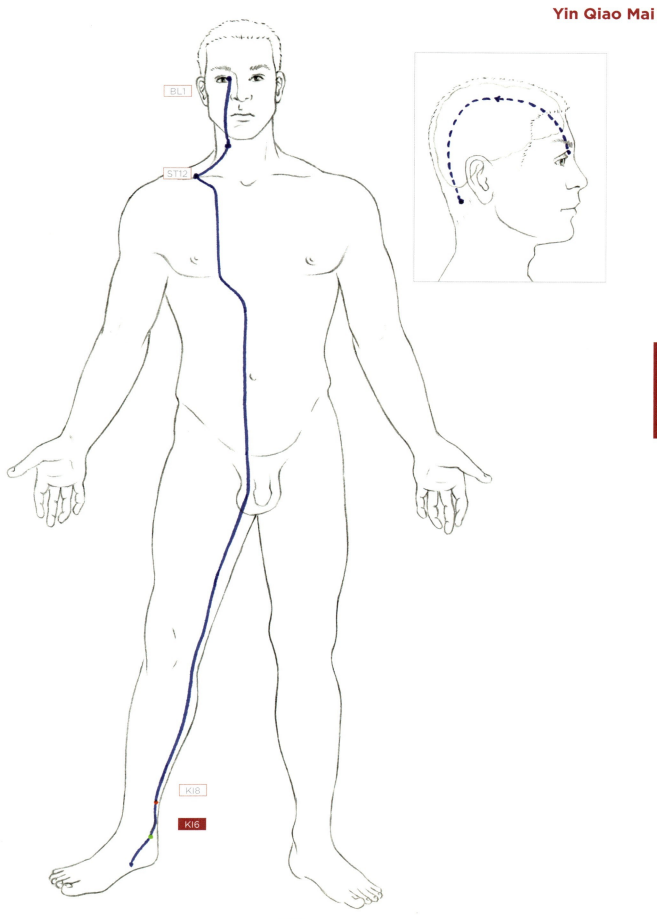

Physical Indications of Yin Qiao Mai

Yin Qiao Mai signs and symptoms arise from the stagnation of excess Yin, or the tensing of Yin.

- Heavy eyes, difficulty opening the eyes.
- Sleeping more than normal, a constant need to sleep, somnolence.
- Tightness of the medial legs, knocked-knee posture, pigeon-toed stance, tight abdominal muscles.
- Obesity, hyperlipidemia.
- Fatigue, lethargy, lassitude, listlessness, lack of engagement, chronic fatigue syndrome.
- Overactive hormones, menopausal hormonal issues.
- Hormonal issues related to the Yin functions of the hormones: the maintenance of fluid volume, blood volume, blood pressure, blood fat level and blood glucose levels.
- Damp and Cold signs: leukorrhea, lower abdominal heaviness or pain, hernias.
- Damp-Cold affecting the structure, icy cold sensations.
- Phlebitis, neuropathy, numbness, Wei atrophy due to Dampness.
- Edema.
- Genital pain, lumbar pain affecting the genitalia.
- Chronic low back pain that moves to the front.
- Chronic unilateral Bi-Obstruction.
- Fibroids, accumulations in the uterus, ovaries.
- Throat pain, neck pain, TMD, impaired eyesight.
- Goiters, breast lumps, emphysema, cysts, abdominal accumulations, brain tumors.
- Overactive parasympathetic nervous system.
- Retention of the placenta.
- Worms (classically, the wandering, sexual and hungry worms), parasites.
- Yin-type epilepsy (with biting and clenching).

Psychological Indications of Yin Qiao Mai

- Being in an overly Yin (slowed) state.
- Low self-esteem, low self-respect, poor self-image, inability to accept the self, a desire to sleep in order to escape the self.
- Depression.
- Narcissism, self-obsession.
- Retreating from the outside world due to disappointment.
- Overweight in order to become numb, eating disorders, reluctance to eat.
- Suicidal tendencies (*Death-Wind*), feeling powerless to create change, feeling desires cannot be fulfilled.

- Inability to meditate, inability to go within, inability to self-examine.
- Reluctance to talk about the self, psychological throat Bi.

Yin Qiao Mai and Yin Luo Channel Connection

Yin Qiao Mai is where pathology from the Yin Luos accumulates. The tenor of the Yin Luo Channels is a lack of interest in the world accompanied by discomfort with oneself.

Points of Yin Qiao Mai

KI-6, KI-2, KI-8, KI-11 to 27, ST-12, ST-9, ST-4, ST-3, ST-1, BL-1, GB-20

Opening Point of Yin Qiao Mai

KI-6   *Shining Sea*   Invites self-reflection, the appreciation of the self.

Xi-Cleft Point of Yin Qiao Mai

KI-8   *Exchange of Faith*   Invites trust in ourselves and the development of trust in the exchange that occurs between the unconscious mind and the manifestation of reality. Treats genital pain, pain during sexual intercourse, sexual identity crises.

Point Translations and Indications - Selected Points of Yin Qiao Mai

KI-6   *Illuminating Ocean, The Mirroring Sea*

Self-introspection and an easiness about identity is articulated and demonstrated to the world by the sparkle in one's eyes. Opening KI-6 activates BL-1 in a Yin Qiao Mai context. Enables one to appreciate oneself, to glimpse the innate perfection of one's inner self and begin to own it. Courses Qi to enable the finding of one's path and in so doing, moves physical pain (Bi) and the pain of being lost, of not being able to navigate one's path. Drains Heat, clears Heat through urine, drains Fire. Lin-strangulary syndrome (urinary tract infections). Opens the throat for loss of voice due to distress, plum pit throat. Inability to articulate one's Heart trauma, clears Heat in the Heart for Shen disturbance, depression, insomnia. When dispersed

		or bled, treats genital itch (heightened desire for sex) in females. Strongly calms the Shen. Tonify to treat somnolence.
KI-2	*Blazing Valley*	(Added to the trajectory by Li Shi Zhen.) To treat Yin Qiao, one must bring Yang energy (fire, passion, desire) into Yin (which contains our identity and is stored in the Kidneys) to motivate the self. KI-2 blazes a fire which transforms one's sense of oneself. This point also connects to SP-8 and hence brings Yang to the limbs for movement. Treats throat Bi and speech issues. Activates larynx for clear self-expression. Dyspnea, shortness of breath. Clears Heat accumulated in Kidneys due to rejection of the self. Rectifies Qi to treat shame and guilt related to the Lower Jiao. Regulates night sweats, wasting and thirsting. When dispersed or bled, treats genital itch (heightened desire for sex) in males, genital swelling and pain, seminal loss. Treats leg pain from excessive standing.
KI-8	*Gateway of Trust, Trust Exchange*	
		Reminds patient that to develop self respect one must have faith in oneself and faith in what one believes. The "exchange" referred to is that which occurs between faith and the fruits of that faith. As the Xi-Cleft of Yin Qiao Mai, it deals with excess and deficiencies related to the Lower Jiao. Treats pain during sex and urination, low back pain, fibroids, ovarian cysts, menstrual pain, prostatitis, testicular and scrotal swellings, Damp-Heat in the Lower Jiao. With strong stimulation, expels dead fetus. Regulates Chong and Ren to resolve Dampness. Treats Yin stagnation and Yin stasis. Difficult elimination (urination or defecation) due to Heat, burning diarrhea, UTIs, the five Lins (urinary difficulties: bloody-, stone-, Qi- (painful), turbid- and exhausting urination).

*The points on the Lower Jiao **KI-11 to KI-15** are moxa'd to invigorate Yang to resolve the Yin stasis characteristic of Yin Qiao Mai.*

KI-11	*The Curved Bone*	Tonifies Chong Mai to resolve Dampness. Strengthens Stomach, promotes urination to disinhibit Damp. Difficult urination, night time urination. Night sweats.
KI-12	*Great Manifestation*	Regulates Chong Mai and Ren Mai to resolve Dampness. Benefits the Kidneys.
KI-13	*Cave of Qi, Palace of the Child, Doorway of the Uterus*	One of the most important points in gynecology. Major fertility point in Lower Jiao. Benefits the Kidneys, rectifies the Qi.
KI-14	*The Four Stases*	Treats fullness of Qi, Blood, fluid and Phlegm. Benefits the Kidneys, helps strengthen Kidney function. Regulates the water passages for resolving fluid accumulation.
KI-15	*Water Pulse*	Nourishes the Kidneys, nourishes Yin, promotes urination, moistens the stools.
KI-16	*Membrane Transport*	Treats permeability of the membranes around organs. Moves and descends Qi. Very powerful analgesic point for pain in the Lower Jiao, e.g., during sex, urination.
KI-17	*Lyric Bell Toll*	Relaxes the exterior. Invigorates the collateral Channels: the Sinew and Luo Channels. Used to tonify. Supplements the Shen. Resolves Dampness by treating the Spleen.

KI-18 to KI-21 *all have a strengthening and supplementing affect on the Spleen and Stomach. They harmonize Spleen and Stomach for nausea and diarrhea and harmonize the Center (Spleen, Stomach and Liver) for epigastric and intestinal pain, gas and vomiting.*

KI-18	*Stone Barrier*	Difficult defecation and urination. Breaks up food stagnation in intestines. Constipation. Treats stagnation in the Bladder.
KI-19	*Yin Metropolis*	Regulates Chong and Ren to resolve Dampness.
KI-20	*Penetrate the Valley*	Breaks up food stasis. Addresses Gu Qi. Opens the chest. Brightens the eyes, opens the spirit outward from the chest.
KI-21	*The Dark Gate*	No moxa. Courses Qi and assists Liver in controlling the smooth flow of Qi. Rectifies Qi. A most powerful point for Liver Qi stagnation or Liver invading the Stomach and Spleen for chronic or constitutional issues.

*The points on the Upper Jiao **KI-22** to **KI-27** are where Yin Qiao Mai meets Yin Wei Mai. They treat Yin deficiency with Yin accumulation, Blood deficiency with Phlegm, Phlegm harassing the Heart with Heart pain, accumulations, rebellious Qi, coughing, vomiting, disinterest in food, the absence of pleasure in eating, depression. They all have the quality of releasing. They all diffuse Lung Qi and unbind the chest, freeing the Lungs to be strong enough to enable the cultivation of forgiveness.*
See Chong Second Trajectory for a discussion of these points, on page 241.

ST-12	*Empty Basin*	The point at which all the Yang Channels enter the torso, except Bladder. Descends Lung Qi to the Kidneys. Treats rebellious Qi: coughing, nausea and vomiting. Strong analgesic point.
ST-9	*Welcome Me, Humanity*	Allows clear articulation of one's understanding of oneself, of one's identity. Treats hyperthyroidism, constant hunger and Heat. Goiters and ocular pressure. Affects sensory orifices. Regulates Qi and Blood.
ST-4	*Earth Granary*	Treats metabolism and establishes homeostasis. Treats constant hunger, constant need to assimilate external stimulation. Treats a feeling of being hollow or empty, causing the patient to compensate externally. For example, by collecting a lot of things or pursuing many interests, believing that an accumulation of things and/or interests will make them an interesting person. Treats gum swelling, headaches, acid reflux.
ST-3	*Gigantic Bone Hole*	Regulates temperature. Treats lingering fevers, unrelenting fever, extreme passion and Heat. Regulates sex drive.
ST-1	*Supporting Tears*	Treats sentimentality, teary red eyes, readiness to cry. Treats a tendency to be judgmental.
BL-1	*Bright Eyes*	Provides clear vision for life's journey. As the termination of both Yin and Yang Qiao Mai, it regulates Yin and Yang. Allows access to the pineal gland (considered in Chinese Medicine to be the true master gland, regulating Yin and Yang), and the pituitary gland (which regulates postnatal Qi and Blood). Both these glands are stimulated to action by the naturally very intense squeezing that occurs

at BL-1 during the journey through the birth canal. BL-1 is the intersection of Stomach and Small Intestine Channels, both of which are responsible for the separation of the pure and the impure, in terms of food and also in terms of consciousness. BL-1 regulates this process, ensuring the transformation of turbidity which, if unchecked, would create stagnation and Dampness. BL-1 in the context of the Qiao Channels controls the secretion of hormones, especially estrogen, prolactin, melatonin, progesterone, and HGH which affects heartbeat, appetite, metabolism, menstruation, lactation, blood sugar and fat levels. Deposits experience in the brain.

GB-20 *Wind Pool* (*Optional*). Assists a patient in synchronizing with time, enabling them to be in the moment even when faced with what could be overwhelming worries and anxieties. Meeting of Qiao and Wei Channels and Triple Heater. The point therefore governs the patient's stance in time. Engages Triple Heater's function of determining how the Jing is to be expressed through the Zang Fu.

Treatment

A Yin Qiao Mai treatment invites the patient to accept themselves and to develop gratitude.

Treatment Principles of Yin Qiao Mai

1. To expel Cold and numbness (including worms)
2. To expel Cold and Dampness
3. To stimulate Yang to resolve Dampness

Needling the Opening Point of Yin Qiao Mai, KI-6

Invert the foot. The point is located where there are several folds in the skin. Find the deep depression and insert perpendicularly. Sometimes, the needle just won't go in perpendicularly but if you insert the needle at 45 degrees toward the sole of the foot, pointing inferiorly, very often you can get the needle to bend laterally into that very deep crevice. The patient will feel a sensation in the throat.

Needling Yin Qiao Mai

- The Kidney points on Yin Qiao Mai are located at a deep level, beneath the Kidney Primary Channel. Needle the Qiao points safely but more deeply than you would the Kidney Primary Channel.
- It is traditional to moxa the first three points on the trajectory: KI-6, KI-2, and KI-8.
- The Kidney points on the Lower Jiao (KI-11 to KI-15) are generally treated with moxa.
- Yin Qiao Mai is needled pointing upwards to bring Yin up to the genitalia, through the chest and up to the eyes which then sparkle with the inner knowing that the self is innately precious and perfect.
- KI-2 often requires deep massage before it is needled. Always press the tube firmly and squeeze the needle in, never tap.
- If KI-11 produces distracting sensations in the genitalia, it is needled too deeply.
- ST-1 and ST-12 are needled transversely.
- If the patient is very somnolent, after moxaing KI-8, needle GB-34 to activate the sinews.

Example of Point Selection for Yin Qiao Mai

KI-6, KI-2 and KI-11, ST-12, BL-1, to stimulate Yang to resolve Dampness affecting Yin Qiao Mai.

Treatment Protocol for Yin Qiao Mai

1. Needle the Opening point, KI-6 (also the first point on the trajectory), right for females, left for males.
2. Needle the landmark points chosen, if any, in ascending order, e.g., KI-11, KI-16, KI-21, ST-12, ST-9, ST-4, BL-1, GB-20.
3. Needle the remaining chosen trajectory points.
4. Moxa KI-6, KI-2 and KI-8.
5. Revisit each point in the order needled and check that the patient feels at least a very subtle vibration in each point.
6. Ask the patient to visualize or to imagine the feeling of the connection of all the points. Often they will report that they already feel this connection vibrating. You might elect to show them a picture of the channel.
7. Take the pulses in the Eight Extra position. If the pulses were absent, they should now be present at the deep level. If they have not, re-vibrate the needles, ensuring that connection with the Yuan level has been made. This is

done by intention rather than literal depth.

8. (*Optional*). Give the patient an affirmation to repeat while they are in treatment. E.g., *I wholly accept and appreciate myself.*
9. Leave needles in for 40 minutes after the insertion of the Opening point.
10. Take the pulses in Eight Extra style, note the change and report it to the patient.
11. Remove the needles in the following order:
    a. Opening point
    b. other needles in the order opposite that of insertion
12. Allow the patient five minutes on the table, preferably alone, to reflect.

If treating unilateral chronic Bi-Obstruction as the chief complaint:

13. Perform steps 1-3 (above), on the side opposite the pain, regardless of gender.
14. Needle the ah shi on the side of the body which has pain.
15. Cup GB-29 and SI-10 on the side of the body which has pain.

Complete the treatment method above beginning at step 4.

YANG QIAO MAI TREATMENTS

The Yang Heel Channel, the Yang Stance Channel, the Yang Motility Channel, the Yang Bridge Channel, the Sea of the Yang Luos

Mechanisms of Yang Qiao Mai

Yang Qiao Mai determines balance, gait and alignment by bringing Yang Qi from Du Mai out to the structure. Its integrity balances the three bony cavities: the skull, the ribcage and the pelvis, and allows us to walk upright. So far in human evolution Yang Qiao Mai has shifted the weight of the head to the spinous processes, away from the arms. The liberation of the arms enables us to look from side to side without compromising the freedom of the shoulders, as LI-15 and SI-10—landmarks of Yang Qiao Mai—are free. Likewise, the nose came away from the ground causing sight, rather than smell, to become our primary sense; hence, BL-1 is a key landmark in Yang Qiao Mai.

When Yang Qiao Mai is tight or loose, issues of balance, gait and structural alignment arise. Yin and Yang Qiao Mai are channels of polarity: when Yang Qiao Mai is tight, Yin Qiao Mai is slack, and when Yang Qiao Mai is slack, Yin Qiao Mai is tight.

Yang Qiao Mai accelerates Yang Qi to the surface and thereby influences the tonicity of the sinews. The alignment of structure (the organization of muscles and bone) is determined by the integrity of the connective tissue. If there is hardening or thickening of the connective tissue, the structure cannot be in alignment. If the connective tissue is released, the structure will eventually reassume correct alignment. The reduction or dispersing of Yang Qiao Mai points enables this release to occur. If the connective tissue is too loose, Yang Qiao Mai points are tonified to enable the return of tonicity in the connective tissues.

If the connective tissue is overly tight for long enough, the body responds with Yang to try to move and loosen it. Over time, this tightness or stagnation combined with the Heat of the Yang Qi begins to consume the tissue, leading to spasms, Bi-Obstruction, and eventually, Wei Atrophy Syndrome. When the connective tissue is affected to this extent, the Heat can begin consuming the Jing which is the origin of Yang Qiao Mai.

GB-29 and SI-10 are keys landmarks of Yang Qiao Mai because they are where Yang Qiao Mai and Yang Wei Mai intersect. It is at these points that our feelings and beliefs about the past and future inform our gait and alignment. This is the mechanism by which our gait and posture reflect our history and the mindset that results.

If we are too focused on the outside world, wanting to change it and rebelling against it, Yang Qiao Mai assumes a state of excess, as Yang is tensed and rebellious Qi signs emerge.

Non-Pathological State of Yang Qiao Mai

When Yang Qiao Mai is in good balance a person feels free and is able to be spontaneous. They are ready and organized in mind and body for anything at any moment. They are in present time in behavior and gesture, and feel that what is most important is what is happening in the moment. The person does not wish to be in a different place or doing something else. They are at peace in and with the world.

Indications of Yang Qiao Mai

Classical Principal Sign: Tight or flaccid muscles along the trajectory. Rebellious Qi with Heat and Wind stirring. Flushed complexion. Unilateral pain.

General pulse picture: Wiry pulses which are excess at the surface. See also, Eight Extra pulse technique on page 228.

Physical Indications of Yang Qiao Mai

Yang Qiao Mai pathology involves rebellious Qi with Heat, and the tensing of Yang.

- Heat responds to move Yang resulting in compounding Heat which consumes mediumship causing Wind to arise.
- Headaches, migraines, insomnia, irritability, high blood pressure, seizures, tics and tremors, vertigo, dizziness, delirium, epilepsy, convulsions, ruddy complexion, fever, nosebleeds, contact dermatitis, spasms in muscles and bones (as rebellious Qi stagnates Yang).
- Rebellious Qi: allergies, chronic bronchitis, cough, nausea, GERD, epigastric pain, Stomach ulcers, gastritis, belching, esophageal reflux (as Yang is hyperactive).
- Abscesses, acne, conjunctivitis, psoriasis.
- Daytime epilepsy, Yang-type epilepsy: seizures with palms and eyes open.
- Chronically tight lateral leg and thigh muscles.
- Lumbar pain as though hit by a sledgehammer, back pain with no swelling. Back pain accompanied by pain in hip and knees.
- Bi-Obstruction: shoulder pain, chest pain, chronic unilateral Bi-Obstruction.
- Calf pain due to the constant need to act.
- Hyperactive Yang in the muscles causes Heat to stagnate which consumes the muscles and leads to symptoms which occur in the following order:
    - spasms
    - pain (Bi-syndrome)
    - Wei atrophy (the consumption of Wei Qi)
    - weak muscles
    - brittle bones as the Marrow is consumed
    - flaccidity and neuropathy
    - Susceptibility to external pathogenic factors as Wei Qi has been consumed.
- Hormonal issues related to the Yang functions of the hormones: maintenance of breath and Heart rate, metabolism, temperature.
- Hyperadrenalism, hyperthyroidism.
- Hyperactivity of the sympathetic nervous system, overactive startle reflex, difficulty sleeping, resting, digesting.
- Neuropathy and coldness of face with high blood pressure as Yin compensates for the exuberance of Yang.

Psychological Indications of Yang Qiao Mai

These signs and symptoms result from rebellion against the external world.
- An inability to accept the world as it is, accompanied by a strong desire to change it, a tendency toward activism.

- Radical, rebellious behavior, righteousness, engaging in causes felt to be noble.
- A strong desire to intervene in external events, a feeling that there's always something to be done which leads to hyperactive, tense muscles, even in the absence of visible action.
- Disagreement about occurrences in the present moment, wishing things were different in the outside world.
- Untempered extroversion.
- Far-sightedness, the inability to notice details.
- Hair-trigger anger.
- Emotional pain due to rebellion, through constantly pushing against the world. The person ponders how to escape the pain of their life. Pain occurs down the sides of the body as there is no escape and they feel walled in.
- Idolatry as a result of unhappiness with self.
- As the desire to change the world wanes and withdrawal from the world seems a better option, Yin Qiao Mai symptoms arise: lethargy, lassitude, listlessness, fatigue, chronic fatigue syndrome.
- Depression rooted in withdrawal from the world due to its perceived imperfections.
- Constantly thinking about what needs to be done (which also causes constant firing of the muscles).

Yang Qiao and Yang Luos Connection

Yang Qiao Mai eventually receives pathology from all the Yang Luo Channels. Therefore the signs and symptoms of Yang Qiao Mai relate to Yang Luo pathology which features stress due to situations in the outside world.

Points of Yang Qiao Mai

BL-62, BL-61, BL-59, GB-29, LI-15, LI-16, ST-4, ST-3, ST-1, BL-1, GB-20.
Li Shi Zhen added GB-39 to the trajectory.

Opening Point of Yang Qiao Mai

BL-62 *Extending Vessel* — Releases and extends the muscles along the channel. Invites a more relaxed engagement with the outside world.

Xi-Cleft Point of Yang Qiao Mai

BL-59 *Leg Yang* — Treats seizures, convulsions, stroke, Bell's palsy.

Yang Qiao Mai

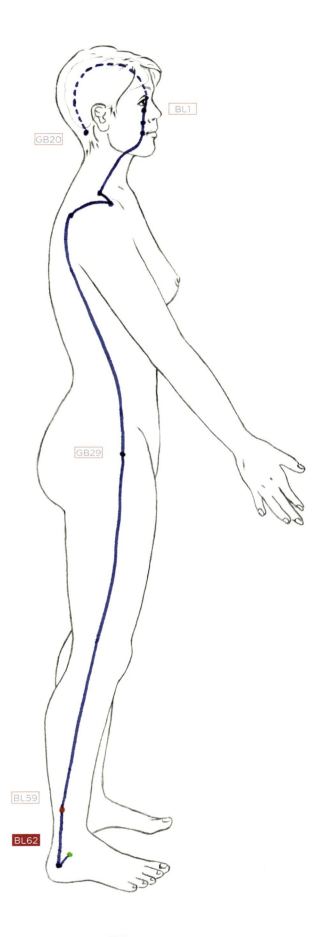

Point Translations and Indications - Selected Points of Yang Qiao Mai

BL-62	*Extending Vessel*	Treats stroke, seizures, convulsions, hysteria, dizziness, agitation, hyperthyroidism, lumbar pain, stiffness, heaviness of the head, hallucinations, mania, coma, unresponsiveness, abscesses, conjunctivitis, loss of voice, spontaneous sweat. Invites extension of the Shen toward heaven, toward divinity.
BL-61	*Subservient Visitor*	Allows patient to accept help, as a guest would. Fosters respect for the helper and relinquishes the lateral tension that arises when receiving help, allowing it to be received with more grace and ease. Treats arrogance, selfishness, headaches from being competitive, glaucoma, eye tension, photosensitivity. Treats a tendency to overcommit and being active beyond one's limitations; having long to-do lists. Eases the feeling that if we want to get something done, we must do it ourselves. Treats chronic pain in the legs, low back pain, heaviness of the head, Damp-Heat in the head, Wei atrophy.
BL-59	*Leg Yang*	Xi-Cleft point. Seizures, convulsions, stroke, Bell's palsy. Supports the instep. Very moving point, treats constipation. Sudden back pain, pain from standing. Heat, high fevers, intermittent fevers. Sudden Turmoil Disorder (simultaneous vomiting and diarrhea). Treats amnesia. Enables us to find our way back home, physically, emotionally and mentally.
GB-29	*Squat Bone*	Affects legs and low back. Meeting of Yang Wei Mai. Point where beliefs about past and future enter Yang Qiao Mai and inform the gait and posture. Opens up hip dramatically. Relaxes the low back, hip, chest and shoulders. Treats Damp in the Lower Jiao, heaviness, constipation and diarrhea. Treats short-term memory loss, absentmindedness. Activates and balances the parasympathetic nervous system. Realigns self-image and one's concept of the role of one's gender in society.
SI-10	*Upper Arm Shu*	Tightness of shoulders, neck, scapulae. Idiopathic shoulder, arm and hand issues, trigger fingers and thumb is-

		sues. Orients patient to the present moment. Opens awareness of greater flexibility, options and choices. Cup for emotional stagnation and physical stiffness. Releases arm for extension into the outside world. Treats deformities and arthritis in the hands, inability to stretch out hands. Moves upper arm. Moves Qi and Blood.
LI-15	*Shoulder Bone*	Urticaria, dermatological conditions, breakouts, spontaneous sweat. Yang-type seizures (with eyes open and mouth foaming). Shoulder pain. Transforms Phlegm and treats goiters. Strongly regulates Qi and Blood.
LI-16	*The Great Bone*	Important point for opening shoulder. Treats head Wind, Bell's palsy, seizures, convulsions, mania, Shen disturbance, malaria. Regulates Qi and Blood. Assists in transforming Phlegm. Treats vomiting or coughing blood.
ST-4	*Earth Granary*	Metabolic, digestive and homeostasis issues, constant hunger, excess stimulation, the constant need to assimilate external stimulation, desiring many different foods, flavors, colors, possessions, fighting many causes, trying to be interesting to compensate for a feeling of incompleteness. Gum swelling, acid reflux, hunger. Facial Wind, deviation of the mouth. Neurological conditions of the sensory orifices. Neuropathy of the legs.
ST-3	*Gigantic Bone Hole*	Lingering and unrelenting fever, unilateral paralysis. Excess passion, sexual overstimulation. Treats sneezing, nasal itch, tearing of the eyes. Swelling of the leg.
ST-1	*Support Tears*	Extreme sentimentality, a tendency to be judgmental. Teary, red, itchy, swollen eyes, visual distortion, floaters. Deviation of the mouth. Tinnitus.
BL-1	*Bright Eyes*	Provides clear vision for life's journey. As the termination of the Qiao's (the channels of polarity) it regulates day and night, Yin and Yang. Allows access to the pineal gland (considered in Chinese Medicine to be the true master gland) which regulates Yin and Yang, and the pituitary gland which regulates postnatal (Qi and Blood). Treats photosensitivity. Activates Wei Qi upon waking.

The intersection of Stomach and Small Intestine Channels which are both responsible for the separation of the pure and the impure in terms of both food and consciousness, ensuring turbidity is in check and digestion is not slowed by Dampness. BL-1 in the context of the Qiao's controls the secretion of hormones, especially estrogen, prolactin, melatonin, progesterone, and HGH which affects heartbeat, appetite, metabolism, menstruation, lactation, blood sugar and fat levels. Deposits experience in the brain.

GB-20 *Wind Pool* (*Optional*). Difficulty being in the moment due to overwhelming worrying and anxiety. Assists a patient in synchronizing with time, enabling them to be in the moment even when faced with what could be overwhelming worries and anxieties. This is where the Qiao Mai, Wei Mai and Triple Heater meet. The point therefore governs the patient's stance in time. Engages Triple Heater's function of determining how the Jing is to be expressed through the Zang Fu.

Treatment Principles of Yang Qiao Mai
1. To release chronic unilateral Bi-Obstruction
2. To subdue exuberant Wind
3. To subdue exuberant Wind for Wind-stroke

Needling the Opening Point of Yang Qiao Mai, BL-62
Evert the ankle. Needle in the center of the tendon bundle nearest the textbook location. The patient will experience a sensation in the low back.

In my practice, I like to get good depth on the Opening points of the Eight extras, unless they are Luo points. When needling BL-62, I approach the point posterior to the tendons, and slip the needle in almost parallel to the line of the foot so the needle goes in almost a full inch behind both tendons. The patient usually feels a sensation travelling deeply in the lateral leg, along the channel.

Pain in the Context of Yang Qiao Mai

While we must always be very sensitive to any communication that a patient may interpret as *blaming* him or her for their illness, it is important to understand that chronic pain, which is a powerful distraction, likely indicates that the patient is not in the present moment. Psychological pain is *always* an indication that the patient is not in the present moment. In the context of Yang Qiao Mai, it is important to cup GB-29 and SI-10, the two major intersections of Yang Wei Mai and Yang Qiao Mai, in order to disengage from the past and future and focus on present time. On the affected, painful side, cup GB-29 and SI-10 and reduce ah shi's. This is a side-lying treatment. The trajectory is needled on the side opposite the pain.

Choosing between Yin and Yang Qiao Mai for Unilateral Bi-Obstruction

Either reduce the channel that is tight, or tonify the channel that is flaccid. Choose the channel based on signs and symptoms. If the person has a predominance of Yang Qiao Mai symptoms and has lateral pain, reduce Yang Qiao Mai. If the patient has lateral pain but has more Yin Qiao Mai symptoms, tonify Yin Qiao Mai; Yang Qiao Mai will automatically be reduced even though it is not being treated directly. Reduction requires fast vibration of the needle. Tonification requires slow vibration of the needle.

Example of Point Selection for Yang Qiao Mai

BL-62, BL-59, GB-29, LI-15, SI-10, ST-4, BL-1, GB-20.

BL-62 on side opposite pain, ah shi on affected side, cup GB-29 and SI-10 on affected side (for unilateral Bi-Obstruction).

BL-62, BL-59, GB-29, gua sha LI-15, BL-1 (Wind-stroke).

When needling LI-15 for shoulder pain, needle the other shoulder while the patient moves the shoulder that is painful.

Treatment Protocol for Yang Qiao Mai

1. Needle the Opening point, BL-62 (this is also the first point on the trajectory), right for females, left for males.
2. Needle the landmark points chosen, if any, in ascending order, e.g., GB-29, LI-15, BL-1, GB-20.
3. Needle the remaining chosen trajectory points.
4. Revisit each point in the order needled and check that the patient feels at least a very subtle vibration in each point.
5. Ask the patient to visualize or to imagine the feeling of the connection of all

the points. Often they will report that they already feel this connection vibrating. In a trajectory that is meandering such as this one, you might elect to show them a picture.

6. Take the pulses in the Eight Extra position. The pulses will have moved deeper into the wrist. If they have not, re-vibrate the needles, ensuring that connection with the Yuan level has been made. This is done by intention rather than literal depth.
7. *(Optional).* Give the patient an affirmation to repeat while they are in treatment. E.g., *I found my place and I am calm.*
8. Leave needles in for 40 minutes after the insertion of the Opening point.
9. Take the pulses in Eight Extra style, note the change and report it to the patient.
10. Remove the needles in the following order:
    a. Opening point
    b. other needles in the order opposite that of insertion
11. Allow the patient five minutes on the table, preferably alone, to reflect.

If treating unilateral chronic Bi-Obstruction as the chief complaint:

1. Perform steps 1-3 (above), on the side opposite the pain, regardless of gender.
2. Needle the ah shi on the side of the body which has pain.
3. Cup GB-29 and SI-10 on the side of the body which has pain.
4. Complete the treatment method above beginning at step 4.

DAI MAI TREATMENTS

The Belt Channel, Consolidating Dai Mai, Original Dai Mai, Classical Dai Mai, Draining Dai Mai

Mechanisms of Dai Mai

Dai Mai, the Belt Channel, is considered the last of the Eight Extra Channels because it links the postnatal and prenatal levels. It connects the Spleen (the centerpiece of the postnatal environment) with the prenatal level. This link occurs via the Gallbladder Primary Channel, a postnatal channel which has access to a curious (Yuan level) organ. Dai Mai uses the pelvis as a basin to absorb or store excesses from the postnatal arena. These excesses include accumulations, concentrations, concretions, and gatherings. The accumulated Damp in Dai Mai is itself an ideal receptacle for the absorption of deeply held emotions and sentiments, emotions of attachment to the past, memories relating to unprocessed events, and violations to the Jing (trauma). Because they are stored in the Jing rather than the Blood, the memories stored in Dai Mai are not easily recalled. There is tremendous taxation on Qi as the patient is weighed down by the Dampness the body has created to allow suppression of these emotions. Enthusiasm for life is then compromised and change is felt to be out of reach. Difficulty with fertility can arise due to the stagnation that occurs.

Dai Mai issues are seen in people who are underweight, overweight or of average weight. Dai Mai will hold pathology (emotional and physiological) in the Jing until one has the resources, the time, strength and mediumship to deal with it. When the channel is saturated with pathology, it leaks, causing discharges.

Dai Mai is a repository of the Qiao Channels. As such it contains emotions related to what we don't like about ourselves. Dai also contains emotions related to actions and activities, often habitual, that we are unable to examine and process. These emotions may or may not have been conscious in the past but proved overwhelming in any case. The body uses Dai Mai to shift the burden of that which cannot be faced, moving it deeper into the constitution where there is limited access to it.

Dai Mai is also seen as the Luo of the Eight Extra Channels in that it is a reservoir. It holds pathology of the Yuan-Source arena at bay, allowing the other Eight Extra Channels to regain a degree of freedom and greater capacity for latency.

Dai Mai absorbs excess Yang. A common Dai Mai scenario is Dampness accumulating in the Dai in response to Heat. Dai Mai could be considered an absorber of perverse Stomach Qi because excess Heat most commonly comes from Stomach Fire which can vent up to the Heart, only to be restrained and descended by Dai Mai. This action occurs in partnership with the Spleen, the Yin-Yang partner of the Stomach, and producer of Dampness. The Dampness is not the pathology, but rather the natural response to pathological Heat. Treatments that aim to drain Dampness without addressing the underlying Heat are likely to fail as the body resists the release of the Damp which is its protection, and the unleashing of latent Heat that would result. This concept is crucial in the formulation of strategies involving Dai Mai.

The Dampness produced can be in a variety of forms: fibroids, endometriosis, prostatitis, cysts, edema, excess fat, etc. In this context, if Dai Mai becomes full, rebellious Stomach Qi will arise, leading to full blown Damp-Heat in the Lower Jiao.

Dai Mai can also contain toxins the body is unable to deal with. These include heavy metals, xenobiotics, the by-products of foods that are difficult to digest, sticky foods eaten in excess (gluten, sugar, dairy), microwaved food and genetically modified organisms which are often indigestible, vaccines, pesticides and pharmaceutical drugs such as antibiotics and steroids. (Pharmaceutical drugs can create Dampness as the body is directed by them to suppress pathology. Damp is produced to create latency for the pathology and for the drug itself.)

Normally the Liver would act to clear these toxins, but when the body is creating accumulations in Dai Mai, the Liver is unable to free them. This is because its Yang partner, the Gallbladder which is charged with the movement of Liver Qi and mediumship, is in a state of stagnation as it holds onto Damp. (Gallbladder points comprise much of Dai Mai, so the stagnation is compounded in Dai Mai.)

Comparison of the Two Dai Mai's

There are two Dai Mai trajectories: *Consolidating Dai Mai* (also known as Original, First or Classical Dai Mai), and *Draining Dai Mai*. If your treatment principle is to "astringe Dai Mai" which means to hold in Fluids, use Consolidating Dai Mai. If your intention is to release or drain Dai Mai, use Draining Dai Mai.

Consolidating Dai Mai

Consolidating Dai Mai is used when seeking the preservation of Fluids leaking from the Lower Jiao. Tonification technique is used to hold Qi in place. (Qi, in turn, holds Fluids in place.) This Dai Mai is the consolidator of the Chong, Ren and Du Channels. It supports them in the connections they make between each other. Dai Mai can assume pathologies from these three channels, thereby relieving their burden and ensuring their interaction is unencumbered. Consolidating Dai Mai connects to prenatal Qi at the Gallbladder (GB-26), Kidneys (BL-23), Ren (CV-8) and Du (GV-4) and with postnatal Qi at the Spleen (SP-15) and Stomach (ST-25). It links the Zang Fu and Curious Organs at GB-26.

Consolidating Dai Mai connects to the Bladder and Kidney Channels at GV-4 and BL-23 where the moving Qi of the Kidneys generates the Triple Heater mechanism. This mechanism distributes Jing upward into the organs, chiefly the Zang organs. The initial distribution of the Jing to the Zang (accomplished during the birth process) determines the personality. Triple Heater inevitably energizes the Zang unevenly and it is this very unevenness that accounts for an individual's unique energetics, the formation of a unique temperament, and challenges within the personality. If the patient cannot arrive at an internal peace or self-acceptance with these conflicts within the personality—if they cannot tolerate aspects of themselves—the body represses these aspects by creating Damp in Consolidating Dai Mai. This Dampness inhibits the distribution of Jing to the Zang to curb expression of the personality.

LR-13, the first point on the Dai Mai trajectory, is also the influential point of the Zang organs. When needled in the context of Consolidating Dai Mai, LR-13 stabilizes the patient's discomfort with their internal conflicts, thus re-establishing freedom in the distribution of Jing.

Conversely, the patient might be having difficulty expressing who they are due to Dampness in Dai Mai that originated in the Middle Jiao, due to poor eating or lifestyle habits. Yuan-Source Qi may be unable to flow freely into the Shu points due to this obstruction in Dai Mai. The Dampness may also cause confusion and poor concentration, further limiting natural expression of the self. Needling into Consolidating Dai Mai activates Kidney Yang to correct this impediment. The sensation of a Consolidating Dai Mai treatment is profoundly comforting and securing.

Dai Mai

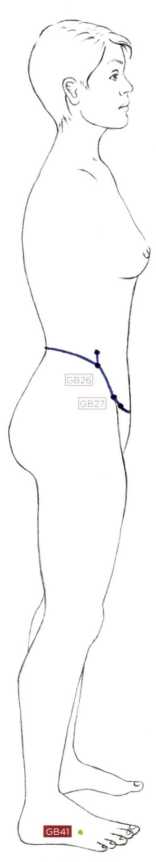

Draining Dai

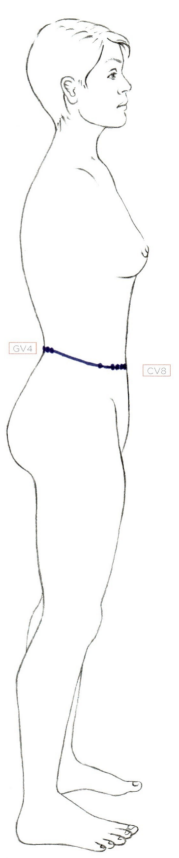

Consolidating Dai

Indications of Consolidating Dai Mai

Issues involving leakage of constitutional Essence: Urogenital issues involving the prostate, reproductive and gynecological issues involving leakage of Blood or Jing Fluids, chronic postnatal issues, especially those related to the Spleen being unable to bank Qi and Blood. Shen disturbance originating in the first cycle of seven and eight. Consolidates the Chong, Ren and Du to treat Blood or Qi deficiency that has a constitutional origin.

Choosing between Consolidating and Draining Dai Mai

Choose Consolidating Dai Mai when you want to stop leakage of the Jing, or to treat a constitutional Blood or Qi deficiency using Dai Mai. Choose Draining Dai Mai to facilitate the release of Damp pathology being held in Dai Mai.

Points of Consolidating Dai Mai

LR-13, GV-4, BL-23, BL-52, GB-26, SP-15, ST-25, KI-16, CV-8 (not needled).

Needling Technique for Consolidating Dai Mai

Generally, all points are tonified, to hold Qi in place.

Needle unilaterally according to gender. Needle LR-13. Then, starting at GV-4, thread the points of the belt together superficially, finishing with a needle inserted at KI-16 and extending under CV-8. This is a side-lying treatment.

Treatment Principles of Consolidating Dai Mai

1. To astringe Fluids in the Lower Jiao, to stop loss.
2. To maintain the integration of the three members of the first ancestry: the Chong, Ren and Du to maintain their upward movement.

Treatment Protocol for Consolidating Dai Mai

All points are needled with vibrating technique, except for GB-41. (See technique for GB-41 on page 329.)

1. With the patient side-lying, hook the needle into the Opening point, GB-41, right for females, left for males.
2. Needle from the spine to the front on the side of gender. E.g., GV-4, BL-23, BL-52, GB-26 (classically found on the lateral midline), SP-15, ST-25, KI-16

curved under the navel. (Insert at KI-16 and needle under the navel.) The points can be threaded or needled distinctly. Alternatively, with the patient supine, needle accessible points beginning with GB-26 and work medially. If the aim is to stimulate Kidney Yang in the context of Dai Mai, begin at KI-16 and work back to GV-4.

3. Revisit each point in the order needled and check that the patient feels at least a very subtle vibration in each point.
4. Ask the patient to visualize or to imagine the feeling of the connection of all the points. Often they will report that they already feel this connection vibrating.
5. Take the pulses in the Eight Extra position. The pulses will have moved deeper into the wrist. If they have not, re-vibrate the needles, ensuring that connection with the Yuan level has been made. This is done by intention rather than literal depth.
6. *(Optional)*. Give the patient an affirmation to repeat while they are in treatment. E.g., *I release all that does not serve me and I accept all that is nurturing to me.*
7. Leave needles in for 40 minutes after the insertion of the Opening point.
8. Take the pulses in Eight Extra style, note the change and report it to the patient.
9. Remove the needles in the following order:
    a. Opening point
    b. other needles in the order opposite that of insertion
10. Allow the patient five minutes on the table, preferably alone, to reflect.

Draining Dai Mai

> *Warning: If Draining Dai Mai is used incorrectly, Jing will be wasted. Many Dampness issues can be successfully treated by strengthening the Spleen. The Jing must be determined to be involved to warrant Dai Mai treatments. If in doubt, treat the Spleen and if there is not appreciable improvement in the pulses, move to Dai Mai.*

Draining Dai Mai is reduced to drain Dampness created in the Middle Jiao (by the Spleen). Very often the Spleen has created the Dampness in response to Heat. LR-13 is the connection between the Spleen and Dai Mai. LR-13 is the Spleen Mu point and, as a Liver point, is elementally related to the Gallbladder whose points are featured in Dai Mai. The Liver Channel as last of the postnatal channels, has the task of depositing unresolved postnatal material into the Jing in the Lower Jiao, to be energetically passed on to the next lifetime for resolution.

When Dai Mai is full it begins to leak. Releasing the Draining Dai Mai causes the elimination of Dampness which allows the resumption of clarity of thought. The release of Draining Dai Mai also results in more room to hold pathology latent, if needed.

Indications of Draining Dai Mai

Classical Principal Sign: The feeling of being submerged to the waist in a basin of cold water. "Red and white discharge": leukorrhea, spermatorrhea. Sudden low back pain, pain upon lifting. Inability to bend backwards and forwards.

General Pulse Picture: Slippery Middle Jiao pulses. Slippery rapid pulses close to the tendon. See also Eight Extra pulse taking technique on page 228.

Physical Indications of the Dai Mai's

When Dai Mai overflows with pathology, it leaks, leading to the following signs and symptoms:

- Diarrhea, mucus in the stools, frequent urination, Damp (mucus) or blood in the urine, urogenital disorders, premature ejaculation, spermatorrhea, prostatitis, testicular pain, impotence, hernias, dysmenorrhea with white discharge, leukorrhea, bloody discharge between periods, pain during or after sex.
- Edema, sagging sensation in the waist.
- Cold-Damp Bi-Obstruction in the abdomen with edema, bloating, Cold or heaviness in the abdomen, intestinal issues featuring Dampness, borborygmus, obesity.
- Inability to arch the back.
- Paralysis of legs, phlebitis, hemiplegia.
- Infertility as the harboring of regrets and negative emotions prevent the creation of new images and expectations. Jing is distracted by having to hold pathology in latency.

Psychological Indications of the Dai Mai's

- Inability to let go of the past.
- Resentment
- Obsession
- Feeling unsupported.
- Deeply held trauma.
- Stubbornness, lack of spontaneity.

Points of Draining Dai Mai

LR-13, GB-26, GB-27, GB-28.

Gallbladder points are reduced. LR-13 is needled with even technique.

Opening Point of Dai Mai

GB-41 *Leg Receptacle of the Tears*

Elicits the exocrine release (crying), or cathartic release necessary for complete discharge of burdens (manifesting as Damp) to which there is an emotional attachment. As a Shu-Stream point, encourages the discharging of Dampness.

Translations and Indications of the Points of Dai Mai

LR-13 *Camphorwood Door* Releases memories resulting in pathology. Releases the Blood being used to store past experiences, thereby taking pressure off the Jing in Dai Mai which is storing past experiences. Drains memories into Gallbladder Channel. Strengthens the Spleen to prevent further accumulation of Damp in the Middle Jiao. Use LR-13 if draining Damp that originated in the postnatal arena.

GB-26 *Belt Channel* Local Opening point of Dai Mai. Stops leakage (if using astringing technique) or releases the belt channel (if using reduction technique).

Note: Classically, GB-26 is located on the lateral midline, at the level of the navel.

GB-27 *The Five Axes* Releases Damp-Heat. An analgesic point. Releases the five ancestral axes: sternocleidomastoid, diaphragm, psoas, the paravertebral muscles and their connection with trapezius and gluteus. Treats leukorrhea, yellow discharge, explosive diarrhea, Heat in the urine and stool, frequent urination, pelvic inflammatory disease.

GB-28 *The Linking Path* Reminds the patient that all that matters is the present moment. Clears pathology held in the Dai Mai so that the Wei Channels can be freed of the weight of their history. Treats the stagnation that creates confusion of being stuck in the past, and reminds the patient that past can be let go. Treats Damp-Cold in the Lower Jiao. Leukorrhea, white discharges, hemorrhoids, early or painful periods, pain in the Lower Jiao, difficult urination, dysmenorrhea.

Pairing Dai Mai with Yang Wei Mai

The coupled pair is applicable when the body has generated enough Heat to move the Dampness up to the sensory orifices or out to the four limbs. Add TH-5 when Dai Mai is presenting with:

- Dampness developing more Heat, causing Damp to rise to the sensory orifices causing cataracts, glaucoma, watery eyes.
- Wind-Hot-Phlegm, shaking hands and feet with numbness as Dampness overflows from Dai Mai causing restricted movement.
- Paralysis of the legs, phlebitis.
- Migraines, red eyes, headaches.

Treatment Principles of Draining Dai Mai

1. To drain Damp-Cold in the Lower Jiao
2. To drain Damp-Heat in the Lower Jiao

Consolidating Prior to Draining Dai Mai

We often think that if Dai Mai is full, we should drain it. Sometimes, however, patients are holding so much unconscious trauma that the Dampness is providing a soft insulating cushion for them, just as a child would hold a security blanket. Draining Dai Mai in these cases feels threatening to a patient. Consider *consolidating* Dai Mai in order to augment a sense of protection until you feel the patient is sufficiently reassured to begin allowing the clutch on his or her defenses to relax.

The Importance of Releasing the Five Pillars before Treating Dai Mai

Dai Mai is intimately connected with the Five Pillars or *Axes,* muscular areas of gross structural support which are active in all full-bodied activity. The axes are muscular areas that the body can use to hold pathology in latency if Wei Qi has failed to eradicate the pathology.

The pillars are as follows: *sternocleidomastoid*, the connection between the cranium and the thorax; the diaphragm which connects between the thorax and spine; psoas, which connects the spine and pelvis; the paravertebral muscles which form the connections between the spine and the first three ancestral sinews (just described); and the muscle responsible for maintenance of the coccyx, the gluteus. (In Japanese acupuncture *rectus abdominis* is included.) The complete release of Dai Mai depends on these axes being released. This can be readily achieved with cupping or gua sha. During the treatment of Dai Mai, GB-27 *The Five Axes,* activates the release of the five muscle groups. These areas are palpated; the tight areas that are found can be treated in various ways.

The following is a list of my preferred release methods for the Axes:
1. SCM can be gua sha'd, or at the very least, released at its attachments with a Sinew treatment.
2. The diaphragm is powerfully released by reduction at BL-17 and LR-14.
3. The paravertebral muscles are strongly released with sliding cupping along their entire length. Trapezius is gua sha'd.
4. The psoas is strongly released by Sinew releases (not described in this book), by treatment of the Stomach Sinew (described in the Sinew chapter), or by reducing ST-30.
5. The gluteus can be released by cupping or deep reduction at GB-30, sliding cupping the local area, or by reduction needling of Bladder points on gastrocnemius, especially BL-57.

Point Selection Method of Dai Mai

GB-26 is essential in any Dai Mai treatment, whether draining or consolidating.
BL-60 is traditionally added to Dai Mai if Dai Mai pathology has affected the Upper Jiao, particularly the sensory orifices, or if there is Heat above and Cold below Dai Mai.
LR-2 is added if there is abdominal pain around the navel.
LR-3 is added if the menses are irregular and migraine headaches occur.

Differentiating between GB-27 and GB-28

GB-27 is chosen in cases of Damp-Heat.
GB-28 is chosen in cases of Damp-Cold.
It is not necessary to needle both GB-27 and GB-28.

Needling the Opening Point of Dai Mai, GB-41

GB-41 is needled with *hooking* technique. Vibration technique is generally not applied here, as long as the hooking technique is used. Starting lateral to the fifth metatarsal, insert the needle pointed medially (across the width of the foot). Don't insert it between the fourth and fifth metatarsals. Hook the needle, making it into a U-shape, under the fifth tendon so that once it passes the tendon the needle continues its path medially close to the surface of the foot. To remove it painlessly, hook the needle as it's coming out.

If Dai Mai has been opened successfully, the patient will feel a permeating warmth in the entire pelvic region. There will also be a very subtle downward pull in the abdomen.

Treatment Protocol for Draining Dai Mai

All points are needled with vibrating technique.

1. Release the Five Pillars (described on page 328) with gua sha, cupping, sliding cupping, or needles.
2. Needle the Opening point, GB-41, right for females, left for males, with hooking technique.
3. Needle the chosen trajectory points in descending order
   a. LR-13, GB-26, GB-27 (Damp-Heat), or
   b. LR-13, GB-26, GB-28 (Damp-Cold).

GB-26 is located on the lateral midline level with the navel.

4. Revisit each point in the order needled and check that the patient feels at least a very subtle vibration in each point.
5. Ask the patient to visualize or to imagine the feeling of the connection of all the points. Often they will report that they already feel this connection vibrating.
6. Take the pulses in the Eight Extra position. The pulses will have moved deeper into the wrist. If they have not, vibrate the needles again, ensuring that connection with the Yuan level has been made. This is done by intention rather than literal depth.
7. *(Optional)*. Give the patient an affirmation to repeat while they are in treatment. E.g., *I release all that does not serve me.*
8. Leave needles in for 40 minutes after the insertion of the Opening point.
9. Take the pulses in Eight Extra style, note the change and report it to the patient.

10. Remove the needles in the following order:
    a. Opening point.
    b. other needles in the order opposite that of insertion.
11. Allow the patient five minutes on the table, preferably alone, to reflect.

Frequently Asked Questions About Dai Mai

1. *Unilateral needling feels powerful on all the Eight Extras except when I'm treating with Draining Dai Mai. Should I needle this channel bilaterally?* Classically, the Dai Mai would be needled unilaterally, but if you look at the treatment on the table and you feel that the funnel shape of Draining Dai Mai is not strongly delineated, go ahead and needle the opposite side also. Your treatment must feel strong in your mind.

2. *My patient has both Damp-Heat and Damp-Cold signs. Should I use GB-27 or GB-28?* Use both. Or determine which one preceded the other and needle according to the earlier pathology.

DA BAO and BAO MAI

Da Bao and Bao Mai connect Blood to the Lower Jiao. Da Bao is a wrap around the chest that features the Great Luo of the Spleen, a key point in the management of Blood. The Great Luo of the Spleen (three cun below the axilla, which today is known as GB-22) treats pain all over the body due to Blood stasis. Along its trajectory, it connects to Bao Mai at CV-15 (the Luo of Ren) which in turn connects to GV-1 (the Luo of Du).

Da Bao and Bao Mai connect Blood to the Yuan-Source level via Source and Luo points that occur on Eight Extra Channels and therefore affect that arena. They are not considered Eight Extra Channels themselves.

It is Bao Mai that carries Blood (which is made by the Spleen) to the Lower Jiao. Emotional holdings in the chest are transported to the Lower Jiao via this trajectory. Rather than allow them to reside in the Luo points of the deepest level of the constitution (CV-15 and GV-1) where they would inform the next incarnation, the body moves the emotional mass to Dai Mai to be stored, and hopefully released.

If the emotionally loaded Blood is transported to the Lower Jiao but Dai Mai is full, there will be pathological leakage of Blood or disturbances in the Blood of the Lower Jiao (e.g., fibroids, endometriosis, dysmenorrhea, pre-menstrual syndrome, prostate issues) accompanied by symptoms of Shen disturbance.

Bao Mai establishes Heart-Kidney communication, compared with Chong which establishes Kidney-Heart communication. The emphasis on Bao Mai is downward to the Kidneys, while the emphasis in Chong's second trajectory is upward, to the Heart. This is useful information if using directional pulse taking to determine which end of the communication is compromised.

Comparison of Draining Da Bao and Consolidating Da Bao

Da Bao has two trajectories (see drawings), one that consolidates, and one that drains.
- **Draining Da Bao** is the great wrap which encircles the chest three cun below the axilla, from GB-22 to GB-22 (the earlier Great Luo of the Spleen). Draining Da Bao is used to move stagnation out of the chest. This trajectory is commonly used in conjunction with Bao Mai.

- **Consolidating Da Bao** is the great wrap which encircles the chest from SP-21 to SP-21, the Great Luo of the Spleen, six cun below the axilla. Consolidating Da Bao is used to hold Qi, Blood or Fluids in the chest. Generally, consolidating Da Bao is not used with Bao Mai.

Bao Mai is the vertical channel which connects the Da Bao to Dai Mai. When Draining Da Bao and Bao Mai are used together, they bring physiological or psychological pathology away from the chest, down into Dai Mai for drainage. For example, if treating Blood stasis due to emotional trauma as a Dai Mai issue, e.g., the patient presents with dysmenorrhea and fibroids and was molested or raped in childhood; Da Bao and Bao Mai are used to shift the emotions to Dai Mai for draining, providing an opportunity for deep healing, opened consciousness, and release.

Signs and Symptoms of Da Bao

Fullness of the chest, chest congestion.
Blood stasis due to emotional trauma.

Signs and Symptoms of Bao Mai

Failure of Heart and Kidneys to communicate, *Running Piglet Qi*, panic attacks, paranoia, anxiety, painful periods, clots, prostatitis, systemic Blood stagnation and Blood stasis. Blood stasis prohibiting pregnancy. Heat signs descending into Dai Mai. Full Luo signs and symptoms transmitted to Dai Mai, resulting in emotional issues.

Points of Da Bao

Draining Da Bao: **GB-22** (three cun below the axilla), **CV-15**, to the opposite **GB-22**.
Consolidating Da Bao: **SP-21** (six cun below the axilla), **CV-15**, to the opposite **SP-21**.

GB-22   *The Great Luo of the Spleen, the Great Wrap*
3 cun below the axilla. Master point of the Luos, treats pain all over the body. Blood stagnation all over the body. Master point of Da Bao.

SP-21   *The Great Luo of the Spleen, the Great Wrap*
6 cun below the axilla. The point at which Blood pathology enters the constitution. Consolidates Blood in the chest.

Da Bao Mai

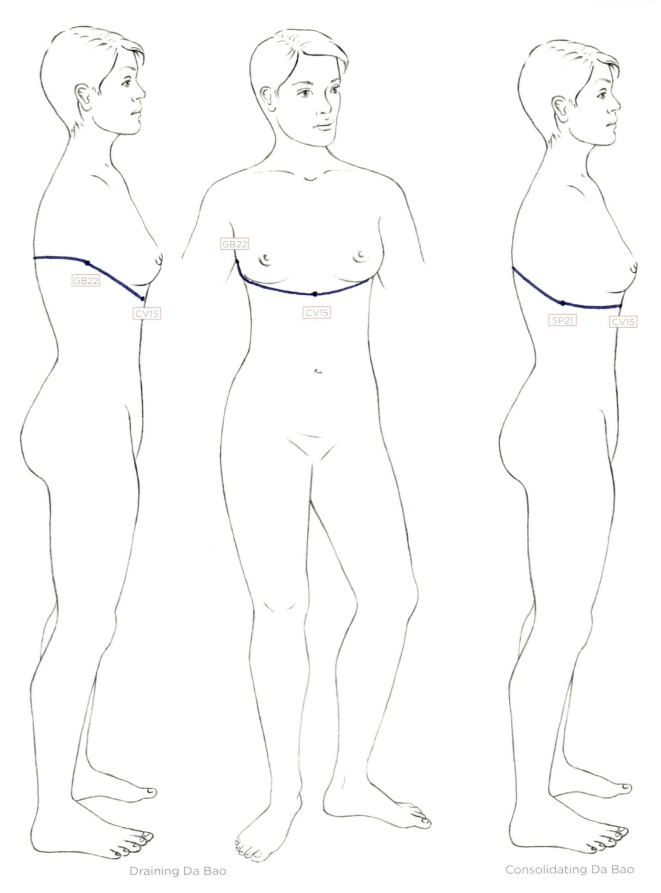

Draining Da Bao

Consolidating Da Bao

Bao Mai

8 EXTRA

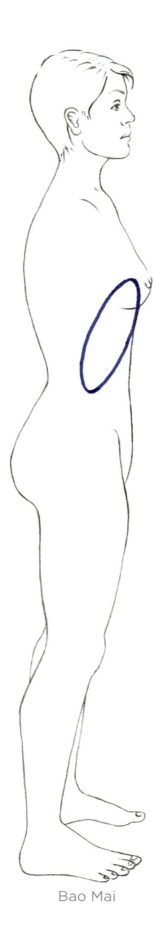

Bao Mai

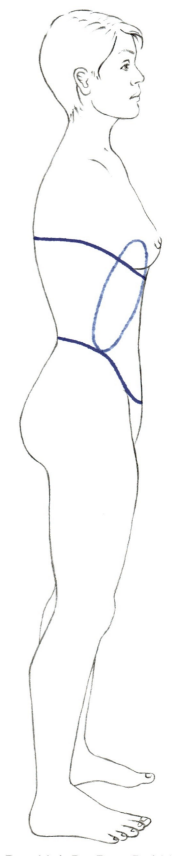

Bao Mai, Da Bao, Dai Mai

The Nan Jing puts SP-21 as three cun below GB-22. The Ling Shu has it three cun below the axilla at what it now known as GB-22.

Points of Bao Mai

CV-15, GV-9, GV-1. (GV-1 and GV-9 indirectly access Bao Mai.)

CV-15	*Turtledove Tail*	A point on both Da Bao and Bao Mai, and the connection between the two. Luo point of the Ren Channel. Source point of all Yin. Nourishes Yin, calms the Shen. Treats abdominal pain due to Blood stagnation. Transforms Phlegm. Moistens dryness. Treats *dian-kuang* (mania and withdrawal). As the tip of the sternum, connects energetically to the tip of the coccyx, the connection between the constitutional Luos, CV-15 and GV-1.
GV-9	*Extreme Yang*	Master point for coughing and wheezing, opens chest. Root of trapezius and master point for the diaphragm. Treats chronic Damp-Heat. Regulates Liver and Gallbladder.
GV-1	*Long Endurance*	Luo point of the Du Channel. Treats Damp-Heat, dysentery, turbid or burning urine, prolapse of anus, hemorrhoids, stiffness of the spine, heaviness of the head. Calms Shen, anchors Yang.

Point Selection, Da Bao and Bao Mai

Select points from Da Bao, Bao Mai and Dai Mai.

A typical point selection would be GB-22, GV-9, CV-15, GB-26, GV-1.

Note: GV-1 can be replaced by BL-57 which opens GV-1.

Salt moxa is useful on CV-8 if BL-57 or GV-1 is removed and the patient moves to supine position.

If the emotions being released from Bao Mai to Dai Mai are Yang in nature (anger, anxiety), add GB-27. If they are Yin in nature (grief, fear, obsessive thinking), add GB-28.

Treatment Principle for the Use of Da Bao, Draining Bao Mai and Dai Mai Together

To move Blood stasis from the Upper Jiao to Dai Mai.

Treatment Protocol for Connecting Da Bao to Bao Mai and then Dai Mai

1. Release the Five Pillars (described on page 328) with gua sha, cupping, sliding cupping, or needles.
2. Bleed GB-22.
3. Bleed CV-15.
4. (*Optional*). Needle GV-9.
5. Bleed GV-1 or needle GV-4 or BL-57.
6. Needle GB-26.
7. Hook needle into GB-41, right side for females, left for males.

(In my practice, a Da Bao to Bao Mai to Dai Mai treatment looks something like this: GB-22, CV-15, GB-26, GB-27, GV-1 (or BL-57 depending on the patient), GB-41.

8. Revisit each point in the order needled and check that the patient feels at least a very subtle vibration in each point.
9. Ask the patient to visualize or to imagine the feeling of the connection of all the points. Often they will report that they already feel this connection vibrating.
10. Take the pulses in the Eight Extra position. The pulses will have moved deeper into the wrist. If they have not, vibrate the needles again, ensuring that connection with the Yuan level has been made. This is done by intention rather than literal depth.
11. (*Optional*). Give the patient an affirmation to repeat while they are in treatment. E.g., *I release all that does not serve me.*
12. Leave needles in for 40 minutes after the insertion of the Opening point.
13. Take the pulses in Eight Extra style, note the change and report it to the patient.
14. Remove the needles from top to bottom, GB-41 last.
15. Allow the patient five minutes on the table, preferably alone, to reflect.

This treatment is still effective if the Luo points are not bled.

APPENDIX I

The Primary Channels

Including their Internal Pathways

Although the scope of this manual does not encompass treatment protocols for the Primary Channels, this book does include illustrations of those channels drawn according to the descriptions in the Classical texts. In this way the channel system is presented in its entirety. The inclusion of the Primary Channels drawn this way will also help in determining Transverse Luo and Emptied Luo diagnoses.

The pathways of the Primary Channels are described in chapter 59 of the *Su Wen* and in more detail in chapter 10 of the *Ling Shu*.

Lung Primary Channel

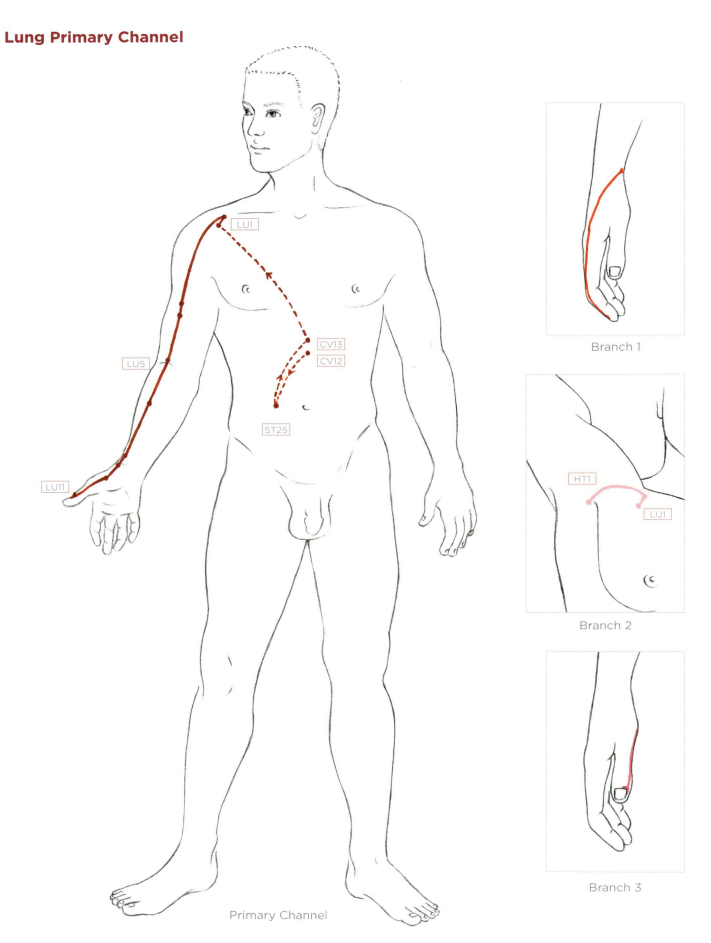

Lung
Primary Channel plus three branches

Primary Channel:
Begins at CV-12 in the Middle Jiao, descends to the Large Intestine Mu at ST-25, ascends to the opening of the Stomach, CV-13, goes through the diaphragm, into the Lung, emerges at LU-1 where it becomes external, and goes down the arm to **terminate at LU-11.**

Branch 1:
Extends from LU-9 to LI-1.

Branch 2:
Begins at LU-1, goes to LU-2, and **terminates at the axilla, at HT-1.**

Branch 3:
Begins at Cun Kou (*Inch Opening*, LU-9), to LU-10 and then **terminates at the thumb**.

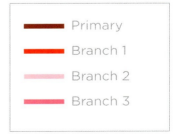

Large Intestine
Primary Channel plus three branches

Primary Channel:

Begins at LI-1, goes to LI-4, goes up past the elbow, connects to LI-15 and **terminates at GV-14.**

Branch 1:

Begins at LI-15, goes to ST-12, goes into the Lung, through the diaphragm and **terminates in the Large Intestine at ST-25.**

Branch 2:

Begins at **ST-12, goes through LI-17, LI-18,** goes to ST-5, encircles the mouth to LI-19 and **terminates at LI-20 on the opposite side.**

Branch 3:

Begins at the Large Intestine at ST-25 and **terminates at the Lower He-Sea point of the Large Intestine, ST-37.**

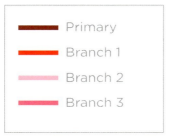

Large Intestine Primary Channel

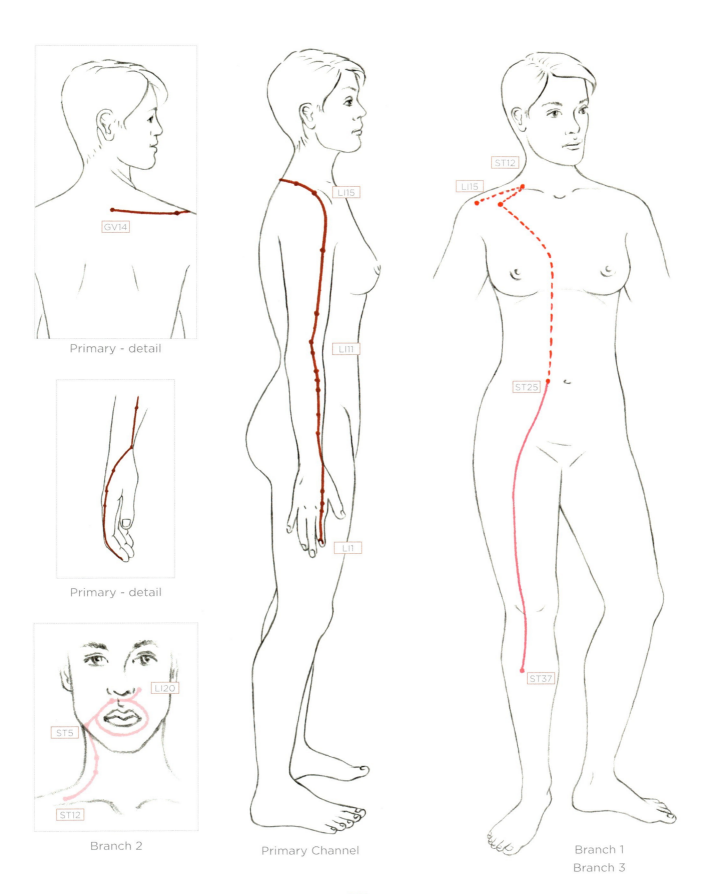

Primary - detail

Primary - detail

Branch 2

Primary Channel

Branch 1
Branch 3

Stomach Primary Channel

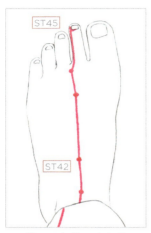

Branch 3 - detail

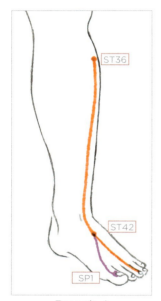

Branch 4
Branch 5

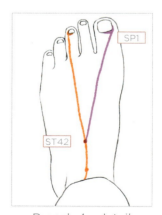

Branch 4 - detail
Branch 5

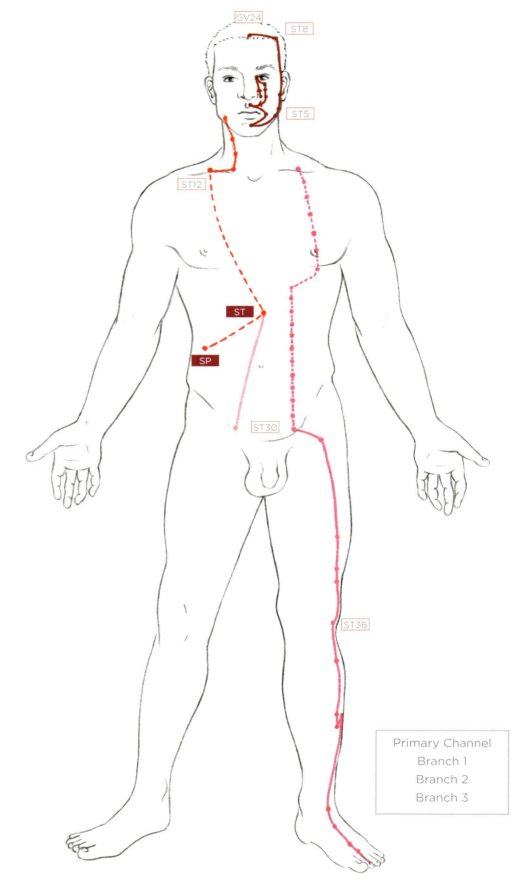

Primary Channel
Branch 1
Branch 2
Branch 3

Stomach
Primary Channel plus five branches

Primary Channel:

Begins at LI-20, ascends to Yin Tang, descends back down the outside of the nose slightly more laterally than its ascent, encircles the mouth, goes to CV-24, ascends to the ears at ST-8 and **terminates at GV-24**.

Branch 1:

Begins at **ST-5**, descends to ST-9, goes to ST-12 where it becomes internal, goes through the diaphragm and **terminates in the Stomach and Spleen**.

Branch 2:

Begins in the Stomach and **terminates at ST-30**.

Branch 3:

Begins at **ST-12**, is internal to ST-30 where it becomes external goes to ST-32, to the knee and **terminates at ST-45**.

Branch 4:

Begins at **ST-36**, goes to ST-42, and **terminates at the middle toe**.

Branch 5:

Begins at **ST-42** and **terminates at SP-1**.

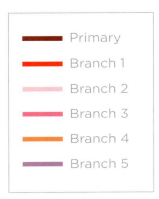

Spleen Primary Channel

SP1

Primary - detail

SP20
SP21
HT
ST
SP
SP1

Primary Channel Branch 1

344

Spleen
Primary Channel plus one branch

Primary Channel:
Begins at SP-1, ascends to SP-12, goes to the Stomach and Spleen, through the diaphragm, through the throat and **terminates at the root of the tongue.**

Branch 1:
Begins in the Stomach, at CV-12 and **terminates in the Heart,** at CV-14.

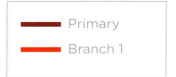

Heart
Primary Channel plus two branches

Primary Channel:

Begins in the Heart, goes through the diaphragm and **terminates in the Small Intestine**.

Branch 1:

Begins in the Heart, goes to the throat, to the tongue at CV-23, to the area behind the eyes enabling the spirit to brighten the eyes, and **terminates in the brain**.

Branch 2:

Begins in the Heart, at CV-14, goes to the Lung, to the armpit, to HT-3 and **terminates at HT-9**.

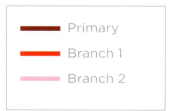

Heart Primary Channel

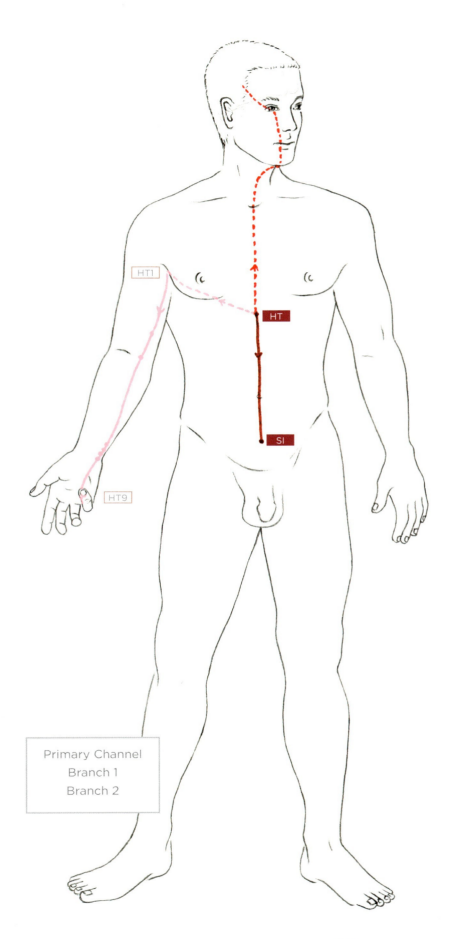

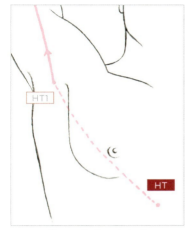

Branch 2 - detail

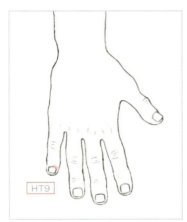

Branch 2 - detail

Primary Channel
Branch 1
Branch 2

Small Intestine
Primary Channel plus one branch

Primary Channel:

Begins at SI-1, ascends to LI-15, then to the scapula, to SI-12, BL-41, BL-12, SI-14, BL-11, SI-15, GV-14, then to ST-12, CV-14, CV-13, CV-12 and **terminates in the Small Intestine at CV-4**.

Branch 1:

Begins at the ST-12, goes to SI-16, ascends to the cheek at SI-18, goes to the outer canthus at GB-1 and **terminates at the ear at SI-19**.

Branch 2:

Begins at SI-18 and **terminates at BL-1**.

Branch 3:

Begins at CV-4 and **terminates at ST-39**.

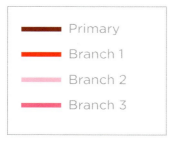

Small Intestine Primary Channel

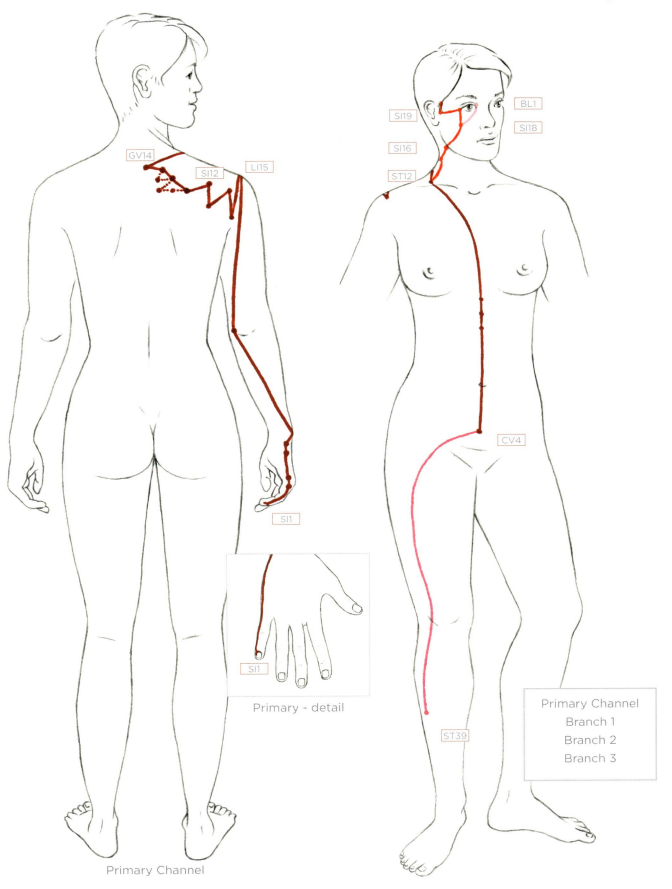

Bladder
Primary Channel plus four branches

Primary Channel:

Begins at BL-1, goes to the junction between the eye and the brain, then to forehead at GV-24, then to GB-15 and **terminates at GV-20**.

Branch 1:

Begins at GV-20 and **terminates above the tip of the ear**.

Branch 2:

Begins at GV-20 goes through the brain, emerges at GV-16, descends to the lumbar region, and **terminates in the Kidney at BL-23 and in the Bladder at CV-3**. This branch creates the inner Bladder Shu line.

Branch 3:

Begins at BL-23, goes to BL-35 and **terminates at BL-40**.

Branch 4:

Begins at GV-17, then goes to GV-14, descends along the outer Bladder Shu line to the hips, goes to BL-40, and **terminates at the little toe at BL-67**.

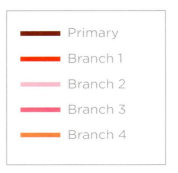

Bladder Primary Channel

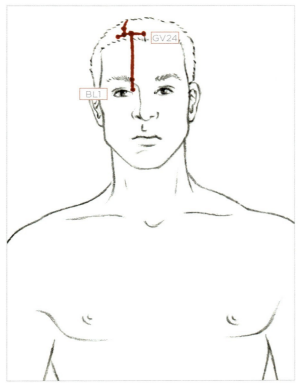

Primary Channel

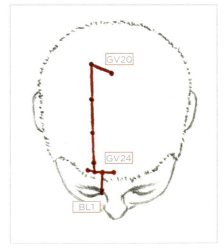

Primary - detail

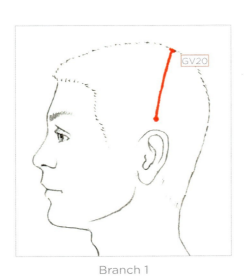

Branch 1

Bladder Primary Channel

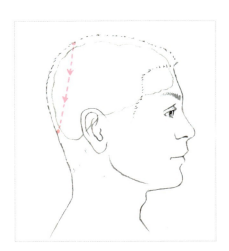

Branch 2 - detail

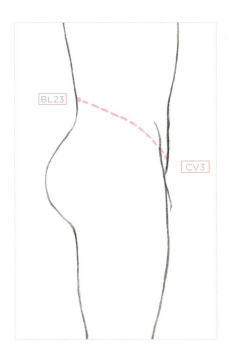

Branch 2 - detail

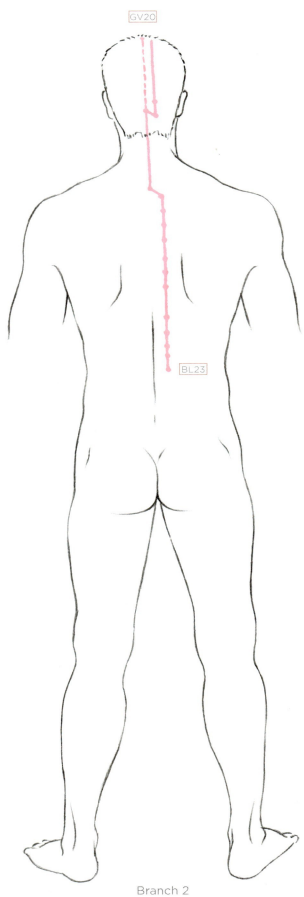

Branch 2

Bladder Primary Channel

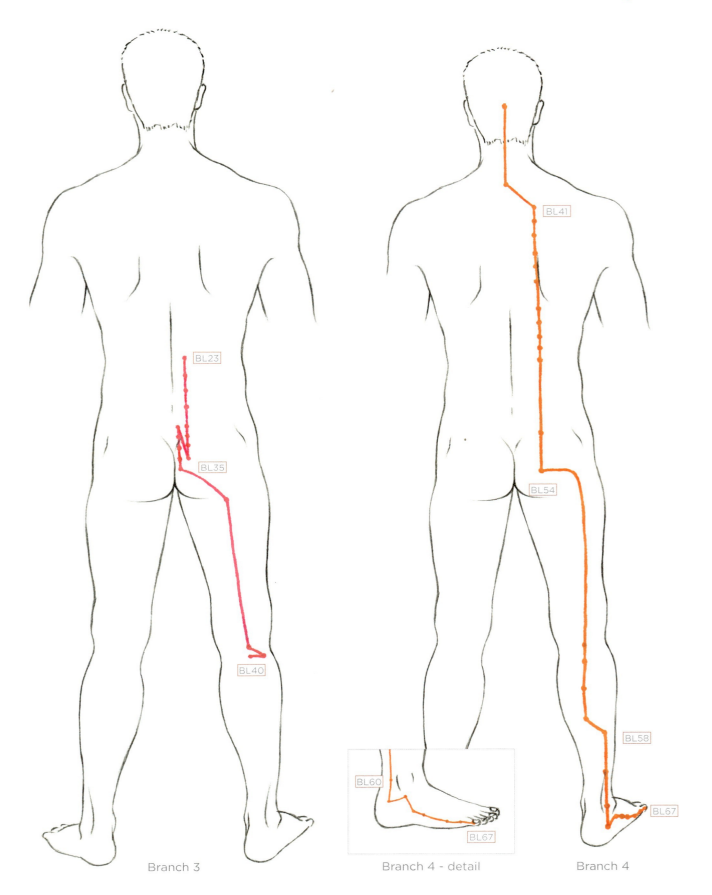

Branch 3

Branch 4 - detail

Branch 4

Kidney
Primary Channel plus two branches

Primary Channel:
Begins in the fleshy pad under the little toe, goes to KI-2, then to KI-10, to GV-1, GV-4, and **terminates in the Kidney at BL-23 and Bladder at CV-3.**

Branch 1:
Begins in the Kidney, goes to the genitalia, up through the diaphragm, to the Lung, to the throat and **terminates at the root of the tongue.**

Branch 2:
Begins in the Lung at LU-1 and terminates in the Heart and disperses in the chest.

Branch 3:
Begins at KI-2 and terminates at SP-8.

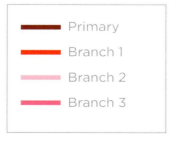

Kidney Primary Channel

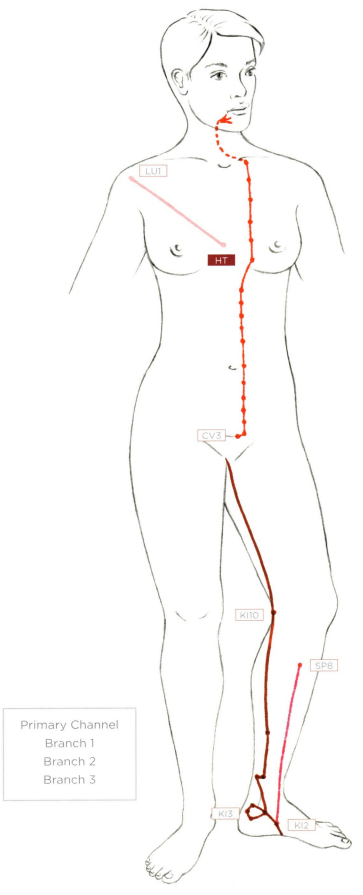

Primary Channel
Branch 1
Branch 2
Branch 3

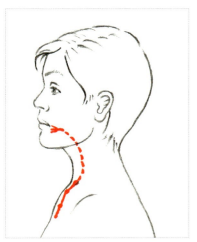

Branch 1 - detail

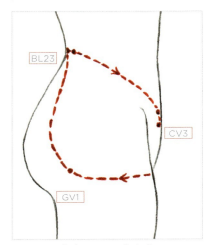

Primary - detail

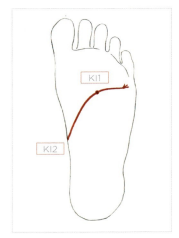

Primary - detail

Pericardium Primary Channel

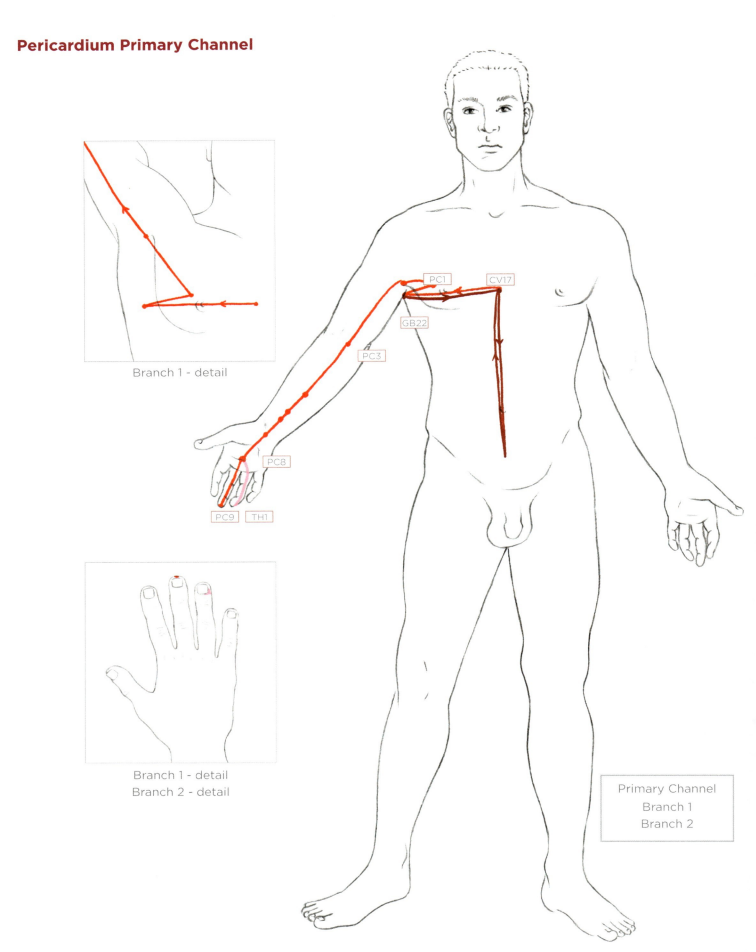

Pericardium
Primary Channel plus two branches

Primary Channel:
Begins at GB-22, then goes to CV-17, through the diaphragm, descends to the Lower Jiao and ascends to the Middle and **terminates in the Upper Jiao.**

Branch 1:
Begins in the chest, goes through the ribs to GB-22, to PC-1, up to the armpit and terminates at the tip of the middle finger.

Branch 2:
Begins in the palm at PC-8 and **terminates at TH-1.**

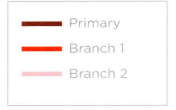

Triple Heater
Primary Channel plus two branches

Primary Channel:

Begins at the tip of the fourth finger, ascends to GV-14, then GB-21, then ST-12 where it becomes internal and spreads in the chest, goes to the Pericardium at PC-1, then KI-16, descends to the Lower Jiao at CV-3, then goes up the spine, distributing Jing to the Bladder Shu points starting at the level of BL-28 and BL-32 and **terminates with the distribution of Jing at BL-13.**

Branch 1:

Begins at CV-17, ascends to ST-12, goes up behind the ear, around the top of the ear and **terminates under the eye.**

Branch 2:

Begins behind the ear, goes into the ear, comes to the front of the ear, goes to GB-3 and **terminates at TH-23.**

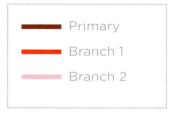

Triple Heater Primary Channel

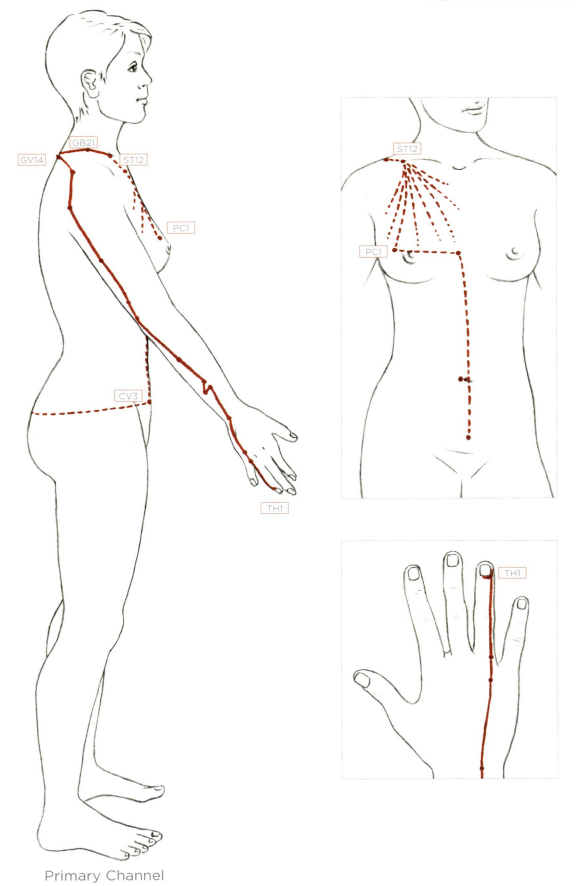

Primary Channel

Triple Heater Primary Channel

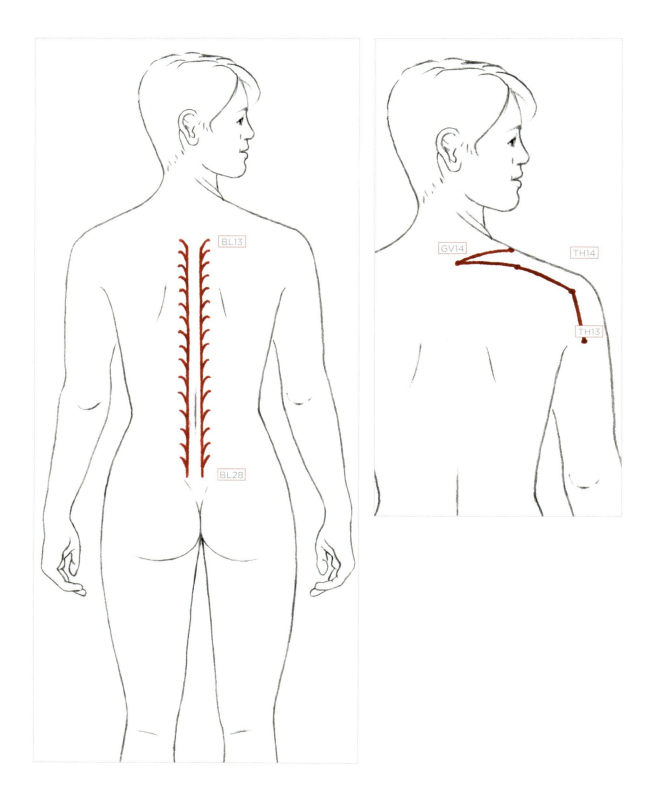

Primary Channel

Triple Heater Primary Channel

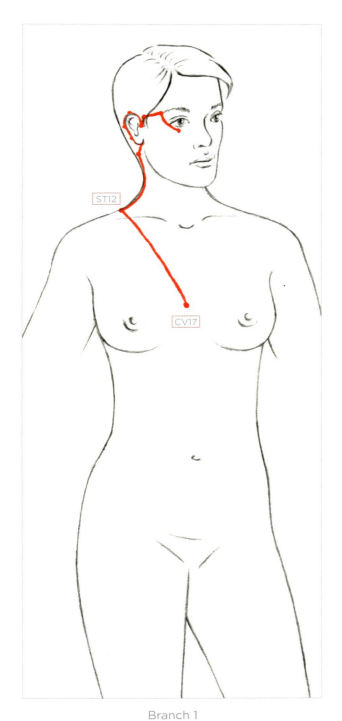

Branch 1

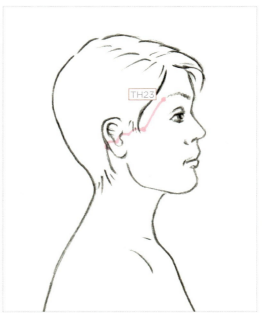

Branch 2

Gallbladder
Primary Channel plus four branches

Primary Channel:

Begins at GB-1, GB-2, ascends to TH-22, GB-3, ST-8, GB-4, descends behind the ear, then to SI-17, GB-13 to GB-20, then GB-21, then GV-14 and **terminates at ST-12 and SI-12 at the same time**.

Branch 1:

Begins at GB-1, descends to ST-5, under the eyes, ST-6, into the mandible and teeth, then to SI-18, descends to ST-12, PC-1, goes to the Liver at LR-14, and Gallbladder at GB-24, descends to ST-30, encircles the genitals and **terminates at GB-30**.

Branch 2:

Begins behind the ear, then TH-17, enters the ear at SI-19, comes to the front of the ear, ST-7 and **terminates at GB-1**.

Branch 3:

Begins at ST-12, goes to the axilla, goes to the chest and ribs at GB-22, LR-13, GB-23, GB-24 and GB-25, goes through NO organs, to the inguinal region, to GB-30, then fans out to all the Bladder Liao points: BL-31, BL-32, BL-33, BL-34, down the thigh and **terminates at GB-44**.

Branch 4:

Begins at GB-41 and **terminates at LR-1 and ST-45** at the same time.

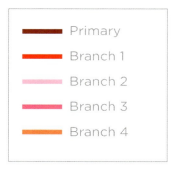

Gallbladder Primary Channel

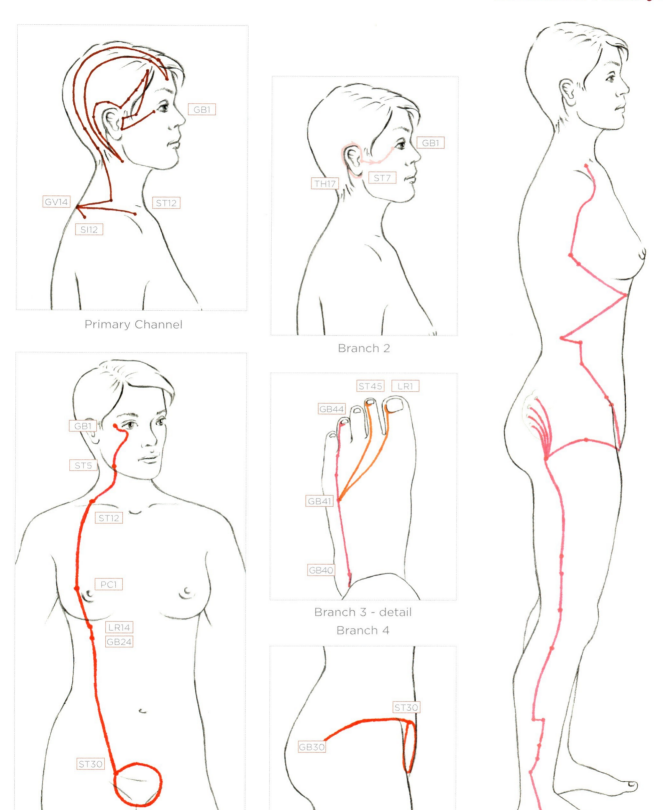

Liver
Primary Channel plus two branches

Primary Channel:

Begins at LR-1, ascends to ST-42, crosses the Spleen Channel eight inches above the medial malleolus, goes to LR-8, the genitals, the Stomach where it becomes internal, then the Liver and Gallbladder, the diaphragm, the throat, the eyes and **terminates at GV-20**.

Branch 1:

Begins at the eyes, descends through the cheeks and encircles the lips then **terminates at the lips**.

Branch 2:

Begins at the Liver, goes through the diaphragm (CV-12), then to PC-1, and **terminates in the Lung, where the cycle of the Primary Channels began**.

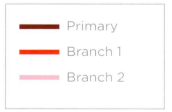

Liver Primary Channel

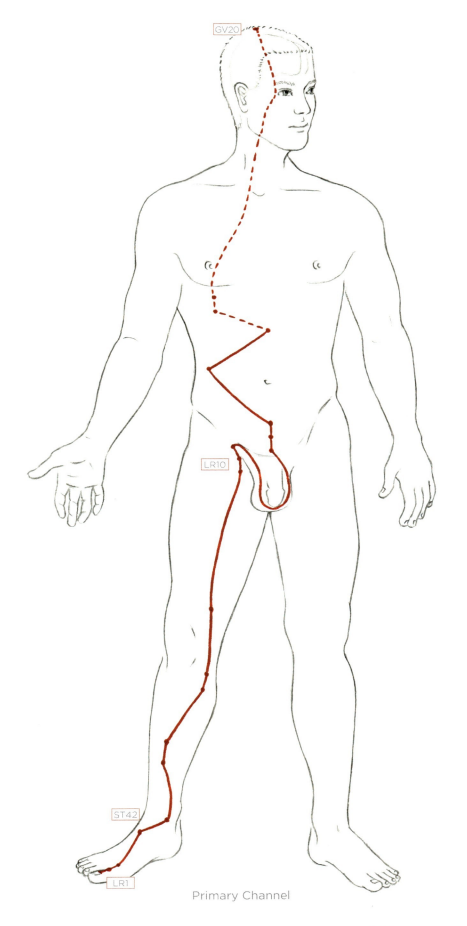

Primary Channel

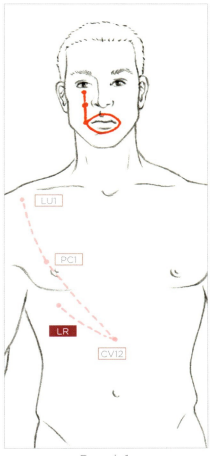

Branch 1
Branch 2

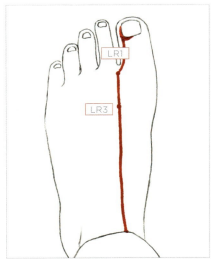

Primary - detail

365

APPENDIX II

Divergent Confluent Point Functions

Needling with intention is only possible with knowledge of point function. In Divergent Channel treatments the most important points are the Confluent points. These points signal to the body that a Divergent treatment is underway and, in most instances, encapsulate the treatment principle being enacted.

Acupuncture points yield different functions depending on the needling technique applied. When needled with Divergent technique, the Confluent point functions are somewhat distinct from the functions of the same points in a Primary Channel context. (Incidentally, the trajectory points are intended to function similarly to the way in which they do in a Primary Channel context. This is why the application of Divergent technique on trajectory points is optional.)

The Divergent Confluent points and Opening points function as described below when Divergent needling technique is used. These functions often differ from the Primary Channel point function.

Note: Bladder and Stomach Divergents open at their lower Confluent point.

Bladder and Kidney Divergent Confluent Points: BL-40, BL-10

BL-40 *Wei Zhong* translates as "crease at the middle of the back of the knee", but with the disease radical added, it translates as Wei Atrophy Syndrome, or "diseased Wei Qi", or "the inability to bend or stretch".

- Soothes and relaxes the Sinews to enable the body to release a lingering or unresolved pathogen.
- Treats the Heat or Damp-Heat that develops when the body is trying to move out a pathogenic factor but is unsuccessful.
- Treats Wind causing neuropathy. Addresses the decline in neurological function that occurs with long-term Damp-Heat and its destruction of Yin and tissues.
- Releases the low back.
- Treats Damp-Heat in the Fu-Bowels where the body has placed the pathology seeking an exit for it.
- Principal point for treating the Blood-Heat and Phlegm-Heat that develops with the accumulation of toxins.
- Treats difficulty in the transportation of toxic waste. Promotes bowel movements.

- Treats digestive issues being held at back of the knees: cracking, spasms, tightness.
- Treats Wei Atrophy resulting from the accumulation of emotional pathology.
- Courses Wind in the treatment of illnesses that often include emotional etiologies (arthritis, rheumatoid arthritis, asthma, hypertension, throat conditions, Hashimoto's thyroiditis, Graves' disease, pain, etc.) to allow for movement in a new direction.
- Clears Blood Heat (only with Divergent style needling) by coursing Wind.
- Induces sweat and promotes urination to drain Dampness and disinhibit pathogenic factors.
- Disinhibits to clear UTIs, cystitis, prostate swelling, benign prostatic hyperplasia.
- Treats painful, cloudy, grainy, bloody, tiring urination (Lin Bi).
- Treats prostate issues.
- Draws pathology from the Zang organs and, secondarily, from Fu organs through its connection to the inner Bladder Shu points.
- Treats Summer Heat.
- Reduces inflammation.

BL-10 *Tian Zhu, Celestial Pillar*
- Soothes and relaxes the Sinews. Relieves pain in the Sinews.
- Expels external Wind, unresolved external pathogenic factors.
- Treats pain along the pathway, for example, stiff neck and sciatica.
- Scatters Cold, clears Heat, courses Wind.
- Regulates excess Yang going to the head and brain leading to hypertension, chronic headaches, wind stroke, dizziness, encephalitis, meningitis, floating Yang.

Kidney Divergent Channel Opening Point
KI-10 *Yin Gu, Yin Valley*
- Treats pathology of the turbid aspect of the Jin-Thin Fluids that occurs when there is disruption to Gu Qi. These disruptions are often caused by tightness of the Sinews that leads to Qi stagnation in the gut and failure to eliminate adequately.
- Treats Dampness, Phlegm, edema, swollen joints. Transforms, dispels, disinhibits and resolves Damp.
- Treats heaviness in the abdomen: uterine bleeding, leukorrhea, flaccidity in Lower Jiao, impotence.
- Treats loss of gait due to vertigo caused by Dampness.
- Disinhibits Damp through the Lower Jiao. Drains stagnation.
- Clears the head.

- Reduces taxation on Yuan-Source Qi by freeing Gu Qi.
- Regulates body Fluids. Nourishes Fluids.

Gallbladder and Liver Divergent Confluent Points: CV-2, GB-1

CV-2 *Qu Gu, Curved bone*
- Secures the Jing-Essence by promoting the storage of Blood.
- Can be moxa'd to warm Kidney Yang in order to hold on to Blood.
- Treats Cold in the Liver.
- Regulates periods, Blood and the Lower Jiao.
- Transforms and regulates turbidity and Dampness. Stops the discharge of Fluids.
- Invigorates Blood, prevents stagnation.

GB-1 *Tong Zi Liao, Virgin Child's Bone Hole*
- Allows for and encourages changes in the way in which the world is perceived. Invites clear-sightedness. Enables the experiencing of the world to occur in a surrendered way. Enables clarity of vision, brightens the eyes. Enlivens. Restores the capacity to feel energized and ready to accept different options, challenges, new ways and new ideas. Relaxes habituation.
- Restores innocence by letting go of the past.
- Encourages reflection, retrospection.
- Courses Wind.
- Disinhibits the Upper Jiao.
- Opens the upper orifices.
- Treats ophthalmological issues.

Gallbladder Divergent Channel Opening Point

GB-30 *Huan Tiao, Continuous Jumping*
- Soothes the Sinews. Opens the Jing-Wells of the toes.
- Opens buttocks, strengthens low back.
- Influential point for the lower limbs.
- Protects Jing-Essence.
- Expels Wind-Damp. Clears Damp-Heat. Extinguishes Wind.
- Dissipates pathology in the joints.
- Enhances endurance.

Liver Divergent Channel Opening Point

LR-5 *Li Gou, Wormwood Canal*
- Travels to genitals to meet with CV-2.
- Rids the body of the "three worms" (entities): the hungry, sexual and wandering worms, which often reside in the Liver or Gallbladder.
- Treats joint Bi.
- Treats rebellious Qi.
- Calms the psyche.
- Moves pathology via the Blood.
- Brings Blood to support Jing-Essence.

Stomach and Spleen Divergent Confluent Points: ST-30, BL-1

ST-30 *Qi Chong, Qi Street*
- Soothes and relaxes the Ancestral Sinews: sternocleidomastoid, diaphragm, rectus abdominis, psoas, paravertebral muscles.
- Soothes and relaxes the Sinews. Treats heightened sensitivity of Wei Qi. If the sinews are not relaxed, Wei Qi can become obstructed in the smooth muscles, causing GERD, colitis, cystitis.
- Moves pathology in the Jing-Essence.
- Regulates Qi and Blood. Regulates menstruation and the uterus.
- Harmonizes Blood and Qi.
- Assists in the production of Blood.
- Treats the failure to digest food properly.
- Treats Running Piglet Qi.

BL-1 *Jing Ming, Eye's Clarity*
- Courses Wind. Treats aversion to Wind and Cold. Aversion to Wind can also mean aversion to change.
- Clears Heat.
- Activates Chong Yang, The Yang of Chong, ST-42, the Yuan-Source point of the Stomach that governs the distribution of Fluids to the sensory orifices. Also activates Chong Channel to bring postnatal Qi to support prenatal Qi. Assists in the maintaining of latency.
- Relieves pain.
- Balances hormones. Treats swollen pituitary gland, thyroid issues, goiter.
- Stimulates movement of water; transports or benefits water.
- Brightens the eyes. Enables the attainment of a clear vision of one's path.

Spleen Divergent Channel Opening Point
SP-12 *Chong Men, Doorway of Chong*
- Disinhibits Damp or Phlegm. Promotes diuresis. Treats breast lumps.
- Treats Dampness trapped in the Lower Jiao, for example, polycystic ovaries. Treats inguinal hernias.
- Clears Heat.
- Moves Qi to move Blood. Increases lactation.
- Rectifies Qi, especially in patients with a tight, wiry, bowstring quality in the cun pulse indicating an inability to let go or to open the chest. If the chest is not open, the Divergent Channels cannot function to bring the pathogen up and out, and treatment will not be effective. Guilt and shame can be a cause of tightness of the chest. SP-12 rectifies this Qi.
- Treats Sudden Turmoil Disorder (simultaneous vomiting and diarrhea).

Small Intestine and Heart Divergent Confluent Points: GB-22, BL-1
GB-22 *Yuan Ye, Canyon of Ye*
- Soothes and relaxes the Sinews. Relaxes Wei Qi.
- Yin arm Sinew Channel Confluent point.
- Invigorates Blood in the channels and collaterals.
- Regulates Blood, especially Blood going to the tongue. Treats dementia.
- Opens or unbinds the chest. Normalizes Qi to create acceptance.
- Activates Bao Mai for communication with the Kidneys.
- Connects us back to our Source. Treats Shen disturbance, mania and shock.

BL-1 *Jing Ming, Eye's Clarity*
- Treats Wind and aversion to change.
- Goes into brain, into the pituitary gland. Treats swollen pituitary gland.
- Affects and balances glandular and hormonal function.
- Treats pain and tension around the eyes.

Small Intestine Divergent Channel Opening Point
SI-10 *Nao Shu, Upper Arm Shu*
- Relaxes the Sinews.
- Clears Heat in the Blood.
- Invigorates the Blood to expel Wind.

- Breaks up Jie-Clumping (mobile or immobile masses, abscesses, clots) in the nodes (also known as the lower abdomen, chest, throat, and sensory orifices).
- Treats chest oppression, throat Bi, abdominal fullness.
- Releases upper limbs.
- Summons inner strength.

Heart Divergent Channel Opening Point

HT-1 *Ji Quan, Ultimate Spring*

- Treats the Nine Heart Pains, (the Nine Palaces), challenges in the curriculum of one's life.
- Rectifies Qi to dispel resistance to the challenges of life. Addresses issues of morality. Deals with the Heart pain associated with not being able to overcome life's challenges.
- Strengthens enthusiasm for life. "Ultimate" also refers to the ultimate or endless possibilities in life and that ultimately, we have the free will to live to the fullest.
- Assists in Kidney-Heart communication. The "Ultimate Spring" also refers to the Kidneys.
- Treats swelling in armpit, swollen lymph nodes, scrofula.
- Opens the chest. Loosens tightness, especially in the chest.

Triple Heater and Pericardium Divergent Confluent Points: TH-16, CV-12

TH-16 *Tian Yu, Celestial Orbit, master Windows to the Sky point*

- Expels rapidly spreading Wind which is causing nerve damage.
- Treats Phlegm.
- Relieves pain.
- Disinhibits Damp, rids swellings and Yin stasis which arise as the capacity for latency is lost. As Yin goes into decline, the body accumulates Dampness as compensation.
- Disperses swellings, disinhibits and transforms or expels Dampness.
- Clears Heat that has gone out of control and become Fire.
- Treats overwhelming Heat, drains Fire by promoting urination.
- Addresses Dampness as it compensates for deficiencies of Jing, Blood, Jin-Thin Fluids and Ye-Thick Fluids.
- Treats cranial and facial swellings and goiters. Opens the throat.
- Treats blockages in the brain and in the sensory orifices, for example, Alzheimer's disease.

CV-12 Zhong Wan, Central Vessel, Mu point of the Stomach
- Treats digestive issues.
- Aids in the separation of pure and turbid Fluids. Deals with the accumulation of turbidity in Middle Jiao.
- Secures the root by tonifying postnatal Qi (strengthening Spleen and Stomach) thereby reducing taxation on Yin and Yang.
- Harmonizes Spleen and Stomach.
- Transforms Dampness.
- Disinhibits Dampness.
- Descends Qi to the Bladder and Small Intestine for absorption by the Kidneys.
- Treats obsession.
- Treats the Nine Heart Pains.

Triple Heater Divergent Channel Opening Point
GV-20 Bai Hui, Hundred Convergences
- Suppresses rebellion.
- Pacifies Wind. Treats seizures, convulsions, epilepsy.
- Subdues Yang.
- Quiets Shen, treats mania and agitation.
- Treats prolapse. Raises Qi. Opens the crown chakra.
- Opens the head and sensory orifices.

Pericardium Divergent Channel Opening Point
PC-1 Tian Chi, Heavenly Pool
- Enables one to reconcile themselves with what Heaven has bestowed (the pool of challenges). Enables moving on, transcendence.
- Treats the Nine Heart Pains, The Nine Challenging Curricula.
- Opens the chest to allow a person to surrender. Opens upper limbs.
- Rectifies the Qi to assuage guilt.
- Diffuses Lung Qi to address stress-related cough, coughing when experiencing difficulty expressing the self, and asthma. Treats foggy-headedness.
- Clears Blood Heat due to pestilent Qi (that came from "Heaven" and "pooled" in the body).
- Treats recklessness, restlessness and delirium.
- Treats breast lumps caused by Blood Heat. Breaks up nodules. Increases lactation.

Large Intestine and Lung Divergent Confluent Points: LI-18, ST-12

LI-18 *Fu Tu, Support the Chimney*
- Regulates Qi and Blood. Treats rebellious Qi, especially coughing, wheezing and vomiting. Regulates blood pressure.
- Moves Qi. Diffuses Qi to prevent further penetration of a pathogenic factor.
- Prevents stagnation.
- Opens and disinhibits the throat. Treats sudden loss of voice.

ST-12 *Que Pen, Broken Dish*
- Regulates Qi and Blood.
- Invigorates the Blood to prevent further decline.
- Diffuses Lung Qi to prevent further internalization of pathogenic factors. (When latency is lost, the "dish" is "broken".)
- Clears Heat in the chest. Treats binding of the chest. Treats irritability and restlessness due to a feeling of stuffiness in the chest.
- Descends Qi. Treats shortness of breath.
- Enables one to let go. Releases the neck and shoulder. Treats scrofula, goiter, throat Bi.
- Treats loss of Yang which is causing chills and the feeling of Cold with or without a fever. Treats low back pain or rigidity stemming from the loss of Yang Qi. Treats life-threatening conditions in which Yang is failing.
- Treats neuropathy or Wei Atrophy Syndrome.

Large Intestine Divergent Channel Opening Point

LI-15 *Jian Yu, Shoulder Bone*
- Transforms Wind-Phlegm and Damp. Dissipates Phlegm.
- Promotes urination to rid Dampness.
- Courses Wind to rid pathogens.
- Regulates Qi and Blood.
- Relieves taxation on the Marrow.
- Assists in anchoring Yang.
- Harmonizes Qi and Blood, for example, when white blood cells are elevated and red blood cells are low.
- Breaks up Blood stagnation in the arm.
- Helps the body to establish homeostasis.
- Releases pathology from the joints, disinhibits the joints (clears joints via urination).

Lung Divergent Channel Opening Point

LU-1 *Zhong Fu, Middle Palace*
- Diffuses Lung Qi.
- Descends Qi to treat coughing and wheezing.
- Transforms and dissipates Phlegm. Clears Dampness and Phlegm from the Middle Jiao.
- Clears Heat.
- Courses Wind. Courses Qi.
- Enables one to let go.
- Opens the neck, treats goiter.
- Treats Running Piglet Qi.

APPENDIX III

Healing Events

Healing events are re-emergences of suppressed, unresolved or latent illnesses that sometimes arise after a healing acupuncture treatment. They are an important part of the peeling back of layers of energetic blockages that conceal natural good health. They last between one and ten days in length. Between six and ten days is considered very severe and is very unusual. Watch these longer events carefully. Healing events are to be welcomed and not feared.

Most often a patient will report puzzlement during a healing event because although the signs and symptoms might appear dramatic, they feel relatively good. Often patients have a strong sense that they are clearing something "old" because they intuitively don't feel very ill although the body might be having strong symptoms. Sleep is relatively unaffected and usually deeper and more peaceful during a healing event. Often the patient will report they feel the best they've felt in years while they are spending days purging copious phlegm, sweating a remarkably stinky fluid, urinating a deep yellow frothy liquid, defecating an unusually foul-smelling stool or even vomiting peculiar mucus.

Healing events are characterized by pulses that are stronger than before the crisis. They are often resolved by a hot Epsom salt or sea salt bath which helps draw the remaining pathogen out of the Yuan level. The patient should be instructed to make the bath a safe, almost-hot temperature.

Healing events can be startling in their manifestations. They are often characterized by copious phlegm emerging from the sensory orifices and sinus cavities. Sometimes this phlegm can be dark green and thick. Often a patient will think they are getting a bad cold. Consider using the Stomach Divergent which opens all the sensory orifices while expelling an EPF (SDS).

Sometimes the patient will say the illness "came out of nowhere". One minute they were fine and the next they are coughing green phlegm.

Healing events are often mistaken for a new illness or for a fresh repeat of an old illness. If your patient does not understand the nature of a healing event or does not know what to expect, and they see a Western doctor and are given antibiotics, the opportunity for clearing pathology is missed. The pathogen is pushed back into the Yuan level once again, ready for the next round of treatments to get the pathogen to emerge once more.

Healing events should be treated. When a healing crisis emerges, be ready to treat it using any type of channel, except the Eight Extras. Most commonly, one would choose Sinew or Luo treatments. If the patient is unable to get to the practitioner, they should be able to do enough at home to encourage the resolution of the crisis. This could be an Epsom salt bath, a sea salt bath, a head-steam bath.

Example: A patient is treated for chronic gastritis using Stomach Divergent Channel. After three days, the gastritis disappears but the patient is immobilized by low back pain. He remembers having a bad injury 20 years earlier, in college. The pathology moved from the third confluence to the first confluence. You're peeling back the layers. Explain to the patient why this is positive progress and treat Bladder Divergent Channel to clear the pathology.

APPENDIX IV

Safety

1. The Ribcage
    a. Needles anywhere on the ribcage should <u>not</u> be inserted perpendicularly.
    b. Needles on the ribcage should be a <u>maximum</u> of one inch in length.
    c. Special care should be taken on all points on the ribcage, especially LR-14 which is in a hollow.
    d. Needle ribcage points very obliquely.

2. Moxibustion
    a. Moxa can easily burn. Keep your fingers present as heat monitors.
    b. Occasionally a patient will *not* report that the moxa is too hot when in fact it is.
    c. Patients with diabetes or neuropathy frequently have compromised sensitivity, especially in the feet. They might not sense moxa heat accurately.
    d. Heat lamps can burn. Heat lamps attempt to approximate the warmth generated by qigong practice. They are not a substitute for moxa. Heat lamps should be far enough from the skin so as not to overheat the skin.
    e. Never leave a patient unattended with moxa *or* a heat lamp.

3. The Face
    a. Needles around the eyes and nose should be half inch and inserted <u>freehand</u>. The margins for error on BL-1 and GB-1 are far smaller than the inside diameter of a tube. Take off the tube and throw it away!

4. Babies and Children
    a. Never needle a baby's or toddler's head.
    b. Never treat GV-4 in any way on a prepubescent child. It will produce premature aging. (TH-4 will not have this effect.)
    c. Needles affect children very quickly and need not be retained.

5. Pregnancy
    a. Never needle in the Lower Jiao.
    b. Never needle the Middle Jiao after the first trimester.
    c. Pregnancy treatments are best done away from the abdomen altogether, and only if required.

6. Universal Prohibitions
    a. Never needle GV-10 or GV-11. Needling these causes Shen disturbance.
    b. Never moxa GV-6. Moxa on GV-6 causes scoliosis.

7. Don't release the exterior if the pulse is weak and thin in the moderate level. Harm will result.

8. Always take the pulses after the treatment. Allow time to rectify issues or omissions that become apparent—visibly or through the pulses—after the treatment.
    a. E.g., the clearing of heat should be immediate. If the pulses became thin or the complexion became pale, the patient had a Qi and Blood deficiency and you cleared Qi along with the Heat. Immediately treat accordingly.
    b. E.g., if the face went from red to pale but the pulse stayed rapid, you forgot to nourish Fluids, or didn't nourish them sufficiently. Immediately treat accordingly.

9. Never needle a Divergent Channel Superficial-Deep-Superficial if there is insufficient mediumship at that level. You will mobilize the pathology but the body won't have the mediumship to expel it.

APPENDIX V

Equipment Essential for Advanced Acupuncture Treatments

1. The most essential piece of equipment in the Classical Acupuncturist's kit is the needle. A Classical Acupuncturist, like all acupuncturists, is interested in poignant, accurate, swift and effective movement of Qi within the treatment session. In order to produce these immediate and potent effects, the needle used must be able to engage the Qi. For these purposes:
    a. It's essential that needles have a eyelet or loop (a hole) at the top of the needle. This allows the Qi to do what it needs to do: circulate, enter, release, or reach equilibrium.
    b. Plastic-handled and/or silicone-coated needles are not used. Complement Channel treatments conducted with plastic handled needles are likely to fail. (There are people performing very powerful treatments with plastic-handled needles, I'm sure. There are even people performing powerful treatments just by doing acupressure with the plastic tube! With deeply cultivated intention, all things are possible. While we find our legs, though, we need the most appropriate equipment available.)
    c. Divergent and Sinew treatments in particular are quite impossible to perform effectively with plastic-handled or silicon-coated needles.
    d. Needles that look dark and shiny or slightly bluish are too slippery for Complement Channel treatments. They will not grip Qi very effectively and they definitely will not engage Wei Qi in a Sinew or Divergent treatment, probably rendering your treatment ineffective. Use bright and shiny stainless steel needles with no silicone.
    e. Lengths. The choice of lengths is a more personal thing. I like to keep things very simple. This is my complete needle list, just as an example:
        i. 34 gauge half inch
        ii. 34 gauge one inch
        iii. 34 gauge two inch
        iv. 30 gauge three inch
        v. Medium (23 gauge) and fine gauge lancets
    f. Consider buying boxes of 500 needles packaged five to a tube. The reduction of waste is enormous. Many people ask how to manage these in the hand. Peel the paper backing down a third of the way, grasp the needles and the tube and pull the whole unit out of the plastic. Take the needles from the tube as

a group and put all the needles as a group back in the tiny plastic packet they came from. Now you have the empty tube in your hand and all the needles in the tiny plastic and paper envelope, ready to load. I buy 100 boxes of 500 needles (50,000) needles at a time which saves a lot of transportation, oil and resources.

2. I recommend having two grades of lancets, medium and fine. Medium lancets are essential to get into very thick-walled Luo Channels. Experiment with brands until you find a fine one, but not the finest. It's essential to have these on hand for the extremely fine Luos and also for very sensitive or deeply traumatized patients who normally have extreme sensitivity. Both grades are available in the pharmacy and from acupuncture supply services. *Lancets must have a top that you have to break off, not a top that is replaceable, so that sterility is unquestioned.*

3. Cotton balls. Two grades: large for major Luo treatments and small for minor incidental bleeding or minimal Luo treatments.

4. Moxa. The best and hottest moxa is the compressed weed itself, the old fashioned moxa stick. I like the Vietnamese ones especially but they're sometimes hard to find. Once I was given a few packets of very wonderful, smooth moxa from Vietnam and I've not been able to locate it again. The best moxa I've ever used was Sun Si Miao's own formulation which I purchased in China when I was on "Acupuncturists' Row" in Beijing with Jeffrey. He pointed it out on the shelf with enthusiasm. It makes a lot of smoke but is particularly healing and wonderful smelling. In our offices, due to the fire code we don't use smoky moxa, however. That leaves "smokeless", which certainly does work. There are a few important things to know about smokeless moxa.
    - It has to be solid (not hollow). The hollow moxa is fragile and often cracks and can break apart. We can't risk moxa falling on the patient.
    - When de-ashing the stick, don't hit or tap the stick on the ash receptacle. It will crack and break if you do. Instead, gently scrape it. I scrape it gently on the sharp resting edge of the moxa extinguisher.
    - If you're heating up a needle with the stick, get as close as you can to the needle without touching the needle. It will heat up beautifully without contact. Touching the needle will cause ash to spill on the skin. I don't use needle-top moxa because you have to wait a long time for the needle to warm up and then the heat is short-lived.

a. An essential part of the tool kit is a jar of the tiny, tiny moxa "cones" also known as thread moxa. These come in flat plastic disc-shaped containers that look like wide lip gloss pots. These are indispensable for stopping bleeding using SP-1 and LR-1. Stick them on with a tiny amount of burn cream and light them with incense. Bleeding stops very quickly with this method.

5. Rubber gloves are absolutely essential for Luo treatments. I buy big boxes from the acupuncture supplier, but the pharmacy brands are fine, too. Some patients are allergic to latex and so buying latex-free is a good idea. I always buy powder-free so that I don't have to wash my already well-washed hands just because I took a glove off.

6. Lighters. I use a huge triple-jet cigar lighter. They light smokeless moxa in seconds, something that can take forever with a single-jet moxa lighter. I have three lighters so that I'm never wasting treatment time refueling in front of a patient.

7. A 2% dilution of Myrrh (20 drops in one ounce of almond oil) is invaluable to dab on bruises that might emerge. Some practitioners here at the Center use homeopathic creams and find them indispensable. Bruises are infrequent, but when they do happen, firm pressure and quick application of some cream or prepared oil can prevent the bruise emerging almost completely. Use a clean cotton ball to take the cream from the tube to the patient, never a finger.

APPENDIX VI

Cultivation

Cultivation is in every aspect of acupuncture: writing the email or text or making the call in response to an inquiry, greeting the patient at the door, doing the intake, taking the pulses, needling the patient, making the recommendations, saying goodbye, all require cultivation.

Cultivation is really a state of detachment where the practitioner is aware of the infinite nature of all things and therefore is aware of the inseparability of the patient from their true (unencumbered) state. When communicating with the patient at any time, there's a feeling that they are already better, that they have already achieved what they came for.

When needling, there's a focused intention and a feeling and sensing that the needle is assisting in the flow of Qi. There's a feeling that the outcome of the treatment is positive even before it has begun. And at the end of the treatment there's a feeling imparted to the patient that all is well, that all will steadily improve as that wellness is already revealed. All these actions and non-actions are products of cultivation.

Ultimately, cultivation is the achievement of the embodiment of this feeling, of the actual knowing that there is one universal connectedness in all things. That's the nitty gritty. The only thing in existence is the Godforce, an all-embracing and all-inclusive Qi that contains and connects everything. Our patients, like us, are connected segments of that Godforce and we are using our Godforce to remind the Godforce of the patient that it is unimpeded. This fact alone makes cultivation essential. We have to get our Qi to be relatively unimpeded. If the integrity of the Godforce in the practitioner is influencing and tuning that of the patient, we'd better have that force in order.

Traditionally in our practice, the best aligners of energy in the body are meditation, tai chi and qigong. All take tremendous concentration and discipline and all of them create an open experiential awareness that there is a permeating connectedness in all things. When that quality is palpably felt, one's practice soars. There is no secret to a successful acupuncture practice, it depends solely on cultivating knowing that the interconnectedness of all things is all that there is. Here are some additional thoughts from Andrew Sterman, musician and teacher of qigong.

Self-Cultivation for Acupuncturists

by Andrew Sterman

Imagine the Dalai Lama deciding he needed some time off, maybe a few days in Vegas playing dice and hanging out with some former showgirls. Or, Gandhi taking a break from being Gandhi, Jesus taking a break from being Jesus. Imagine Buddha letting his students' meditations go awry while he munched on chicken wings with sauce.... Unimaginable, all of that, of course. Maimonides—the great Western scholar of the Middle Ages, who codified vast collections of Hebrew writings into one authoritative text, all the while memorizing the entirety of known ancient Greek and Arabic medicine—imagine him feeling that his knowledge was a burden on his shoulders, and wouldn't it be nice to have a vacation from being himself! A rest, perhaps, but not an escape. Imagine Ge Hong, the great Daoist alchemist, going for a vacation before taking the alchemical pill he had developed, or just before settling down to write *One hundred Remedies To Have Up Your Sleeve*. The point is that for these masters, and countless others, there is no conflict between what they believe and how they really want to live. The path of the spirit no longer has any conflict with the path of the body. Nor with the path of human relations. Simply put, conflict has been overcome. Overcome by willpower? Perhaps at first, but discipline alone leads to burnout, and it is impossible to think of someone like Buddha having burnout.

I imagine some people may be thinking, we are not Buddha, or Jesus, or Gandhi, or any great master or saint. We are not Mother Theresa, or even a famous philanthropist. We are just us. Perhaps it is not our destiny to be a Daoist Immortal, a Christian saint, a Buddhist bodhisattva, or a Jewish tzadik, but destiny is not potential; we have the same potential as any buddha or saint, and that is where self-cultivation comes in. Self-cultivation, very simply, is working with ourselves to unfold our potential. Furthermore, self-cultivation always includes all parts of our being: broadly speaking, the physical body, the emotional realm, and our mental/spiritual aspects.

There are many, many methods of self-cultivation. The term itself is from the language of Daoism, but even within that system, the term refers to a wide array of practices, including meditation and physical practices such as qigong. Qigong practices include martial arts development, medical/healing work, and religious or spiritual development. Self-cultivation is broad, but in any system, (traditional or home-made), self-cultivation is always working with our Essence, with our Jing. Self-cultivation is always cultivating our constitutional Essence. The "self" we are "cultivating" is our essential self, our deepest identity, our pure life-force. "Working with" means both conserving and developing.

For the acupuncturist or other healing clinician, the first point is to have some kind of self-cultivation practice, whether meditation, qigong, tai chi (tai ji), yoga. Health practices, such as conscious cooking, are a nearly essential part of self-cultivation, but very rarely are a complete cultivation practice on their own. Likewise with certain hobbies. That being said, it might be important to understand a few more aspects of what is meant by self-cultivation. In self-cultivation, we don't simply act as good people, ethical and responsible, for example, or the warmest friend or best clinician anyone could have. Those are fine things to be, but in self-cultivation the idea is that we do some kind of awakening, or at least some kind of growth, some kind of transformation, in a daily practice. We walk the paths of our lives, forward. We walk toward our personal destinies. We develop the concurrence of our Jing and our Shen. We employ practices to overcome our personal blocks and put to rest the conflicts within our personalities. We use self-cultivation techniques to overcome our illnesses and to gather enough vitality (Qi) to discover and claim our callings, to become sovereign masters of our own lives.

Self-cultivation requires integration of body, breathing and consciousness. Typically, the body requires work with postures, breathing requires work with conscious breathing practices (as in qigong or yoga/pranayama), and consciousness means working with meditation in some way. Self-cultivation requires integrating all three levels of practice.

Further, self-cultivation has aspects of letting go (purification) and building-up. Letting go can be learning to free tension while repeating a qigong movement, lengthening exhalation, freeing the knots of the mind while doing sitting practice, or simply standing while balancing looseness with alignment in ever increasing efficiency and naturalness. Building-up could include strengthening tendons (as in some styles of qigong), increasing inhalation and concentration, physical endurance, and so forth. Further, there is the idea that you develop your inherent energies. By developing your energies through various specific practices (you also feed them with food, water, sunlight and all the influences of the outside world), it is possible to transform your fundamental inherited vital energies into more and more refined energetic forms. This is the famous transformation of Jing into Qi into Shen. Medically speaking everyone has Jing, Qi and Shen, but the practitioner of Daoist self-cultivation does something different, reaching into the depths of their energies and developing them in special ways.

An easy way to think of Jing, Qi, Shen is the analogy of a candle: the wax is our Jing (inherited bodily capacity, substantial, thick, essential), the flame is our Qi (manifestly energetic, warm, not quite substantial), and the light the flame emits is our Shen (far less substantial even than the flame, the "reason" the candle exists, more refined than the wax or even the flame).

It is here, at this level, that what practices you use, what lineage you follow, becomes significant. Martial qigong develops the Jing differently than medical qigong, spiritual qigong or meditation. Tibetan meditation cultivates the energies somewhat differently than Daoist meditation. In fact, each different technique approaches cultivation differently, being different in goal, methods and results.

Is working-out at home or a gym self-cultivation? No. Exercise may be good for you, but it's only self-cultivation if you are developing conscious breathing, integrating the physical, human experiential and spiritual levels, working in an informed way with transforming inherent qualities, in a path of self-evolution. Professional sports training comes a bit closer, as it often includes serious mental and emotional training, but nonetheless it remains very different. The very first point to consider would be whether you entertain your mind as you exercise, with, for example, an iPod, television or reading. Exercise may be a good thing for an individual, but it is very different from self-cultivation.

Nonetheless, sophisticated techniques are not necessarily superior to simple ones. Whether classical practices or home-made methods, the main points are to:
- have a steady, daily practice in your life.
- use a practice you enjoy.
- understand that for self-cultivation, you are cultivating your Essence, your constitutional "gift" (ancestral inheritance).
- include some degree of conserving your life (not "burning the candle" too fast).
- get energized by your practice (cultivate Qi).
- awaken some degree of internal wisdom (Shen).
- integrate your constitutional, energetic and spirit/consciousness levels (Jing/Qi/Shen).
- integrate your cultivation practice throughout your daily life.

Within qigong, there are specific techniques for building Qi into the hands, developing intuition, and so forth. Individual acupuncture practitioners may choose to practice these techniques daily and especially before each working day. There also exist letting go techniques to insure no negativities from patients attach to our own energetics. There are many such techniques, from different traditions, some formal, some informal. It is not necessary to know all of them, but very useful to use some.

It is easy to think that self-cultivation is having a daily practice to become at least a little more like the masters we admire, but ultimately this will always be a false path, contrary to the innermost principles of genuine self-cultivation. It is our own essential self that we cultivate, and that needs no improvement, evolution or correction. It is already present within us in complete and thorough perfection. The "cultivation" is not to change or improve our essence, rather to cultivate our relationship with our own essence, to bring awareness of our truest nature into our daily lives, into the way we walk, breathe, love, eat, socialize, work, create, joke, drive and all the other aspects of our lives. True self-cultivation attempts no altering of what is. We do what we do as a celebration of who we are.

One thing that self-cultivation is not, however, is the commitment to build up enormous Qi energy and transmit it into patients, giving them magical treatments or highly entertaining sessions. Rather, the idea is that as a clinician, you have traveled on your path in a way that lends authenticity to your unpretentious assistance of your patients so that they can do the same for themselves. The idea is that beyond knowledge and acquired skill, you have explored within your being what is the true foundation of your daily work as a clinician. Each day, before touching a patient's pulse, needles or moxa, you have at least briefly tended the vast essential world of your own life, cultivating connection of body, energy and spirit. Then, you are ready to work with others.

BIBLIOGRAPHY

Huang-Fu Mi, *The Systematic Classic of Acupuncture and Moxibustion* (Boulder: Blue Poppy Press, 1993).

Li Shi Zhen, *Pulse Diagnosis* (Brookline: Paradigm Publications, 1985).

Maoshing Ni, *The Yellow Emperor's Classic of Medicine* (Boston: Shambhala, 1995).

Paul Unschuld, translator, *Nan Ching, Classic of Difficult Issues* (Berkeley: University of California Press, 1986).

Paul Unschuld, general editor and translator, Hermann Tessenow, translator, *Huang Di Nei Jing Su Wen: An Annotated Translation of Huang Di's Inner Classic* (Berkeley: University of California Press, 2011).

Wang Shu-He, and Shou-Zhong, Yang, *The Pulse Classic, A Translation of the Mai Jing*, (Boulder: Blue Poppy, 1997).

Wu Jing-Nuan, translator, *Ling Shu or The Spiritual Pivot* (Honolulu: University of Hawaii Press, 1993).

Nelson Liansheng Wu, Andrew Qi Wu, translators, *Yellow Emperor's Canon Internal Medicine*, (Beijing: China Science and Technology Press, 1999).

Dr. Jeffrey Yuen, oral transmission. One of the primary sources of oral transmission of Classical Chinese Medicine at an international level is Jeffrey Yuen, the 88th generation of his Taoist lineage: *Yu Ching Huang Lao Pai*, (Jade Purity School, Yellow Emperor/Lao Tzu sect); 26th generation of *Chuan Chen Lung Men Pai* (Complete Reality School, Dragon Gate Sect).

Zhang, Ye, Wiseman, Mitchell, Feng, *Shang Han Lun, On Cold Damage*, (Brookline: Paradigm, 1999).

INDEX

The Table of Contents can be found on pages iii to xxi.

Western diagnostic terms appear in this index but it must be noted that Chinese medicine does not treat diseases or conditions. Chinese medicine only treats the individual. The encounter between practitioner and patient with the taking of pulses and the examination of the tongue enables the practitioner to determine which channel is best used to free the individual's unique blockage, thereby assisting the patient's body and mind to remember how to achieve or return to the state of health the patient desires. The practitioner is ever mindful of the inherent capacity in each patient to return to his or her desired state of health.

In the Chinese medical setting, the Western diagnosis can be immaterial. For example, the Western medical diagnosis of Multiple Sclerosis could be given to twenty individuals, but the number of unique Chinese medical diagnoses in that same group could number 20. The root cause of that disease could range from a Wind invasion, to Thin- or Thick-Fluid deficiency, Blood deficiency, Jing stasis, Rebellious Qi, internal Wind, internal Heat, internal Cold, systemic Damp, Wind-Damp, Hot Phlegm, combinations of these, and others. Even armed with full knowledge of all the signs and symptoms presenting, the Chinese medical diagnosis is unknown until the diagnostic procedures of pulse and tongue examination are performed on that patient.

With that said, I have included an index containing Western medical diagnoses. This is expressly not to assist in making Chinese medical diagnoses. The Western terms are included for the sole purpose of providing a starting point for the contemplation of a case by a practitioner learning the Complement Channels. Although it can be very tempting to try to link a Western medical diagnosis with a particular channel, the channels indexed with a given Western medical diagnosis should only be used if the tongue and pulses are in alignment with a Chinese medical diagnosis for which that channel is appropriate.

A

Abbreviations, xxi
Abdomen,
> Chong, 234
> distention, 91, 148, 234
> pain, 179, 187, 325
> tight, painful, 183
> heaviness, 325
> itch, 100
> lumps, 206
> muscles, 235
> Rebellious Qi, 261, 262, 267, 272
> post-surgery, 19
> spider veins (Luo vessels), 101

Abortion,
> spontaneous, 247

Abscesses, 311, 371
> Divergents, 149, 204, 206
> Yin depletion, 147

Absentmindedness, 314
Acceptance, 370
Accumulations, 319-20
> abdominal, 302
> compensatory, 256
> cysts, 261, 282
> emotions, 367
> fibroids, 170, 261, 282, 302
> five, 234, 282
> Fluid, 179, 286, 305
> goiter, 170
> hernia, 282
> interests, 306
> Luo Channel, 81
> karma, 100-1
> moving, 239
> obesity, 286
> obsession, 282
> ovaries, 302
> Phlegm, 197
> prostatitis, 282
> possessions, 306
> toxins, 366
> trauma, 235

> tumors, 261, 282
> turbidity, 372
> uterus, 302
> Yin, 260, 306
> Zang organ, 234, 282

Accumulation (Mu) points,
> as shown in drawings, 109, 110
> Divergent theory, 149, 171
> Divergent treatments, 138

Achievement, over-, 267, 289
Acne, 311
Activism, 311
Abnormal growth, 222-3
Addictions,
> Luo, 91
> Eight Extras, 258
> to talking, 258

Addison's Disease, 187, 247
Advanced Acupuncture, xxvii
Adventure, 283
Aging,
> Chong, 234
> Eight Extras, 221
> iatrogenic, 219
> resistance to, 281, 283
> safety, 377

Agricultural practices, 223
Ah shi,
> in ancient practice, 214
> definition, 42
> in Divergents, 138
> finding, 44
> unilateral Bi, 302, 311, 316-7
> Yang Qiao, 309

AIDS, 221
Alcohol,
> in utero environment, 221
> jaundice, 253

Alignment, 40, 309-10, 384
Allergies, 40, 94, 171, 176, 191, 206, 221, 237, 267, 270, 311
> acute, 171, 179
> chronic, 179, 180, 206

food, 183, 234, 237, 257
originating in childhood, 237
stress, 296
tearing, 297
Alopecia, 204
Alternating chills and fever, 171, 291
Alternating hot and cold, 119
Alzheimer's Disease, 220, 247, 282, 371
Amenorrhea, 260
Amnesia, 267
An Qiao, 5
Analgesic, 286, 295-6, 305-6, 326
Ancestral Qi, (Zong-Gathering/Chest Qi), 221, 241, 244, 262
Ancestral sinews, (Five Axes, Five Pillars), 157, 326-8, 369
Ancestry, 222-3, 254, 266, 281, 323
Andropause, 222, 289
Angina, Heart pain, 96, 112-3, 148, 235, 243, 289, 306
chest oppression, 92, 285
disappointment, 281-2
failure to express self, 287
Liver Blood deficiency, 283
Rebellious Qi Lower Jiao, 267, 272
sternum fullness, 241
Anemia, 208
Anger, 50, 119, 120-2, 148, 312, 335
Angiogenesis, 55
Animation, 92, 244, 268, 276
Anuria, 95, 112
Anus, 160, 257, 268, 335
Anxiety, 50, 96, 121-2, 191, 235, 243, 269, 286-7, 316, 332, 335
about disease, 283
about future, 283
about past, 283
in relationship, 255
in society and work, 286
Appetite, 307, 316
loss or poor, 112, 195, 239, 244, 263
Arms,
evolution, 309
inflammation, 62
lifting, 148, 195
rotating, 41
Arrhythmia, 119, 282
Arrogance, 270, 314
Arthritis, 171, 197, 220, 367
and cold packs, 122
hip, 171
origin xxviii
rheumatoid, 197, 367
Asbestos, 50, 132
Ascites, 91, 204, 261, 269
Aspartame, 220
Asthma, 171, 176, 204, 221, 249, 257, 295, 367, 372
Attention Deficit Hyperactivity Disorder (ADHD), 267
Autism, 89, 183
Autobiography, 281, 289
Autoimmune diseases, 20
Autointoxication, 145, 191
Aversion,
change, 369-70
cold, 289, 291, 369
commitment, 267
responsbility, 267
wind, 369
Axes, Five, 326-8
Axilla, 41, 187, 199, 200, 208

B

Baby, 86, 234, 254-6, 260, 263
needling, 377
seizures, 266
Back (Bladder) Transporting (Shu) Points,
Chong, 247
creation, 350
distribution, 358
distance from midline, 160, 164
vs. Hua To points, 160, 164
needling children, 278
order, 243
Triple Heater, 109
Zang organs, 367
Bacteria, xxviii, 50, 53, 132

Belching, 311
Bell's Palsy, 183, 266, 290, 291, 312
Betrayal, 96
Bi-Obstruction, 310, see also *Pain*
    abdominal, 325
    Blood stasis, 247
    cause, 131, 310
    Dai Mai, 325
    discerning between the Qiaos, 317
    Luo, 122
    technique, 6
    throat, xxviii, 373
    unilateral, 302, 309-11, 316-18
    Yang Qiao Mai, 310-11
Bilateral needling, 17, 226
Bile, 119
Binding Nexuses, 42
Birth,
    and Lung activation, 85
    bonding compromised, 85
    canal, 307
    defects, 234
    deficient Qi at, 237
    environment, 255-6
    moment of birth, 254
    Ren activation, 255
    re-humanizing, 256
    separation at, 255
    trauma, 234, 237
    treatment of issues, 221
    Triple Heater mechanism, 120, 265, 321
Bitter taste, 291
Bitterness, 244
Bladder, 191, 247, 305
Bladder Shu Points,
    Chong, 247
    creation, 350
    distribution, 358
    distance from midline, 160, 164
    needling children, 278
    order, 243
    Triple Heater, 109
    vs. Hua To points, 160, 164

    Zang organs, 367
Bleeding,
    from genitals, 175
    gums, 187
    reckless blood, 253
    coughing, hemoptysis, 149, 187, 208
    nose, 95, 187, 311
    ulcers, 187
    uterus, 367
Blemishes, 90
Blindness, loss of vision, 187
    acute, 179
Bloating, 114, 119, 325
Blockage, 157, 375
    brain, 372
    lower orifices, 95, 202, 239
    upper orifices, 247, 291
Blood,
    deficiency, see *Blood Deficiency*
    fat level, 302
    glucose level, 302
    harmonizing, 373
    Heat, 62, 366-7, 370, 372
    ice affecting, 158
    invigorate, 368, 370
    latency, supporting, 146-7
    loss, 150, 199
    Mansion, 126
    at Mu points, 149
    tests for pathogen are negative, 158
    pressure, 373
    pulse status, 171, 175
    red cells, 373
    in sputum, 63
    in stool, 63, 287
    stagnation, see *Blood stagnation*
    stasis, 46, 191, 202, 241, 247, 249, 269, 331-2, 336
    thinners, 126
    toxins, 175
    in urine, 63, 325
    vessels, 26, 52, 54, 57, 220-1, 227
    volume, 175, 302
    in vomit, 11, 63, 315

white cells, 373
and Wind, 164
Blood deficiency, 239
    after treatment, 126, 378
    constitutional, 323
    in Divergents, 146
    face, head, eyes, 191
    headaches, 283
    Liver tightness, 247
    Luo treatments, 126
    menstruation, 283
    pain, 247
    with phlegm, 306
    Shen disturbance, 283, 370
    visceral dryness, 283
    Zang, 283
Blood Mansion, 126
Blood Stagnation, 171, 373
    acute, 171
    Bao Mai symptom, 332
    Chong 2nd trajectory symptom, 241, 243
    Chong 3rd trajectory symptom, 247
    Chong 5th trajectory symptom, 253
    as Luo pathology, 55
    with Qi Stagnation, 123
    in Sinews, 122
    Yin Qiao Mai symptom, 300
Blood thinners, 126
Blood toxins, 175
Blueprint of Life, 101, 117, 218-9, 233
Bond, bonding, 85-6, 88, 254-5, 257-8, 268
Bone,
    fracture, 40, 247
    broken, 40
    Marrow, 102, 194-5, 221, 227, 251, 269-70, 290, 292, 297, 311, 373
Borborygmus, 234-5, 253, 325
Boundaries,
    Bladder Luo, 94
    Chong, 234
    failure, 268
Bowel issues,
    chronic, 112
    constipation, 63, 95, 139, 148, 183, 191, 239, 256-7, 286-7, 295-6, 305, 314
    diarrhea, 22, 63, 84, 112-3, 119, 148, 160, 183, 187, 191, 204, 234-5, 237, 253, 256, 261, 269, 287, 295, 304-5, 314, 325-6, 370
    frequent, 119
    irritable, 187, 247
    tiredness, 204
Bowel movements, 119, 204, 366
Brain,
    access, 370
    blockage, 371
    dehydration, 187, 296
    Du, 274
    Eight extra connection, 227
    evolution, 220
    experience, 297, 307
    fog, 291
    function, 180
    Gallbladder Divergent, 174
    Gallbladder Primary, 291
    Heat, 297
    Primary Channels, 346, 350
    tumor, 302
    wasting, 195
    Wei Qi, 186-7
    Wind, 269-70, 297
    Yin Wei Mai, 285
    Yang Wei Mai, 289
Breastfeeding, 85-6, 254-5
Breathing, 85, 254
    at birth, 255
    difficult, 148, 191, 243
    hormones, 311
    irregular, 103
    labored, 148
    Luo treatment, 81
    needling, 9
    rapid, 149, 208
    Ren, 254, 260
    resuscitation, 294
    shortness, 195, 204, 304, 373
    when looking upward, 148

when lying down, 148, 191
Yin Wei Mai, 288
Bright lights, 256
Bright Yang, see *Yang Ming*
Brittle bones, 311
Bruises, 52, 381
Buffalo hump, 257
Bulimia, 258
Burns, 40
    moxa, 82, 377
        Luo treatment sensation, 83
Bunions, 40
Buttocks, 368

C

Calm, 295
    affirmations, 240, 254, 279, 288, 299, 318
    birth, 255
    digestion, 261
    practitioner, 225
    Shen, 261-2, 268-70, 288, 295, 297, 304, 335, 369-70, 372
        Lung distress, 262
Cancer, 195, 197, 220-3
Capillaries, 57, 81, 191
Carcinogens, 220
Career, 283, 289
Cardiac,
    failure, 208, 294
    reflux, 119, 187
Cardiovascular issues, 191, 258, 278
Carpal Tunnel Syndrome, 149, 200
Case studies, 47, 131
Cataracts, 179, 297, 327
Catatonic, 99, 287
Celiac disease, gluten intolerance, 237, 253, 257, 320
Cellulitis, 208
Central Axis, 233
Cerebral spinal fluid, 191
Channel of Bonding, 254
Channel System, 23
Chest,
    Heat, 373

oppression 63, 92, 112, 149, 199, 200, 208, 241, 257, 371, 373
Childhood, 20, 221, 237, 255, 258, 332
Children, 85, 223
    diarrhea, 269
    needling safety, 278, 377
    nine heart pains, 283
    Wind, 279
Chills, 289, 295, 373
    and fever, 171, 174, 195, 208, 291
Chiseling, 2, 10, 11, 42, 47
Cholecystitis, 109
Chromosomal abnormalities, 234

Chronic Degenerative Diseases, xxvii, 130
Chronic Fatigue Syndrome, 102, 302, 312
Circulatory issues, 113
Classic of Difficulties, the Nan Jing, xxxiii, 8, 51, 60, 117, 125, 218, 232, 268, 335
Classical Chinese Medicine, xxvii, 379
Clear Heat, 270, 295, 297
    chest, 62
    face, 270
    Heart, 269, 285, 287, 303
    Kidneys, 304
    throat, 62, 269, 297
    through urine, 303
Climatic factors, 50, 122
Club fingers and toes, 257
Clots, 237, 332, 371
Cold,
    aversion to, 289, 291
    Blood, 241
    common cold, xxviii, 114, 143
    Damp-, 230, 261, 302, 327-330
    Du Mai symptom, 266
    during eight extra treatment, 232
    feet, 99
    food and drinks, 157
    hands, 113
    limbs, 99
    in Liver, 260, 368
    moxa on Ren, 264

packs, 27, 45, 122
Ren Mai symptom, 257, 262, 268
treatment warning, 219
scatter, 232, 265, 367
sores, 180
Wind-Cold, xxviii, 2, 45, 62, 64, 208, 237
Yin Qiao Mai symptom, 302
Colic, 257
Colitis, 109, 179, 235, 253, 369
Collapse,
Yang, 202, 208, 211, 294
Collecting Points, see *Mu Points*
Coma, 314
Commitment, 258, 267, 292
Complement Channels, xxviff, xxxv
ease of use, 20
map, 23
Complete Reality School, 387
Complexion, 62, 310-1
Conception, 101, 117, 220, 22
Conditional love, 234
Cones, 227, 264, 381
Confidence, 234
Confluent Points, 136, 366
Confusion, 199, 295, 321, 326
Conjunctivitis, 183
Congenital defects, 221
Congestive Heart failure, 103
Consciousness,
group, 258
loss, 291, 297
mobilization, 299
open, 270, 332
resuscitation, 270, 296
separation of pure and impure, 307, 316
stimulation, 261
Consolidate,
Blood, 146, 332
Chong, 323
Dai Mai, 327
Jing-Essence, 160, 166
Yin, 195, 265
Yang, 290, 292

Constipation, 63, 95, 148, 183
life-long, 257
post-delivery, 256
Constitution, 4, 22, 24, 305
changes, 197, 200
conduits, 219
damage, 234, 287
deficiency, 323
emotions, 111, 120-2, 319
leakage, 323
Luos, 87, 232, 331-2, 335
pathology, 52, 117, 278, 332
Divergent predisposition, 114
warning, 219
Consumption,
Marrow, 292
Wei Qi, 311
Convulsions, 11, 208, 221, 311-2, 314-5, 372
Cough, xxix, 22, 62, 112, 148-9, 171, 243, 261, 269, 306, 311, 335, 372-4
blood, 63, 315
dry, 208
when expressing self, 372
healing event, 84
stress-related, 297, 372
Courage, 98
Course,
Qi, 374
Wind, 367-9, 373-4
Cramp,
elbow, 98
jaw, 183
Creativity, 99, 283, 297
Criticism, 93-4
Crohn's Disease, 204, 247
Crossing point, 156
Crown, 372
Cultural Revolution, xxv
Cup,
chronic Bi, 309, 317-8
cutaneous regions, 214-5
Damp-Heat, 298
emotional stagnation, 315, 317

394

releasing the Five Axes, 328
seizures, 296
Sinews, 155
sliding, 44, 46
steaming bone syndrome, 269
Divergent, 161, 167, 174, 178, 182, 184, 190, 194, 198, 203, 207
Zonal Divergent, 213-4
Dai Mai, 328-329, 336

Curiosity, 265-6, 268
Curious Organs, 321
Curriculum, 233, 268, 371
Cutaneous regions, 24, 133, 138, 155, 157, 214-6
Cutting and slashing, 102
Cycle of seven and eight, 120, 220-3, 233, 235, 263, 278, 281, 323
Cynicism, 283
Cystitis, 109, 166, 179, 367, 369
Cysts, 302, 320
- Luos, 55-7, 107, 128
- Divergents, 148
- ovarian, 166, 176, 257, 261, 282, 304
- shoulder, 204

D

Damp,
- accumulations, 286-7, 299, 300, 307-8, 320-1, 323-30
- cause of disease, xxviii
- chest oppression, 257
- constant, 257
- Dai Mai, 319
- Damp-Cold, 261, 302, 327-30
- Damp-Heat, 298, 326
    - blockages, 239
    - chronic, 197, 269, 335
    - clearing, 368
    - eyes, 297
    - Fu-Bowels, 366
    - gut, 253
    - head, 314
    - joints, 197, 367
    - Lungs, 296
    - Luos, 62
    - Lower Jiao, 166, 247, 260-1, 268, 304, 320, 327-30
    - rising, 291
    - Wei atrophy, 197
- disinhibit, 305, 367-8, 370-3
- Divergents, 132, 191, 195, 197
- Du Mai, 268
- Luos, 50, 54, 56, 62
- Ren, 261-2, 264, 268-9
- resolve, 239, 298, 304-5, 307-8, 367
- Shao Yang, 291
- Sinews, 26, 27, 40, 43-5
- Spleen, 239
- treatment, 278
- Wind-Damp, 62-63, 296
- Yang Qiao, 314, 316
- Yang Wei, 295
- excess Yin, 258
- Yin Qiao, 302, 304-5

Daoism, xxx, xxxi, 218
Daydreaming, 100
Deafness, 112
- long-term, 149
- sudden, acute, 89

Death, 84
- accepting, 292
- wish (Death-Wind), 95, 302
- of important people, 258, 289

De Qi, 4
Defecation, bowel movement,
- difficulty, 267, 272, 304-5
- healing crises, 84
- pain, 237

Decision-making, 93, 98, 258, 291, 295
Decline of Jing, 22, 149, 160, 194, 221
Defensive Qi, see *Wei Qi*
Deficiency,
- Blood 191, 371
- in divergent theory, 132, 145
- in Luo treatments, 114, 124, 126
- Fluids, 183, 371
- Jing, 371

Qi, 199
Underlying, 98
Wei, 27, 40-41, 53, 122
Yin, 187, 195
Dehydration, 239, 257
Deja vu, 290
Delirium, 149, 197, 269, 311, 372
Delivery, 256, 296
Dementia, 247, 370
Depression, 95, 102, 112-3, 243, 269, 297, 302-3, 307
    and Mania, 199
    and fatigue, 237
    and fear, 282
    with judgment, 312
    post-partum, 256
    severe, 99, 102
    with stagnant Yang, 292
Dermatological conditions, 155, 213, 221, 267, 315
    contact dermatitis, 311
Despair, 98
Destiny, 218-19, 221, 233-4, 256, 286
Detoxification, 286
Development, 220
    curiosity, 265
    emotional, 85, 96
    reflexes, 265
    society, 286
    trust, 303
Deviated septum, 296
Diabetes, 188, 377
Diagnosis, 14
Dian-kuang, 262, 335
Diaper rash, 90, 257
Diaphragm,
    constriction, 112
    distention, fullness, 63, 148
    Five Axes, 326, 328, 369
    Master point, 269, 335
    numbness, 89
    release, 328
    Shu, 247
    Zong Qi, 241
Diarrhea, 63, 112-3, 119, 148, 183, 187, 191, 234, 253, 256, 261, 269, 287, 305, 314, 325
    chronic, 295
    cockcrow, 204, 235, 237
    explosive, 326
    frequent, hot, 160, 304
    healing event, 84
    pathogenic encounter, 22
Diet, 50, 53-4, 132, 159
Digestion, 63, 183, 239, 261, 316, 367, 372
Dignity, 93
Disappointment, 255, 281-3, 289, 292, 302
Disc herniations, 247
Discouragement, 97
Disease Nemesis Theory, xxvii, xxx, 130
Disease Progression, xxvii, 14, 52, 55-6, 85, 88, 114, 133, 144, 194
Disinhibit, 305
Disinterest
    in food, 306
    in learning, 272
    in life, 88, 99
Disorientation, 291
Disperse
    Lung Qi, 43, 47
    needling technique, 8, 9, 11, 264
    Wei Qi, 41
Distention,
    abdomen, 10, 91, 148, 234, 261, 286
    chest, 62, 206
    diaphragm, 63
    epigastric, 112, 114
Distinct, xxxv, 130-1
Disturbed,
    Shen, 62, 197, 199, 262, 266, 278
    sleep, 148, 191
Diuresis, 370
Divorce, 289
Dizziness, 119, 148, 166, 171, 291, 311, 314, 367
    on exertion, 191
    Luo treatments, 126
    standing, 269
    visual, 282, 291, 296
DNA, 218, 220-1

Doorways to the Earth, 197, 200, 202
Down's Syndrome, 256-7, 278
Dragon Gate Sect, 387
Dreams, 84, 92, 292
    Daydreaming, 100
Drinking, 180
Drowning, 260
Dwarfism, 249
Dry, 257
    Blood, 183
    cough 208
    Damp, 262, 264
    eyes, 187
    heaving, 10
    lips, 112, 197
    mouth, 148, 197
    stools, 148
    throat, 112, 187, 200, 267, 272
    visceral, 283
Ducts, clogged, 296
Dying process, 221, 243
Dysentery, 204, 268, 287, 335
Dyslexia, 92
Dysmenorrhea, 175, 287, 325, 327, 331-2
Dysrhythmias, 191
Dyspnea, 62, 149, 204, 234, 304

E

Ear,
    ache, 174, 195
    infections, 291
    issues, 112, 171, 179, 291
    lesions, 180
    open, 62
    pressure, 204
    ringing, 296
Earth, 236, 244, 262, 306, 315
Eating disorders, 239, 302
Ecological factors, 50, 132
Eczema, 176, 180
Edema, 179, 239, 302, 320, 325, 367
    facial, 208

Elbow
    atrophy, 93
    dislocation, 98
    stiff, 98
Elderly, 126, 222
Electromagnetic fields, 223
Elimination,
    bowel movements, 139, 261, 286, 304, 325, 367
    route of, 139
Emotions
    anger, 50, 119-122, 148, 312
        hair-trigger anger, 122
    anxiety, 50, 96, 121-122, 191, 235, 255, 283, 332
    as a cause of disease, 111
    Dai Mai, 335
    fear, 50, 121-122, 294, 335
        of commitment, 258
        extreme, 95
        with back pain, 282
        being left alone, 95, 268
        of future, 281, 292
        paralyzing, 292
        of sex, 176
        swayback, 291
    frustration 86, 98
    grief, 120
        early weaning, 257
    sadness, 86, 121
    worry or pensiveness, 50
    obsessive thinking, 50, 91, 93, 120, 335
    obsessive compulsive, 95
Empathy, 96-7
Emphysema, 297, 302
Encephalitis, 191, 221, 291, 297, 367
End stage disease, 150, 204, 208, 292
Endocrine, 132, 150, 186, 188
Endometriosis, 175, 239, 247, 257, 320, 331
Endurance, 368
Energy transfer, 114, 118
Enteritis, 109
Enthusiasm, 268, 276, 283, 319
Entitic Invasion, 11

Epigastric,
    distention, 112, 114
    pain, 305, 311
Epilepsy, 63, 208, 221, 266, 268-9, 274, 291, 296, 297, 372
    daytime (Yang-type), 311
    nighttime (Yin-type), 302
Epistaxis, 62, 179
Esophagus,
    issues, 257
    pain, 179, 183
    reflux, 187, 235, 253, 311
Epsom salt, 45-46, 375-6
Escaping Yang, 208
Essence, Jing-Essence, 63, 132, 135, 140-2, 146-7, 149
    Blood supporting, 369
    pathology, 369
Estrogen, 307, 316
Ethics, 92, 218
Ethnicity, 220, 222, 258, 263
Evolution, 220-1
    channel, 289
    human, 309
    self, xxvii, 385
Exertion, 191
Exocrine, 132, 149, 179, 326
Exterior, 22, 43, 46, 52-3, 94, 108, 121, 127, 135, 143, 145, 149, 155, 160, 219, 268, 285, 289, 291, 305, 378
External Pathogenic Factor, 22, 26, 53, 200, 296, 311, 366-7
Extroversion, 312
Eye,
    Blood deficiency, 191
    brightens, 369
    cataracts, 179, 297, 327
    Damp-Heat, 297
    degeneration, 179
    difficulty opening, 300, 302
    discharge, 112
    dry, 187
    fluids, 63
    glaucoma, 112, 179, 297, 327
    glowing, 221, 303, 308
    heaviness, 300, 302
    inability to close, 62
    issues, 171, 179, 297
    itchy, 262, 296-7, 315
    lost sparkle, 113
    mother contact, 254
    opens, 270
    pain, 370
    pressure, 297
    red, 179, 262, 274, 297, 306, 315, 327
    self-mutilation, 102
    Sinews, 26
    sphincter issues, 257
    stye, 180
    swollen, 179, 262, 266, 274, 297, 315
    tearing eyes, 112, 262, 297, 306, 315
    tension, 314, 370
    tics, 183
    visual distortion, 262
    watery, 112, 306, 327
    yellowing, 112-3

F

Face, 42
    bleeding, 270
    Blood deficiency, 191, 241, 244
    capillaries, 191
    Cold, 311
    Du Mai, 268
    Heat, red, 270
    hypersensitive, 191
    moisture, 179
    needling, 377
    neuropathy, 311
    pale, 241
    post-treatment, 378
    swelling, 270
    Wind, 183, 262, 270
Fainting, 6, 113, 126, 294
    sudden, 282, 291
Fatal, 108, 131
Fatigue, 102, 112, 237, 239, 302, 312
Fatty deposits, 234, 257, 282
Fear, see *Emotions*

Feeble-mindedness, 267
Fei Yang, 282
Feelings, see *Emotions*
Fetishes, 94
Fermentation, 191, 253
Fetus, 221
    expel, 304
Fever,
    case example, 114
    with chills, 171, 174, 195, 208, 291, 295
    to expel pathogen, xxviii
    high, 112, 266, 289, 291, 314
    intermittent, 291
    long, unrelenting, 306, 315
    low grade, 291
    Luos, 53, 62
    needling technique, 9
    Sinews, 26
    with sweat, 112
    with Wind, 269, 311
Fibrillations, 103, 282
Fibrocystic breasts, 243
Fibroids, 148, 166, 176, 237, 247, 257, 261, 282, 302, 304, 320, 331-2
Fibromyalgia, 102, 197
Fire,
    drain, 303, 371
    Heart, 187, 261
    Kidney, 304
    Liver, 291
    regulation, 222
    Stomach, 118, 261-2, 267, 270, 320
    technique, 5, 9
    -toxins, 55, 195, 294
Finances, 283
Five accumulations, 234, 282
Five Axes, Five Pillars, 157, 326-8, 369
Flaccid, 26, 42, 44, 98, 310-1, 317
Flatliner, 294
Flatulence, gas, 114, 119, 305
Floaters, 262, 315
Fluids,
    Divergent choice, 145
    mobilization for latency, 143, 146-150
    Thin Fluids, 132, 141, 142, 145-7, 149, 183
        assimilation, 180
        Chong, 241
        depletion, 142, 146, 159, 180
        Divergent choices, 145
        hydration, 180
        pathology, 367
        pulse status, 179
        Pure Yang of the Stomach, 241
        Stomach and Spleen Divergent Channels, 179
        supporting Jing-Essence, 141
        Thick Fluid supporting, 186
        as transporter of pathology, 141
    Thick Fluids, 186
        choosing confluence, 145
        depletion, 142, 146, 159, 190
            spectrum of depletion, 190
        and latency, 142, 147, 150, 186
        Loss, 150
        and loss of latency, 191
        Divergent theory, 132
        Heart and Small Intestine Divergent Channels, 186
        mobilization, 150
        pulse, 186
        signs, 147
        supporting Jing-Essence, 142
    regulation, 368
    separation, 372
    sequence, 143
Foggy headedness, 372
Fright-Wind, 295, 297
Frigidity, 261, 266
Front (Kidney) Transporting (Shu) Points, 138
    distance from midline, 160
    stagnation, 170
    organ relationship, 170
    locating, 232
    and the Great Luo Channels, 241
    reverse order of, 243

Food,
- allergies, 183, 234, 257, 263
- dairy, 320
- digestion, 251, 266, 315-6, 320
- disinterest, 306
- early weaning, 89, 257
- fried, 119
- genetically modified, 320
- gluten, 320
- ice cream, 157
- microwaved, 320
- poisoning, 54, 253
- raw, 45, 157
- salad, 157
- Sea of Food and Drinks, 179, 251, 253
- sensitivity, 263
- smoothies, 157
- stasis, 183, 187, 235, 239, 253, 256, 260, 305
- sticky, 320
- sugar, 320
- undigested, 113, 237, 261, 287
- Wei Qi, 26

Four Great Signs of Yang Ming, 112

Fright, 50, 63, 95, 285, 292
- Fright-Wind (insanity), 295, 297
- stagefright, 90

Frustration, 86, 98

Fu Qi, Latent Qi, Hidden Qi, xxx

Fu-Bowels, 237, 261, 366, see also *Zang Fu*

Fu Mai, Hidden Pulses, 144

Function,
- Complement Channels, 22
- Confluent points, 136
- crossing point, 156
- coupled pairs, 225
- Divergent Channels, 131
- Divergent trajectory points, 137
- Eight Extraordinary Channels, 219
- Hua To, 164
- Jing-Wells in Divergents, 155
- Luo Channels, 50
- Opening points in Eight Extra, 223
- Primary Channels, 85-99, 133
- Sinew Channels, 26

Fungus, 132

Future, 220, 255, 281-2, 285, 287, 290, 292, 295, 297, 300, 310, 314, 317

G

Gait, 117, 220, 267, 295
- loss of, 367

GB-22 location, 59-61, 64, 83, 102-3, 125-6, 331-2, 335

Gallstones, 296

Gas, 114, 119, 305

Gastritis, 109, 131, 179, 187, 197, 311, 376

Gastroesophageal Reflux Disease (GERD), 179, 191, 311, 369

Gender, 314
- gender-specific channels, 289
- identity, 220, 222, 233, 236, 258, 263
- Luo point sides, 60, 128
- Eight Extra sides, 224, 227, 264, 279
- pulses, 263

Genetic, 218, 219, 233
- diseases, 221

Genetically modified organisms, 320

Genital,
- bleeding, 175
- blockages, 202
- dysfunction, 257
- herpes, 175
- issues, 247, 278, 323
- itch, 100, 175, 237, 260, 304
- pain, 96, 148, 175, 237, 302, 303
- sweaty, 260
- swellings, 100, 175, 260, 304

Genitalia, 61

Gestation time, 235

Gesture, 268, 310

Ghost,
- point, 270
- hungry, sexual, wandering, 296, 369

Glaucoma, 112, 179, 297, 314, 327

Glomus Qi, 282

Gluten sensitivities, 257, 320

Gluteus, 157-8, 276, 326, 328

Goiter, 63, 136, 166, 170, 206, 208, 262, 302, 306, 315, 369, 371, 373
Gold, 11
Graves' Disease, 367
Great Luo of Shao Yin, 234, 241
Great Luos, 241
Growth,
    issues, 220-3, 249
    pathological, 220-3
Grudges, 286
Gu Qi, 26, 262, 305
    disruption, 367
Gua sha
    Axes, 327-9
    cutaneous regions, 133, 138, 153, 155, 157, 214
    in Luo treatments, 62, 81-3
    Windows to the Sky, 200
    Zonal Divergent, 213, 215
Guilt, 97, 262, 272, 283, 304, 370, 372
Gums,
    bleeding, 187, 270
    receding, 187
Gynecology, 305

H

Habituation, 91, 235, 258, 269, 319, 368
Hair,
    failure to grow, 204
    loss, 204
Halitosis, 62
Hallucinations, 314
Hand,
    arthritis, 295, 315
    Cold, 113
    hot, 200
    issues, 295, 314
    pain, 292
    shaking, 327
    tight, 295, 315
Harmonize,
    Blood, 83, 369
    the Center, 305
    Stomach and Spleen, 63, 239, 305
Hashimoto's Disease 187, 367

Head,
    bleeding, 270
    Blood deficiency, 191
    clear, 367
    Damp-Heat, 314
    difficulty lifting, 148, 195
    heaviness, 101, 171, 268, 314, 335
    numbness, 197
    pain, 97
    rigidity, 97
    shaking, 101, 296
    swelling, 63-4, 270
    Wei Qi, 291
    Wind, 262, 266, 270, 274, 291, 315
    Yin and Yang moving, 202
Headache, 94, 119, 311, 327
    chronic, 367
    menstrual, 283
    occipital, 112, 160
    temporal, 291
    throbbing, 191
    with veins showing, 191
Healing crisis/event, 375
    Divergents, 143, 155, 157
    Luos, 84
    Sinews, 46
Hearing,
    decreased, 187
    voices, 99
Heart,
    accumulation, 234, 282
    angina, 285
    attack, 125
    beat, 59, 64, 103, 241, 254, 287, 307, 316
    Blood stasis, 241
    break, 92
    congestive failure, 103
    defects, 221
    deficient Qi, 118
    failure, 208
    feelings in, 89
    fire, 187, 261, 269, 303, 320
    issues, 171

-Kidney communication, 170, 233-5, 241, 244, 331-2, 371
Nine Heart Pains, 283
pain, angina, 96, 112-3, 148, 235, 243, 289, 306
    chest oppression, 92, 285
    disappointment, 281-2
    failure to express self, 287
    Liver Blood deficiency, 283
    rebellious Qi Lower Jiao, 267, 272
    sternum fullness, 241
pathology, 55
Phlegm, 306
pressure, 243
rate, 311
Shen, 233
sovereign ruler, 233
trauma, 303
valves, 244, 257

Heart-Kidney communication, 170, 233-5, 241, 244, 331-2, 371
Heavy metals, 50, 132, 220, 320
Hematoma, 123, 125
Hemiplegia, 266, 325
Hemoptysis, 187, 208
Hemorrhage, 200, 239
Hemorrhoids, 112, 183, 235, 253, 256, 267-9, 272, 276, 327, 335
Hepatitis, 109, 111, 197, 253
Hernia, 176, 276, 282, 302, 325
    hiatal, 183
    inguinal, 370
    disc, 247
Herpes, 291
    genital, 100, 175
He-Sea points, 22, 54, 133, 138, 150, 188, 227
    lower, 206
Hidden beam, 234-5, 241, 243, 282
Hidden Qi, Fu Qi, Latent Qi, xxx
Hip,
    arthritis, 171
    latency, 131, 135, 159
    locating point, 15
    needling, 175
    open, 314
    pain, 295, 311
        on flexion, 148, 171
        on Rotation, 41
    Sinew bindings, 42
HIV, 221
Hives, 204, 297
Home, 274, 283, 286, 296, 314
Homeostasis, 306, 315, 373
Hopelessness, 98
Hormones, 307, 311, 316
    in agriculture, 223
    issues, 191, 302
    overactive, 302
    regulation of endocrine fluids, 186, 369-70
Hospice, 292
HPV, 175
Hua Shan, xxv
Hua To Jia Ji points, 47, 108, 148, 160, 164, 274, 276
Humanity, xxvii, 23, 220
Hunger, 62, 306, 315
Hydration, 262
    before treatment, 153
    dehydration, xxviii, 239, 257
Hyperactivity, 266-7
    immune system, 158
    muscles, 312
    Yang, 311
Hyperadrenalism, 311
Hyperlipidemia, 302
Hypertension, 160, 166, 176, 291, 367
Hyperthyroidism, 306, 311, 314
Hypothyroidism, 166, 180, 188
Hysteria, 90, 314

I

Iatrogenic events, 219
Incarnation, ii, 101, 117, 331
Ice, 27, 45, 47, 122, 158
Ice cream, 157
Identity, 220, 222, 233, 236, 258, 261, 285, 287, 299, 303-4, 306
Idolatry, 312

Iliopsoas, 158
Impotence, 166, 221, 266, 325, 367
Immune syetem, 158
Incontinence, 112, 237, 247, 267, 272
Indecisiveness, 296
Independence, 258, 265-8, 274
Individuality, 265
Infections, 200
    acute, 142-4
    difficult to treat, 197
    ear, 291
    fungal, 93
    opportunistic, 200
    organ, 109, 127, 144
    respiratory tract, 171, 179, 208
    sinus, 132
    urinary tract, 164, 303
    viral, 131
    yeast, 247
Infertility, fertility,
    Blood stasis, 269
    Blood deficiency, 175
    Chong, 233
    Eight Extras, 220-1
    emotional, 325
    fear, 176
    low motility, 266
    principal/major points, 261, 305
    stagnation, 319
    Wei Qi overactive, 175
    Yang, 266, 272
Inflammation, 109
    arms, 62
    chronic, 112
    joint, 158
    organ, 109, 127, 197
    pelvic, 175, 326
    reduction, 367
    shoulder, 62
    Wei Qi trapped, 147
Influential points, 138, 227
    Blood, 247
    bone, 248, 269

bowels, 261
lower, limbs, 368
Qi, 262
Zang, 321
Ingenuity, 97
Inhibition, 281, 321
Injury,
    acute, 40
    chronic, 40
    determining Sinew affected, 40
    and Divergent loop, 154
    emotional origin, 123
    frequency of treatment, 45
    theory of healing, 27
    post-traumatic stress disorder injury, 292
    wei accumulation, 27
    unexplained, 122
Inner strength, 371
Innocence, 368
Insanity, 90, 297
Insomnia, 191, 199, 303, 311
Intelligence, 93, 96
Intention, xxvi, 225
    Divergent 134, 137, 151
    Divergent needling, xxxi
    Eight Extra, 227
    focussing, xxxviii
    needling, 3, 4
    transverse Luo, 113
    Zonal Divergent, 215
Intercostal pain, 295
Interior,
    emotions affecting, 50
    Heat clearing, 109
    Transverse luos, 111-2, 118
    warming, 260, 263-4
    warming technique, 9
    balancing with exterior, 289, 291
    Sinew failure, 53
    Yuan-Source failure, 114
    returning Wei to Yang, 134
Internal Pathogenic Factor, 53-4, 123
Introspection, retrospection, 303, 368

Introversion, 98-9, 113
Intuition, 97
Irritability, 112, 114, 148, 197, 199, 244, 287, 311, 373
Irritable bowel, 187, 247
Isolation, 98
Itch, 204
    abdominal, 100
    eyes, 262, 296-7, 315
    fungal, 93
    genital, 100, 175, 237, 260, 304
    nasal, 315
    palms, 88
In utero, 223, 234, 255
Invigorate,
    Blood, 232, 244, 247
    collaterals, 305
    Kidney Yang, 244, 247, 304

J

Jade Purity, xxv, xxxi, 387
Jaundice, 269, 291, 296
    the Five, 253
    limbic, 253
Jaw and TMD (TMD disorder), 11, 62, 166, 171, 183
Jet-lag, 287
Jia and Ju (accumulations and concentrations), 282
Jie-Clumping, 371
Jin-Thin Fluids, see *Fluids*
Jin-Ye (pure and turbid fluids),
    separation, 372
Jing-Essence,
    Blood supporting, 147
    depleted, 132, 146, 149
    distribution, 232
    latency, 132, 140-2, 220
    link to humors, 241
    securing, 368
Joint,
    achy, 112
    atrophy, 93
    cold, xxviii
    disinhibit, 373
    dislocation, 44, 93
    latency, xxix, 118, 131-2
    looseness, 102
    Luo's bypassing, 51
    misalignment, 40
    pain, (Bi), 247, 369
    pathology, 368
    swelling, 367
Judgment, 90, 93, 285, 306, 315
Juices, 157

K

Karma, 100-1
Kidney, 64, 140, 249, 285, 304, 321
    ancient sages, 218
    containing self, 94
    curriculum, 233
    -Heart and Heart-Kidney communication, 170, 233-5, 241, 244, 274, 331-2, 371
    left, 232
    moving Qi of, 321
    pain, 96
    right, 232
Kidney Prime, 249
    needling, 251
Kidney Shu points, 138
    distance from midline, 160
    stagnation, 170
    organ relationship, 170
    locating, 232
    and the Great Luo Channels, 241
    reverse order of, 243
Knocked-knee, 302

L

Lactation, 86, 262, 289, 307, 316, 370, 372
Lament, 286
Lancing, 2, 10, 12, 17, 58, 124
Landmarks, 231, 309, 310
Laryngitis, 171
Larynx, 221, 304
Lassitude, 302, 312
Latency, 22-3, 54-6, 131-5, 145, 147

achieved, xxix, xxxv, 55, 109, 149
failure, xxix, 52, 56, 86, 114, 138, 146, 150, 155, 371
pulses, 145
regions, 158
shifting, 116, 131-2, 134-5, 142-3, 153-4
Latent Qi, Hidden Qi, Fu Qi, xxx
Laughter, 149
Leaking, Leakage, 138
Blood, 323, 325, 331
Fluids, 323
Jing-Essence, 323
gut, 234, 239, 247
lower orifices, 64, 247, 326
prevention, 265
of Qi, 295
Leaky gut, 234, 239, 247
Lethargy, 90, 113, 236, 244, 295, 302, 312
Leukemia, 208
Leukorrhea, 237, 247, 302, 325-7, 367
Li Shi Zhen, 17, 219, 226, 268, 294, 304, 312
Libido, 266
Lifestyle choices, xxix, 50, 53, 131, 159, 321
Life-threatening illness, xxvii, xxxvi, 23, 221, 373
Limbs,
atrophy, 197
cold, 113
Damp-Heat, 197
difficulty lifting, 148, 195
frozen, 99
jaundice, 253
numbness, 113, 266, 274, 327
paralysis, 197
stiff, 276
spasm, 276
weakness, 276
wei qi trapped in, 191
Wind-phlegm, 183
Lin Bi, 367
Liniments, 45
Lineage, xxv, xxvi, xxx, xxxi, 14
Lips, 112, 197, 270
Listlessness, 90, 302, 312
Liver,

Blood, 175, 247, 251
Blood stasis, 241
pulse, 126, 145, 171
regulation, 239
swollen, 171
tight, 247
Wei Qi, 26, 41, 121
Liver Qi stagnation,
due to cold, 247
due to Blood deficiency, 247
Lockjaw, 62
Loneliness, 99
Longevity, 218, 260
Longing, 283
Loss of
animation, 244
appetite, 112, 195, 244
appetite control, 263
Blood, 150, 199
certainty, 98
consciousness, 291, 297
elbow tonus, 98
Fluids, 199
ability to love, 286
Interest in life, 86, 88
latency, 150, 191, 194
loved one, 258, 295
motivation, 99
movement, 41
sensitivity, 27, 270
speech, 92, 191
Thick fluids, 150, 191
vision, 187
voice, 62, 90, 262, 266-7, 270, 303, 314
Yang, 249
Loving touch, 234
Lumbago, 256
Lumps, 147, 206
abdominal, 204, 206
breast, 204, 206, 243, 302, 370, 372
Lung,
accumulation, 234, 282
birth, 255-6

Blood, 125
Damp-Heat, 296
descension, 306
diffusion, 243, 296, 306
disperse, 41, 43, 47
Heat, 204, 269
infection, 143
pulse, 41
Qi deficiency, 269
rebellious Qi, xxix, 261-2
Qi stagnation, 125
Wei Qi, 26, 121
Lupus, 180
Lymph node, 187, 208

M

Madness, 62, 90, 208
Malabsorption, 191, 234, 291
Malar flush, ruddy, 62, 187, 191, 197, 199, 311
Malaria, 266, 315
Mania, 199, 262, 269, 297, 314-5, 335, 370, 372
Mania and withdrawal, Dian-Kuang, 262, 335
Marriage, 289
Marrow,
    breaking down, 102, 194-5, 292, 311
    Eight Extra use, 221, 227, 251
    Gallbladder, 290
    inherited, 221
    relieving, 373
    Sea of, 270
    Wind, 269, 297
Martyrdom, 102
Masses, lumps, 147, 206
    abdominal, 204, 206
    breast, 204, 206, 243, 302, 370
Maternal death, 221
Maternal matrix, 85, 265
Maturity, 220-1
Melatonin, 307, 316
Membrane, 109, 127, 239, 305
Memory,
    loss, 295-6, 314
    poor, 187, 247, 270, 282

PTSD, 292
    somatized, 298
    storage, 247
Meeting Points, 136
Meningitis, 221, 291, 297, 367
Menopause, 222, 289
Menses, menstruation, periods,
    clots, 237, 332
    discharge between, 325
    irregular, 179, 287, 328
    long, 235
    painful, 327, 332
    regulate, 64, 368-9
Mental function, 247, 314
Mental retardation, 256
Metabolism, 306-7, 311, 315
Microwave, 320
Migraine, 174, 291, 311, 327-8
    one-sided, 291
    stress, 295
Mind, ii,
    absentmindedness, 295, 314
    changes, 280, 297, 369
    clear, 270, 295
    control, 102
    feeble, 267
    mindset, 310
    rational, 90
    unconscious, 303
Ming-Destiny, 218
Miscarriage, 221, 247, 296
Mitral valve prolapse, 257, 282
    valve regurgitation, 187
Moisture, 179
Mold, xxviii
Mood, 58, 120, 176
Morals, 92, 272, 371
Motility, sperm, 266
Motivation, 99, 268, 276, 283, 287, 296
Mouth,
    addiction, 258
    baby's, 254-5
    bitter taste, 291

deviation, 262, 315
dry, 112, 148, 187, 197, 200
inability to close, 62
issues, 179
pain, 183
sphincter issues, 257
swellings, 270
Movement,
impairment, 26
assessment, 40-1, 123
Moxa, moxibustion,
Confluent points, 139
Eight Extra treatments, 227, 249, 299, 304
Ren, 264
forbidden points, 262, 269, 270, 278, 305, 378
indication, 123
Jing-Well, 123
GV-1, 102
Luo treatments, 58, 81-3
Luo, transverse, 113-4
origin, 2
quality, 380
safety, 377
Sinew treatments, 27, 44, 46-8
supplies, 381
Yang collapse, 211
Mu Points,
in Divergents, 138
organ representatives, 109, 110
pathogen, 149, 171
sides, 174
Mucosa, 187
Mucus,
excess, 179, 187, 197, 204
in stool, 237, 287, 325
in urine, 325
Multiple Personalities, 99, 100
Multiple Sclerosis, 183, 197, 291
Mung beans as pulse weight, 144, 228
Muscles,
abdominal, 302
atrophy, 191
"burned", 291

five pillars/axes, 157, 326-8
firing, 292, 312
flaccid, 98, 310
hidden beam, 235
integrity, 299, 309
issues, 291
Luo, 50, 122-3
orbicular, 257
pain, 123
relax, 286, 296, 312, 328
smooth, 247
spasms, 311
sphincters, 257
tight, stiff, 40, 310-12
weak, 40, 311
worsening condition, 133
Myocarditis, 109

N

Narcissism, 302
Nasal,
congestion, 94, 208, 297
discharge, 95, 148, 179, 187, 197, 204
itch, 315
polyps, 180, 183, 296
post nasal drip, 206
Nausea, 112, 119, 187, 204, 235, 253, 261, 291, 305-6, 311
Neck,
blockages, 157
lost latency, 195
nodules, 256
pain, 112, 148, 197, 302
release, 47, 197, 199, 200, 202, 373-4
retracted, 256
ruddy, 191
stiff, rigid, 64, 97, 166, 296, 367
tight, 153, 314
Neediness, 86, 256, 258
Nerve receptors, 104, 212, 229
damage, 371
Neurological signs, 183, 266, 278, 291, 297, 315
Neuropathy, 40, 113, 187, 191, 195, 302, 311, 315, 366, 373, 377

Nightmares, 187
Nine Heart Pains, (Nine Palaces), 283, 371-2
Nipple, 206, 254, 296
Nodes, (Roots and Terminations), 109, 371
Nodules 7, 50, 54-7, 83, 86-103, 107, 114, 128, 195, 204, 256, 372
Nose, see also *Nasal*
    bleeds, 11, 95, 148, 187, 296, 311
    evolution, 309
    irritated, 171, 179, 291
    open, 296
    runny, 296-7
    swelling, 270
Numbness, 266, 302, 307, 327
    diaphragmatic, 89
    head, 197
    leg, 113
    limbs, 266, 274
    psychological, 98
    Sinews, 27, 40
    throat, 90
    Wei deficiency, 27
Nurturing, 234
Nutritive Qi, Ying Qi, 22, 24, 50, 52, 54-5, 85, 111, 113, 134
    emotions, 121-2
    latency, 132
    pulses, 229

O

Obesity, overweight, 286, 302, 319, 325
Obsession, 283, 286, 325, 372
    about past and future, 281-3, 285, 292
    self-, 302
    time, 287
Obsessive compulsive behavior, 95
Obsessive thinking, 50, 91, 335
Ocular pressure, 306
Opening points,
    Divergents, 137
    Eight extras, 223-5, 232

Oppression,
    chest, 63, 92, 112, 149, 199, 200, 208, 241, 257, 371
Ophthalmological issues, 368
Oral,
    cavity, 90, 265
    tradition, xxxi-iii, 130
Orbicularis oris and oculi, 257
Orifices,
    blockage, 95
    lower, 247
    sensory, 109, 141, 179, 195, 202, 234, 241, 244, 247, 253, 262, 263, 267, 270, 291, 295-6, 306, 315, 327-8, 368, 369, 371-2, 375
    stagnation, 95
    upper, 187, 368
Organ,
    failure, 197
    inflammation, 127, 197
Original Qi, see *Yuan-Source Qi*
Osteoporosis, 220
Otitis media, 291
Ovaries,
    ovarian cysts, 148, 176, 257, 261, 282, 304, 320
        ruptured, 166
    polycystic, 183, 370

P

Pain, 40, 247
    abdominal, 302
    all over, 331
    axillary, 187, 199, 208
    back, 257, 267
    on bearing weight, 41, 98
    Blood stagnation, 247
    calf, 311
    chest, 311
    chronic, 298, 317
    constant, 41, 295
    emotional, 283, 312 (due to rebellion), 317
    epigastric, 311
    esophageal, 179, 183, 187, 235, 253, 311, see also *Reflux*
    due to fear, 291
    Heart, 267, 272, 281-3, 285, 306, 371
    hip, 41, 148, 171, 311

injury, 27
intercostal, 148, 282
intestinal, 305
jaw, 166, 171, 183
joint, 247
knee, 311
GB-22, 44
genital, 302, 325
    pain, sudden, 148
leg, 179
leg tightness, 302, 311
upon lifting, 325
Liver constraint, 247
longing, 283
low back, lumbar, 282, 291, 311, 373
Lower Jiao stabbing pain, 247
mouth, 183
moving, 302
navel, 253, 328
neck, 302, 367
Nine Heart Pains, 283
ovulation, 183
periods, 332
PTSD, 292
Qiao's, 308
Qi stagnation, 281, 285
relief, 369
rib, 171, 191, 282
side, 312, 317
Sinews, 367
stagnant Yin and Yang, 282
sexual intercourse, 325
shoulder, 311
sternum, 235
sudden,
    back, 148
    in Divergent treatments, 158
    genitalia, 148, 175
testicular, 257
thigh, 148, 171, 179, 311
throat, 302, 371, 373
tongue, 183
unilateral, 310

urination, 191, 267-8, 272, 304-5, 327
wrist, 149
Pain nature of,
    dull, 43
    moving, 43
    radiating, 43
    sharp, 43
    stabbing, 27, 247
    stiff, xxix, 40, 63-4, 84, 90, 98, 101, 112, 157-8, 160, 171, 247, 266, 268, 276, 282, 291, 314-5, 335, 367
    shooting, 171
Pain upon,
    abduction, 41
    extension, 41, 294-5, 315
    flexion, 41, 171
    rotation, 41, 47-8
Palms,
    hot, 86, 88, 113, 149, 199, 208
    itchy, 88
Palpation, xxvii, 15, 276
Palpitations, 63, 96, 103, 119, 148-9, 199, 269, 282
Pancreatitis, 109, 197
Panic, panic attacks, 94-5, 235, 241, 243, 294-5, 332
Panting, 282
Paralysis, 3, 6, 41, 99, 197, 287, 315
    lower limbs, 99, 325
Paranoia, 95, 332
Paraplegia, 287
Parasite, 50, 132, 302
    worms, 302, 307
Paravertebral muscles, 61, 157-8, 161, 326, 328, 369
Parkinson's Disease, 183, 266, 274
Pathogenic factors, 22, 26-7
    Divergents, 130-5, 143, 146, 149, 160, 166, 187, 194-5, 200, 204, 208, 210, 214
    Eight Extras, 220, 222, 296, 311
    Luo, 40, 44, 50, 53-7
    Transverse Luo, 109, 114, 123
Pelvic inflammatory conditions, 175, 326
Pelvis,
    alignment, 309
    arthritis, 171
    blockages, 157

Doorway to the Earth points, 202
opening, 200
pain, 179
psoas, 328
releasing, 197, 199
storage, 319
Yin, 202
Penetrating Channel, 233
Pensiveness, 50, 122, 283
Pericarditis, 109, 200
Peristalsis, 160, 179, 187, 261
Permeability, 305
Perpetuation of the species, 221
Pessimism, 269, 283
Pestilent Qi, 372
Petroleum derivatives, 220
Pharmaceutical drugs, 320
Philosophy, xxx
Phlebitis, 302, 325, 327
Phlegm, 112, 149, 152, 183, 197, 210, 261, 305, 371, 373
    breast, 296
    chest, 262
    chronic, 267
    copious, 63, 143, 375
    dissipate, 374
    after eating, 239
    harassing Heart, 306
    -Heat, 366
    hot, 197, 199, 327
    Lung, 296
    nipple, 296
    over-nourishment, 258
    sensory orifices, 296
    sinuses, 270
    stagnation, 300
    stools, 237
    throat, 244, 262
    transforming, 63, 262, 287, 315, 335, 373-4
    Triple Heater, 195
    voice, 262
    Wind-, 63, 183, 296
Phonetics, 265
Photosensitivity, 314-5

Pigeon-toed, 302
Pineal gland, 180, 306, 315
Pituitary gland, 180, 306, 315, 369-70
Placenta, 302
    retention, 256
Plastics, 220, 223, 379
Pleurisy, 109
Plum-blossom, 12, 58
Plum pit Qi, 303
Pneumonia, xxix, 208
Poisoning,
    food, 54, 183, 253
Pollution, 50, 132
Polycystic ovaries, 183, 370
Polyps, 204, 267, 270
    nasal, 180, 183, 296
    intestinal, 180, 206
Postnatal Qi, 170, 218, 222-4, 233-4, 237, 239, 240, 243, 251, 266, 299, 306, 315, 369
    tonifying, 372
Postnasal drip, 206
Post-partum depression, 256
Post-traumatic stress disorder, 94, 96, 287, 292
Posture, 117, 249, 265, 268, 272, 295, 310, 314
    knock-knee, 302
Pregnancy, 220
    death, 221
    detoxification, 286
Premature aging, 222, 377
Premature growth, 222
Premenstrual syndrome, 247
Prenatal Qi, 222, 224, 234, 239, 240, 243, 281, 321, 369
Prickly heat, 297
Progesterone, 307, 316
Projectile vomiting, 296
Prolactin, 307, 316
Prolapse, 183, 247, 249, 267, 276, 372
    Mitral valve, 257, 282
Prosperity, 283
Prostate,
    benign prostatic hyperplasia, 367
    prostatitis, 237, 239, 247, 282, 304, 320, 325, 332
Psoas, 369

Psoriasis, 176, 311
Psychiatric, 55, 111
Psychosomatic, 176, 243
Puberty, 223, 269, 278, 289
Pulmonary failure, 208
Pure Yang of the Stomach, 234, 241, 244, 253, 262
Pyelonephritis, 109

Q

Qi,
- Ancestral, (Zong-Gathering/Chest), 221, 241, 244, 262
- Chopstick, 235
- Coursing, 374
- De, 4
- Defensive, see *Wei Qi*
- Fu, Latent, Hidden, xxx
- Glomus, 282
- Gu, 26, 262, 305, 367
- Influential point of, 262
- Leakage of, 295
- Moving Qi of the Kidneys, 321
- Nutritive, Ying Qi, 22, 24, 50, 52, 54-5, 85, 111, 113, 134
  - emotions, 121-2
  - latency, 132
  - pulses, 229
- Rebellious, 261, 262, 267, 272
- Original, see *Yuan-Source Qi*
- Pestilent, 54, 372
- Plum pit, 303
- Postnatal, 170, 218, 222-4, 233-4, 237, 239, 240, 243, 251, 266, 299, 306, 315, 369, 372
- Prenatal, 222, 224, 234, 239, 240, 243, 281, 321, 369
- Rebellious, xxix, 63
  - Divergents, 183, 369, 373
  - Eight Extras, 236, 244, 261-2, 267, 272, 306, 310-11
  - Luos, 50-1, 83, 90, 119
- Regulation of, 62, 199, 253, 262, 286-8
- Running Piglet, 234-5, 241, 369, 374
- Sea of Post Natal, 233
- Sea of Qi and Blood, 251
- Sea of Zang Fu and Postnatal Qi, 251
- Stasis of, 283, 288
- Wei, Defensive Qi,
  - blockage, 139, 157, 291
  - brain, 186-7
  - bowels, 139
  - Confluent points, 136
  - course of treatment, 139
  - controlled by, 121
  - crossing over, 137
  - cutaneous regions, 138, 214
  - deficient Yang, 267
  - deficiency, 27, 41, 122, 291
  - Divergents, 12
  - Eight Extra, 274
  - excess, 291
  - failure, xxviii, 327
  - freeing, 153
  - Gua sha, 215
  - ice and cold packs, 122, 158
  - infertility, 175
  - inflammation, 147, 158
  - insertion style, 3
  - needle type, 379
  - needling technique, 47, 134
  - origin, 26, 266
  - pain, 156, 159
  - relaxing, 370
  - returning Wei to Yang, 134
  - sensitivity, 369
  - Shao Yang conditions, 291
  - signs, 147, 291
  - Sinews, 26
  - urination, 88
  - Wei Atrophy Syndrome, 310-11
  - Yang Wei Mai mechanism, 289
- Ying, Nutritive Qi,
  - as buffer, 54
  - congealing, components, 55
  - deficiency, 132
  - Eight Extra pulses, 228
  - location of emotions, 121
  - Luo intention, 113

points, 122
taxation on Ying, 22
Transverse Luo, 52
Yuan, Source Qi,
ascension and descension, 236
differing states, 222
disrespecting, 219
distribution, 108
Divergent needling, 134
and Gu Qi, 368
opening points, 224
role in Chong, 233
status in Transverse Luos, 111
Zong-Gathering-Ancestral, 221, 241, 244, 262

R

Rapid,
breathing, 103, 149, 208
and floating pulses, 146, 186, 191, 194, 291
heartbeat, 287
and slippery pulses, 291, 325
and thin pulses, 256
Yuan pulses, 109, 113
Rebellious Qi, xxix,
Divergents, 183, 369, 373
Eight Extras, 236, 244, 261-2, 267, 272, 306, 310-11
Luos, 50-1, 83, 90, 119
Rectify Qi, 371-2
Rectus Abdominis, 157, 234, 240, 328, 369
Reduce, reduction,
technique, 6-8
Reflux, 62, 187, 204, 235, 253, 257, 311
cardiac, 119, 187
Refrigerated water, 157
Regret, 281, 325
Regulate,
Blood, 126, 179, 253
Blood and Essence, 261
Blood and Qi, 62, 199, 306, 315, 373
Chong, Ren, 260, 304-5
Damp, 305, 368
Damp-Heat, 239
digestive system, 62, 261, 307

fluids, 175, 237, 253, 305
hormones, 186, 369-70
intestines, 261
Liver, 239
Liver and Gallbladder, 269, 335
menses, 64
night sweats, 304
Qi, 62, 199, 253, 262, 286-8
responses, 179
sex drive, 306
temperature, 306
Yin and Yang, 234, 306, 315
Reinforcing, see *Tonification*
Relactation, 86
Relationships,
anxiety, 255
confidence, 234
control, 92, 258
dependence, 258
fear, 258
formation, 234, 256, 258
improvement, 84
inappropriate, 258
Nine Heart Pains, 283
sabotage, 94
stressful, 255
Remorse, 286
Renal insufficiency, 96, 235
Repetitive action, 89
Reproduction, Reproductive,
development, 223
issues, 188, 263, 278, 323
organs, 220
RNA, 220
Resentment, 325
Resolve Damp/Phlegm, 239, 298, 304-5, 307, 308
Respiratory failure, 208
Respiratory tract infections, 171, 179, 208
Restlessness, 88, 112, 148, 149, 191, 197, 199, 208, 266, 282, 372-3
Retention of lochia/placenta, 256
Retirement, 289
Retracted,

    neck, 256
    tongue, 148
Retrospection, 368
Retroviral diseases, 221
Rheumatism, 51, 122
Rhinitis, 296
Rigidity, stubbornness, 97
    head, 97
    lower Jiao, 202
    neck, 97, 166, 367
Ring around the chest, 102, 161, 190, 214-5
Ring around the collar, 182, 214
Ripening, 261, 266
RNA, 220
Roots and terminations, 109
Rotting and ripening, 261, 266
Routes of elimination, 139
Ruddy complexion, malar flush, 62, 187, 191, 197, 199, 311
Resuscitate,
    consciousness, 270, 296
    drowning, 260
Running Piglet Qi, 234-5, 241, 369, 374

S

Sabotage, 94
Saccharine, 220
Sacrum, 133, 158
Sadness, 50, 86, 121-2
Safety, 377
Salads, 157
San Jiao, see *Triple Heater*
Scars, 18, 139
Scatter cold, 232, 265
Scattered, 292
Schizophrenia, 99, 102
Schooling, 289
Sciatica, 367
Scoliosis, 160, 278, 378
Scrofula, 373
Sea of Blood, 233, 241, 247
Sea of the Five Zang and Six Fu, 233, 237
Sea of Food and Drink, 251, 253

Sea of Marrow, 251, 270
Sea of Post Natal Qi, 233
Sea of Qi and Blood, 251
Sea of the 12 Primary Channels, 233, 237
Sea of the Yang Luos, 309
Sea of the Yin Luos, 299
Sea of Yin, 254
Sea of Zang Fu and Postnatal Qi, 251
Sea salt, 45-6, 375-6
Secondary, xxvi, xxxv
Secure the root, 151
Seizures, 183, 187, 191, 208, 267, 269, 274, 295-7, 311-12, 314, 315, 372
    chronic, 197
    infantile, 221, 266
    with palms and eyes open, 311
    with vomiting, 296
    Yang type, 315
Self-,
    acceptance, 222, 321
    containment, 260
    cultivation, 383
    deprecation, 299
    discovery, 239
    embodiment, 222
    examination, 285, 303
    expression, 287, 304
    esteem, 298, 302
    introspection, 303
    loathing, hatred, 299
    image, 302, 314
    mutilation, 97
    obsession, 302
    reflection, 303
    respect, 302
Selfishness, 314
Seminal loss, 63, 304
Sensitivity,
    gut hypersensitivity, 200
    loss of, 27
    over, 27, 40
    photosensitivity, 314-5
Sensory-motor tract, 265, 274

Sensory orifices, organs, 109, 141, 179, 195, 202, 234, 241, 244, 247, 253, 262-3, 267, 270, 295, 296, 306, 315, 327-8
    distribution of fluids, 369
    opening, 372
Sensory perception, 241, 244
Sentimentality, 306, 315
Separate Channels, 131
Sexual,
    abuse, 234
    arousal, 100, 175
    drive, 304, 306, 315
    excess, 253
    fear of, 176
    fluids, 221
    function, 220, 266
    identity, 220, 233, 236, 303
    intercourse, 303
    pain during/after, 304-5, 325
    worms, Sexually Transmitted Diseases (STDs), 175, 296, 302
Shaking, 101, 296, 327
Shame, 283, 304, 370
Shen,
    anchor, 262, 264
    animation, 265
    calm, 261-2, 268-70, 288, 294-5, 297, 304, 335, 369, 372
    disturbed, 62, 197, 199, 235, 253, 261-2, 266, 278, 282-3, 303, 315, 323, 331, 378
    Heart, 233
    issues, 263
    lifted, 270, 314
    as Yang humor,
Shingles, 204
Shock, 50, 234, 287, 370
Shoulder,
    bindings, 42
    blockages, 157
    cysts, 204
    evolution, 309
    Heat, 63
    inflamed, 62, 204, 208
    issues, 191, 295
    latency, 159
    pain, 133, 148, 191, 204, 311, 315, 317
    pathogen, 131, 135
    relaxing, 314
    tight, 314
    Wind-Damp, 62
Shyness, 268, 272
Silver, 11
Sinew release, 47, 199, 215, 328
Sinusitis, 94, 179-80, 204, 296
Sjogren's Syndrome, 180, 191
Skin conditions, 171, 291, 297
Skull, 309
    evolution, 220
    tension, 166
Sleep
    blankets, 258
    difficulty, disturbed, 148, 191, 311
    issues, 235
    lack, xxviii
    patterns, 254
    somnolence, 300, 302
Small Intestine, 93, 268
Smell, 309
Smoothies, 157
Sneezing, 84, 148, 315
Society, 256, 285-6, 299, 314
Sociopath, 97
Somnolence, 300, 302, 304
Sores,
    cold, 180
    non-healing, 197
Sorrow, 286
Soul mate, 258
Source points, 54, 108
SP-21 location, 59-61, 64, 83, 102-3, 125-6, 331-2, 335
Spasms, 5, 27, 98, 171, 183, 276, 295, 297, 310-11, 367
Speech,
    issues, 112, 187, 191, 296, 304
    lack, 268
    loss, 92, 191
    stimulation, 269

stuttering, 92, 149, 183, 267-8
Sperm, motility, 266
Spermatorrhea, 325
Sphincters, 257
Spider veins, 50, 55-7, 81, 127-8
Spinal tumors, 256
Spirit, 4
    loss of animation, 244
    Blood as residence, 100
    and Jing, 221, 244
    Heart as residence, 233, 243
    revealing, opens, 244, 305
    shining, 221, 233
    trauma to, 96
Spleen,
    ascending, 237, 249, 266, 276
    boundaries in relationship, 234
    connection to prenatal level, 319
    failure to bank Qi and Blood, 323
    harmonized with Stomach, 239, 372
    Heat, 183
    and prolapse, 269
    Qi deficiency, 99, 113, 234, 237, 253
    Spleen Yang, 239, 240, 244, 249
    swollen, 171
    supporting Lungs and Heart, 244
Splenomegaly, 171, 241
Split personalities, 96
Stagefright, 90
Stainless steel, 11
Stance, 220, 299, 307, 309
    in time, 307, 316
Startle reflex, 94, 311
Stasis, 300
    Blood, 46, 191, 202, 241, 247, 249, 269, 331, 332
    emotional, 288
    food, 183, 187, 235, 253, 256, 261, 305
    Jing, 166, 175
    Qi, 283, 288
    Yin, 256-8, 260-4, 300, 304, 371
Steaming Bone Syndrome, 269
Stenosis, 257
Sterility, 266

Sternocleidomastoid, 158, 326, 328, 369
Sternum, 335
    latency, 158
    Kidney Shus, 170
    pain below, 235, 241
Steroids, 158, 320
Stiffness, 40, 112, 266, 282, 291, 314-5
    after treatment, 157
    back, 247, 282
    elbow, 98
    feet, 90
    sudden, healing crises, 84
    after dietary cold, 157
    knees, 160, 367
    limbs, 99
    in morning, xxix
    neck, 64, 367
    pain, 171
    spine, 63, 101, 268, 276, 335
    tongue, 187
Stomach,
    Cold, 53
    harmonized with Spleen, 63, 239
    Heat, 62, 191
    flu, 131
    Fluids, 26, 41, 43, 47, 183, 195
    opening, 261
    origin of Blood and Fluids, 241
    pestilent Qi, 54
    Pure Yang of the, 234, 241, 244, 253
    rebellious Qi, 63, 261
    ulcers, 179, 180, 187, 197, 311
    Yin, 253
Stool,
    dry, 148
    blood in, 63, 237, 287
    Heat, 326
    loose, 112, 269, 291
    mucus in, 237, 287, 325
    pebbly, 93, 139
    Phlegm, 237
    undigested food, 237, 287
    watery, 237

Stress, xxviii,
    ability to deal with, 96
    allergies, 176, 296
    at birth, 255
    and eating, 261
    emotional, 239
    headaches, 295
    lifestyle, xxix
    lumps, 243
    managing, 96
    organ, 54
    PTSD, 94, 287, 292
    relationships, 255
    response, 239, 269, 295, 297, 312, 372
    skin issues, 176, 297
    work, 286
Stroke, 100, 183, 187, 191, 266, 316-7, 367
Stubbornness, 97, 325
Stunted growth, 249
Stuttering, 92, 149, 183, 267-8
Sudden Turmoil Disorder, 119, 314, 370
Suicide, 99, 100, 102, 295, 302
Suffering, 102
Suffocation, 92
Summer Heat, 367
Sun Luo, 132
Sun Si Miao, xxv, 226, 380
Surgery, 18, 40
Surrender, 372
Swallowing, 148, 179, 197, 257
Sweat,
    in healing events, 84, 375
    in expulsion of pathogen, xxviii, 22, 26, 133, 159
    failure, xxviii, 159
    and fever, 112, 114
    function in pathology, 26
    genitalia, 260
    night, 304-5
    profuse, 62, 257
    spontaneous, 148, 171, 208, 295, 314
Swelling, swollen, 371
    axillary, 187, 200, 371
    breast, 208
    case study, 47
    cranial, 372
    cysts, 57, 107
    eyes, 179, 262, 266, 274, 297, 315
    facial, 371
    fungal infections, 93
    head, 63, 270
    injury, 27
    genital, 100, 175, 257, 260, 304
    glands, 166
    gum, 270, 306, 315
    leg, 315
    lip, 270
    Liver, 171
    lumbar, 291
    Luo channels, 50, 54
    lymph node, 187, 208, 371
    necessary, 122
    nipple, 296
    nodules, 57, 107, 128, 195
    orifices, 270
    salivary glands, 112
    scrotal, 100, 257, 304
    Spleen, 171, 241
    sub-maxillary, 112
    testicular, 100
    throat, 148
    tumors, 57
    uterine, 100, 175
    vaginal, 100
    Yin accumulation as response, 147
Styes, 180
Symbiotic bond, 254
Synchronicity, 254, 287, 307, 316
Synovial fluid, 191

T

Tachycardia, 103, 119, 191, 282
Talking,
    addiction, 258
    to oneself, 99
Tantrums, 90

Taste, 291
Teeth, 89, 114, 148, 179
Television, 89
Temperament, 97-8, 120-2, 233, 295, 321
Temperature, 40, 83, 123, 255, 306, 311
Terminal illness, 113
Terminations, 109
Testicles, 257
Thirst, 62-3, 112, 180, 187, 200, 256, 304
Throat, 63
    dry, 112, 187, 200, 267, 272
    expression, 221
    Heat, 269, 297
    Hot phlegm, 195
    issues, 166, 195, 267, 278, 291, 367
    lumps, 206
    numb, 90
    opening, 244, 262, 303, 371
    pain (Bi), xxviii, 62, 148, 166, 171, 179, 266-7, 270, 283, 302-4
    Phlegm, 244, 262
    plum pit, 303
    raw, 191
    slashing, 102
    swollen, 148
    tight, 197
Thrusting Vessel, 233
Thyroid, 369
    goiter, 63, 136, 166, 170, 206, 208, 262, 302, 306, 315, 369, 371, 373-4
    Hashimoto's thyroiditis, 187, 367
    thyroiditis, 176
Tics, 311
    eye, 183
    facial, 183
Time, 144, 219, 223, 281, 283, 287, 290, 307, 310, 316-7
Timidity, 268
Tinnitus 112, 179, 180, 187, 191, 195, 262, 297, 315
Tissues, 197, 310
TMD, temporomandibular joint disorder, 112, 183, 291, 302, see also *Pain, jaw*
Toilet train, 257

Tongue,
    Chong, 235
    chopstick Qi, 235
    cracks, 131, 187
    dry, 112
    hidden beam, 235
    pain, 112, 183
    pale, 241
    purple, blue, 204
    regulate Blood at, 370
    retracted, 148
    stiff, 187
    thick coat, 119
    ulceration, 11, 187
Tonification, 7-9, 11
    Dai Mai, 321
    definition, 239
    Qiaos, 300, 317
    Yuan-Source, 113, 226
Toothache, 62, 89, 114
Tooth decay, 179, 200
Tortoise Technique, 83
Tourette's Syndrome, 92, 183, 291
Toxins, 50, 132, 320, 366
    Blood, 175
    Fire, 55, 195, 294
    Jing, 175
Tranquilizers, 58
Transcendence, 372
Transform, 372
Transitions, 132, 281, 289, 294
Transmission,
    of tradition, xxx
    oral teaching, 387
    order of transmission of pathology, 112
    to zonal pair, 215
Trauma, 283, 292
    birth, 221, 234, 237
    Dai Mai, 325
    diagnosis, 235
    emotional, 332
    injury, 122
    physical, 294

PTSD, 94, 283, 287, 292
refusal to examine, 297
scar, 18
Sexual, 234
somatized, 298
spirit, psychological, 96, 283, 297, 303, 319, 327
throat Bi, 283
Tremors,
Yang Qiao, Mai, 311
Yang Wei Mai, 296
Trigger fingers, 295, 314
Triple Heater, Triple Burner,
Eight Extra treatments, 227
floating pulse, 22
generation of, 265, 321
GB-20, 296, 307, 316
personality and temperament, 321
Transverse luos, 108-110
and Yin Wei Mai, 283
Yuan-Source points, 232
Trust, 263, 303-4
Tui Na, 5, 6, 14
Tumors, 257
brain, 302
breast, 257
knees, 160
Lower Jiao, 261, 282
Luo diagnosis, 128
ovaries, 257
prostate, 257
testicles, 257
thyroid, 257
spine, 160, 256
uterus, 257, 261, 282
Turbid,
fluids, 372
Middle Jiao, 372

U

Ulcerative colitis, 109, 179, 235, 253, 369
Ulcers,
colon, 179, 253
Stomach, 179, 180, 187, 197, 311

tongue, 11, 187
Umbilicus, 254, 260
Umbilical cord, 254-5
Undigested food, 113, 237, 261, 287
Unilateral needling, 17
Eight Extras, 226
Luo points, 60
physiological responses, 17
trajectory points of Divergents, 138
Union of Yin and Yang, 233
Unresponsiveness, 314
Upper Jiao (burner),
Dai Mai, 328, 336
disinhibit, 152
heat, 206
points in Ren, 263
points in Yin Qiao Mai, 306
poor growth, 206
Upper respiratory tract infections, 171, 179
Urination,
anuria, 95, 112, 119
blockage, 63, 239
bloody, 63, 304, 367
burning, 268, 335
cloudy, 367
dark, 84
difficult, 191, 267, 272, 304-5, 327
exhausting, 304
frequent, 22, 88, 119, 268, 325-6
Heat, 303, 326
issues, 160, 367
lack of, 119
Lin Bi, painful, cloudy, grainy, bloody, tiring urination, 367
night time, 305
painful, 268, 304-5, 367
promotion, 261, 305, 373
stone, grainy, 304, 367
tiring, 367
turbid, 304, 367
Urinary Tract Infections, 164, 303, 367
Urine, see *Urination*
Urogenital issues, 247, 278, 323, 325

Urticaria, 315
Uterus,
    Chong Mai, 247
    Du Mai, 269
    Eight Extras, 221, 227
    evolution, 220
    regulate, 369
    Ren Mai, 257, 260
    Wei Qi, 175
    Yang Wei Mai, 296
    Yin Qiao Mai, 302, 305

V

Vaccines, 220, 223, 234, 320
Vaginal discharge, 247
Vaginitis, 166, 175
Varicosities, 50, 52, 81, 86, 127, 183
Veins,
    disappearance, 55
    reappearance, 56
    spider, 50, 52, 55, 57, 81, 128
    varicose, 50, 52, 81, 86, 127, 183
Vertigo, 311, 367
Vibrating,
    Divergent needling, 12-13
    Eight Extra needling, 13, 224-6, 230, 232
    Opening points, 224
    pulses, 144
    reduction, tonification, 226
    patient awareness of, 240
Victim, 102, 244, 258
Violations,
    acupuncture principles, 219
    unwelcome use of Eight Extras, 223
    Jing, 223, 319
Virus, xxviii, 50, 53, 132
    hepatitis, 111
    retrovirus, 221
Visceral dryness, 283
Vision, eyesight,
    clarity, 368-9
    impaired, 257, 302
    loss, 187
Vocal cord, 171
Vocation, 283
Voice,
    hearing, 91, 99
    inner, 92
    loss of, 62, 90, 266-7, 373
Vomiting, 22, 63, 84, 112, 119, 187, 235, 241, 253, 256, 291, 305-6, 373, 375
Vulnerability, 94

W

Wai Ke, 47
Waist, 268, 325
Wandering,
    corpse, 99
    ghost, worms, 296, 302
Wasting diseases, 208, 234, 256
Waterways, xxviii, 133, 218, 237
Weaning, 89, 257, 265
Weather, xxviii, 40, 258
Wei Atrophy Syndrome, 150, 191, 197, 291, 302, 310-11, 366-7, 373
Wei Qi, Defensive Qi,
    blockage, 139, 157, 291
    bowels, 139
    Confluent points, 136
    course of treatment, 139
    controlled by, 121
    crossing over, 137
    cutaneous regions, 138, 214
    deficient Yang, 267
    deficiency, 27, 41, 122, 291
    Divergents, 12
    Eight Extra, 274
    excess, 291
    failure, xxviii, 327
    freeing, 153
    Gua sha, 215
    ice and cold packs, 122, 158
    inflammation, 158
    insertion style, 3
    needle type, 379
    needling technique, 47, 134
    origin, 26, 266

pain, 156, 159
relaxing, 370
returning Wei to Yang, 134
sensitivity, 369
Shao Yang conditions, 291
signs, 147, 291
Sinews, 26
urination, 88
Wei Atrophy Syndrome, 310-11
Yang Wei Mai mechanism, 289
Wheeze, 112, 119, 149, 204, 206, 208, 373
Wind,
 -Cold, xxviii, 2, 45, 62, 64, 208, 237
 coursing, 367-9, 373-4
 -Damp, 2, 45, 62-3, 268, 296, 368
 Death-, 302
 expel, 164, 269-70, 297, 367, 370-1
 exuberant, 266, 316
 Fright-, 295, 297
 intestinal, 253
 internal, 62, 183, 268, 269
 pacify, 372
 -Phlegm, 296, 373
 subdue in portals, 276
Windows to the Sky, 197, 202 (list)
Withdrawal,
 Divergent order, 154, 157
 needling technique, 8, 9
 from world, 113, 312
Work stress, 286
Worms, 302, 307
Worry, 50, 316
Wrist,
 damp, 300
 pain, 149

X

Xenobiotics, 220, 234, 320
Xi-Cleft points,
 in Divergents, 138
 in Eight Extras, 286
 locating, 15
 Yin Wei Mai, 285
 Yang Wei Mai, 294
 Yin Qiao Mai, 303
 Yang Qiao Mai, 312
Xu Feng, 223

Y

Yang,
 anchoring, 373
 collapse, 202, 208, 211, 294
 escaping, 208
 excess, 367
 loss, 373
 returning Wei to Yang, 134
 rising, floating, 367
 subdue, 372
Yang Bridge Channel, 309
Yang Heel Channel, 309
Yang Ming,
 cutaneous region, 181-2, 205, 207, 214
 movement assessment, 41
 essential oil, 45
 Sinew, 26
 Transverse Luo, 109, 112, 118
Yang Motility Channel, 309
Yang Sheng, 218
Yang Stance Channel, 309
Yang Ji Zhou, 225
Yawning, 88, 119
Yeast, xxviii, 247
Yellow Emperor/Lao Tzu sect, 387
Ye-Thick fluids, see *Fluids*
Yi, 91
Yin,
 accumulation, 256, 260-1, 264, 306
 anchor, 147, 187, 194-5, 257, 264, 311
 ascending, 202
 conservation, 236, 281
 consolidation, 195
 containment of Heat and Wind, 191
 deficiency, 258, 262, 306
  diarrhea, 187
  in Eight Extras, 222, 256
  in Divergents, 146, 195

in Luos, 126
resulting in Wind, 195
descending, 202
Divergents, 166, 186
epilepsy, 302
excess, 202, 258
exhaustion, 159
foundation, 222
humors, 288
hormone function, 302
imbalance of Yin and Yang, 222
inability to support, 200
Kidney, 251
latency, 191, 197
Luo channels, 55
nourish, 63, 260, 262, 305, 335
origin, 247
pathological, 107, 256, 265, 278
regulating Yang, 234, 306, 315
state, 302
sensory orifices, 263
separation, 235
sides, 224
sinking, 222
Source point of all Yin, 262, 335
stagnation, 256, 288, 300, 304
stasis, 256, 258, 260-3, 264, 300, 304, 371
Stomach, 253
supporting Jing, 186, 191
transforming, 263
unfolding, 222
Yin Bridge Channel, 299
Yin Heel Channel, 299
Yin Motility Channel, 299
Yin Stance Channel, 299
Ying Qi, Nutritive Qi,
as buffer, 54
congealing, components, 55
deficiency, 132
Eight Extra pulses, 228
location of emotions, 121
Luo intention, 113
points, 122

taxation on Ying, 22
Transverse Luo, 52
Yuan-Source Qi,
ascension and descension, 236
differing states, 222
disrespecting, 219
distribution, 108
Divergent needling, 134
and Gu Qi, 368
opening points, 224
role in Chong, 233
status in Transverse Luos, 111
Yuan-Source points,
containing pathology, 114-7
Divergents, 138
Luo theory, 54-8
Luo treatment, 81
in Primary channel treatments, 232
Transverse Luo, 56
Yuen, Jeffrey, ii, xxv, xxxi
Yu Wen, xxv

Z

Zang Fu,
Curious Organ link, 321
Divergent theory, 130-1
entrance of pathology, 150
distribution of Essence, 232
diversion of pathology, xxvii, 22, 164
evolution, 220
inflammation, 109, 197
removing pathology, 164
Triple Heater provision of pathology, 194
Zhen Jiu Da Cheng, 225
Zheng and Jia (concretions and gatherings), 282
Zhu Xi, 218
Zones,
as cutaneous regions, 214-5
cutaneous region connection, 133
eradication of Heat, 109
transmission, 27
in Transverse theory 112
Zong-Gathering-Ancestral Qi, 221, 241, 244, 262

POINT INDEX

LU-1,	15, 61, 111, 137, 150, 152-3, 188, 208, 210-11, 248, 339, 354, 374
LU-2,	61, 62, 339
LU-3,	200, 202
LU-4,	81, 88, 114-5
LU-5,	188
LU-6,	47
LU-7,	6, 47, 59, 60, 62, 86, 88, 114-5, 119, 122, 224-5, 230-1, 260, 264, 274
LU-9,	114-5, 122, 339
LU-10,	60, 62, 339
LU-11,	211, 339
LI-1,	149, 207, 339, 340
LI-4,	4, 6, 114, 340
LI-5,	15
LI-6,	59, 60, 62, 89, 114-5, 119, 122
LI-11,	60, 276
LI-12,	81, 89, 114-5
LI-14,	231, 294-5, 298
LI-15,	15, 60-3, 137, 146, 152-3, 206-7, 231, 309, 312, 315
LI-16,	312, 315
LI-18,	136-7, 202, 206-7, 210, 214, 373
LI-20,	153, 174, 180, 182, 212
ST-1,	61, 180, 231, 243-5, 260, 262-4, 274, 303, 306, 308, 312, 315
ST-3,	303, 306, 312, 315
ST-4,	62, 153, 180, 182, 231, 260, 262-3, 274, 303, 306, 308, 312, 315, 317
ST-5,	60-2, 153, 172, 174, 176, 178, 362
ST-6,	362
ST-7,	362
ST-8,	43, 109, 343, 362
ST-9,	61-2, 152-3, 180, 182-4, 186, 202, 214, 303, 306, 308, 343
ST-11,	61-3
ST-12,	22-3, 137, 152, 172, 174, 176, 178, 180, 182, 187-8, 190, 197-200, 203, 206-8, 210-11, 214, 231, 303, 306, 308, 340, 343, 348, 358, 362, 373
ST-13,	61-2
ST-15,	206-7
ST-16.5,	206
ST-17,	61
ST-25,	7, 15, 111, 139, 152, 166-7, 206, 211, 321, 323, 339-40
ST-30,	15, 137, 151-2, 179-80, 182-4, 186, 202, 231, 236-7, 239-40, 245, 247-8, 251, 253, 260, 328, 343, 362, 369
ST-31,	62
ST-32,	343
ST-34,	15
ST-35,	81, 90, 115, 125
ST-36,	188, 231, 251, 253, 343
ST-37,	206, 253, 340
ST-39,	253, 348
ST-40,	17, 52, 59-62, 90, 107, 114-6, 118-9, 122
ST-42,	22, 23, 47, 52, 61, 63, 87, 108, 115-6, 151, 152, 179, 183, 231, 253, 343, 364, 369
ST-44,	148
ST-45,	19, 109, 148, 182, 343, 362
SP-1,	109, 186, 253, 343, 345, 381
SP-3,	52, 107, 114-6, 118, 183
SP-4,	59-62, 91, 108, 115-6, 119, 122, 224-5, 229, 231, 236, 239, 240, 245, 248-9, 253
SP-6,	3
SP-8,	304, 354
SP-9,	188
SP-10,	6, 81, 83, 91, 101-3, 115, 124
SP-12,	137, 183-4, 186, 200, 202, 237, 289, 345, 370
SP-13,	285-6
SP-15,	152, 166-7, 231, 285-6, 288, 321, 323
SP-16,	285-7, 289
SP-21,	59, 60, 64, 83, 125-6, 332, 335
HT-1,	61-3, 126, 137, 152, 187-8, 190, 192, 194, 206-7, 339, 371
HT-2,	81, 92, 93, 115
HT-3,	346
HT-5,	59-62, 92-3, 115, 119
HT-7,	115, 118
HT-9,	346
SI-1,	190, 215, 348
SI-3,	224, 225, 230, 231, 248, 268, 272, 274, 276, 278-9
SI-4,	115, 186
SI-7,	59-61, 63, 93-4, 115, 118, 119, 122

SI-8,	61	**BL-62,**	47-8, 224-5, 230-1, 312, 314, 316-7
SI-9,	81, 94, 115	**BL-63,**	148, 216, 231, 294, 298
SI-10,	115, 137, 151-2, 187-8, 190, 231, 280, 294-5, 298, 309-10, 314, 317, 318, 370	**BL-64,**	115
SI-12,	214, 348, 362	**BL-67,**	19, 48, 109, 124, 148, 160, 215, 350
SI-14,	348	**Kidney Prime,**	249, 251
SI-16,	202, 214	**KI-1,**	109, 148, 170, 249, 287
SI-17,	202, 362	**KI-2,**	148, 303-4, 308, 354
SI-18,	48, 124, 152, 187-8, 190, 215, 348, 362	**KI-3,**	3, 9, 114-5, 249
SI-19,	60, 62, 348, 362	**KI-4,**	59-61, 63, 95-6, 115, 119, 122
BL-1,	12, 15, 26, 61-3, 109, 135, 137, 152-3, 155, 179-80, 182-4, 186-8, 190, 192, 194, 212, 229, 231, 266, 274, 276, 303, 306-9, 312, 315-7, 348, 350, 369, 370, 377	**KI-6,**	224-5, 230-1, 249, 303, 307-8
		KI-8,	303-4, 308
		KI-9,	231, 285-6, 288
		KI-10,	137, 152, 166-7, 170, 188, 231, 249, 354, 367
BL-2,	180	**KI-11,**	81, 96, 115, 202, 231, 237, 239, 249, 303-5, 308
BL-10,	15, 61, 64, 136, 151-2, 160-1, 164-7, 170, 202, 366-7	**KI-12,**	237, 304-5, 308
BL-11,	248, 269, 348	**KI-13,**	237, 304-5, 308
BL-12,	15, 272, 348	**KI-14,**	237, 304-5, 308
BL-13,	210, 358	**KI-15,**	237, 239, 304-5, 308
BL-15,	152, 160-1, 164, 214	**KI-16,**	151-2, 166-7, 231, 237, 239-40, 305, 308, 323-4, 358
BL-17,	47, 126, 152, 247, 248, 328	**KI-17,**	237, 239, 305
BL-18,	126	**KI-18,**	237, 239, 305
BL-20,	126	**KI-19,**	237, 239, 305
BL-23,	151, 160-1, 164, 166-7, 272, 274, 276, 321, 323, 350, 354	**KI-20,**	237, 239, 305
		KI-21,	61, 63, 231, 237, 239-40, 305, 308
BL-28,	151, 160, 166-7, 358	**KI-22,**	170, 231, 243
BL-31,	362	**KI-23,**	170, 243
BL-32,	152, 160, 166-7, 358, 362	**KI-24,**	170, 243
BL-33,	362	**KI-25,**	170, 243-4
BL-34,	152, 362	**KI-26,**	170, 243-4
BL-35,	202, 276, 350	**KI-27,**	166-7, 170, 231, 243-5, 306
BL-36,	151-2, 160-1, 164, 166-7	**PC-1,**	61, 63, 149, 152, 172, 174, 176, 178, 200, 202-3, 214, 357-8, 362, 364, 372
BL-38,	81, 95, 115, 125	**PC-2,**	81, 97, 116
BL-39,	125	**PC-6,**	59-61, 63, 96-7, 116, 119, 122, 224-5, 229-32, 236, 244-5, 285, 288
BL-40,	15, 125, 133, 136-7, 151-3, 160 -1, 165-67, 170, 202, 231, 249, 350, 366		
		PC-7,	116
BL-41,	210, 348	**PC-8,**	60, 62, 225, 357
BL-44,	160, 214	**PC-9,**	149, 203
BL-52,	272, 323	**TH-1,**	148, 199, 357
BL-57,	294, 328, 335-6	**TH-10,**	15
BL-58,	59-61, 63, 94-5, 114-5, 119, 122, 282	**TH-11,**	81, 98, 116
BL-59,	47, 312, 314, 317	**TH-13,**	294
BL-60,	328	**TH-14,**	294
BL-61,	312, 314		

TH-15,	294, 296	**GB-44,**	48, 109, 148, 174, 362
TH-16,	152-3, 174, 197-200, 202-3, 214, 371	**LR-1,**	109, 148, 178, 253, 362, 364, 381
TH-17,	174, 362	**LR-2,**	328
TH-18,	214	**LR-3,**	114, 116, 118-9, 126, 171, 175, 328
TH-19,	214	**LR-5,**	3, 17, 59-61, 64, 87, 99, 100, 116, 119, 122, 137, 152-3, 176, 178, 369
GB-1,	12, 135-6, 152, 155, 172, 174, 176, 178, 348, 362, 368, 377	**LR-6,**	47
GB-2,	362	**LR-8,**	126, 364
GB-3,	358, 362	**LR-9,**	81, 100, 116
GB-4,	362	**LR-12,**	202
GB-8,	22, 23, 109, 208, 210	**LR-13,**	126, 152, 172, 174, 176, 178, 188, 214, 231, 321, 323-4, 326, 329, 362
GB-12,	153, 197-200, 214	**LR-14,**	47, 152, 172, 174, 176, 178, 188, 285, 287, 328, 362, 377
GB-13,	43, 152, 231, 294, 297, 298, 362		
GB-14,	294, 297		
GB-15,	294, 297, 350		
GB-16,	294, 297		
GB-17,	294, 296		
GB-18,	294, 296		
GB-19,	294, 296		
GB-20,	294, 231, 290, 294, 296, 298, 303, 307-8, 312, 316-7, 362		
GB-21,	61, 214, 231, 294, 296, 298, 358, 362		
GB-22,	22, 23, 44, 59, 102-3, 125, 137, 151-2, 155, 174, 178, 187-8, 190, 192, 194, 199, 200, 203, 208, 210, 211, 214-5, 248, 331-2, 335-6, 357, 362, 370		
GB-23,	362		
GB-24,	152-3, 172, 174, 176, 178, 362		
GB-25,	151, 172, 174, 176, 178, 188, 214, 362		
GB-26,	152, 166-7, 247-8, 321, 323-4, 326, 328-9, 335-6		
GB-27,	231, 326, 328-30, 335-6		
GB-28,	231, 326, 328-30, 335		
GB-29,	231, 280, 294-5, 298, 309-10, 312, 314, 317-8		
GB-30,	15, 137, 148, 152, 172, 174-5, 199, 200, 202, 328, 362, 368		
GB-33,	81, 99, 116, 124		
GB-34,	123-4, 276, 308		
GB-35,	231, 294-5, 298		
GB-37,	15, 59-61, 63, 87, 98, 99, 114, 116, 118-9, 122, 124		
GB-39,	312		
GB-40,	116, 119		
GB-41,	2, 224-5, 230-1, 248, 323, 326, 329, 336, 362		
GB-42,	128		